P9-ARS-166

Physical Best

Physical Education for Lifelong Fitness and Health

4TH EDITION

Jackie Conkle

EDITOR

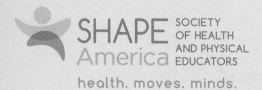

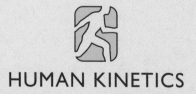

Library of Congress Cataloging-in-Publication Data

Names: Physical Best (Program), author. | Conkle, Jackie, 1982- editor. |
  SHAPE America (Organization) issuing body.
Title: Physical Best : physical education for lifelong fitness and health /
  SHAPE America ; Jackie Conkle, editor.
Other titles: Physical education for lifelong fitness and health
Description: Fourth Edition. | Champaign, Illinois : Human Kinetics, Inc.,
  [2020] | Revised edition of: Physical education for lifelong fitness : the
  Physical Best teacher's guide. 3rd ed. c2011. | Includes bibliographical
  references and index.
Identifiers: LCCN 2018051078 (print) | LCCN 2019001131 (ebook) | ISBN
  9781492589761 (epub) | ISBN 9781492545316 (PDF) | ISBN 9781492545309
  (print)
Subjects: LCSH: Physical education and training--Study and teaching--United
  States. | Physical fitness--Study and teaching--United States.
Classification: LCC GV365 (ebook) | LCC GV365 .P4992 2019 (print) | DDC
  796.071--dc23
LC record available at https://lccn.loc.gov/2018051078

ISBN: 978-1-4925-4530-9 (print)

Copyright © 2020 by SHAPE America – Society of Health and Physical Educators

All rights reserved. Except for use in a review, the reproduction or utilization of this work in any form or by any electronic, mechanical, or other means, now known or hereafter invented, including xerography, photocopying, and recording, and in any information storage and retrieval system, is forbidden without the written permission of the publisher.

The web addresses cited in this text were current as of October 2018, unless otherwise noted.

Acquisitions Editor: Scott Wikgren; **Developmental Editor:** Jacqueline Eaton Blakley; **Managing Editor:** Derek Campbell; **SHAPE America Editor:** Thomas Lawson; **Copyeditor:** Tom Tiller; **Indexer:** Nancy Ball; **Permissions Manager:** Dalene Reeder; **Graphic Designer:** Dawn Sills; **Cover Designer:** Keri Evans; **Cover Design Associate:** Susan Rothermel Allen; **Photograph (cover):** FatCamera/E+/Getty Images; **Photographs (interior):** © Human Kinetics, unless otherwise noted; © Brand X Pictures (chapter 1 opener: pp. iii, 3, and 15; chapter 7 opener: pp. iv, 161, and 181), © iStockphoto.com/EMLENNYs Sudden Jet Lag (chapter 2 opener: pp. iii, 17, and 42), © Monkey Business/fotolia.com (chapter 4 opener: pp. iii, 61, and 95); **Photo Asset Manager:** Laura Fitch; **Photo Production Manager:** Jason Allen; **Senior Art Manager:** Kelly Hendren; **Illustrations:** © Human Kinetics, unless otherwise noted; **Printer:** Walsworth

SHAPE America – Society of Health and Physical Educators
1900 Association Drive
Reston, VA 20191
800-213-7193
www.shapeamerica.org

Printed in the United States of America   10   9   8   7   6   5   4   3   2   1

The paper in this book was manufactured using responsible forestry methods.

Human Kinetics
P.O. Box 5076
Champaign, IL 61825-5076
Website: www.HumanKinetics.com

In the United States, email info@hkusa.com or call 800-747-4457.
In Canada, email info@hkcanada.com.
In the United Kingdom/Europe, email hk@hkeurope.com.

For information about Human Kinetics' coverage in other areas of the world,
please visit our website: **www.HumanKinetics.com**

E6983

Contents

PART I   Foundations of Health-Related Fitness and Physical Activity

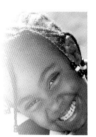

CHAPTER 1
Introduction to Physical Best   3

Suzan F. Ayers and Mary Jo Sariscsany

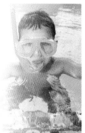

CHAPTER 2
Creating Physical Activity Behaviors
That Last a Lifetime   17

Hannah Brewer, Ethan Hull, and Randy Nichols

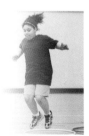

CHAPTER 3
Basic Training Principles   43

Sean Bulger and Brooke Towner

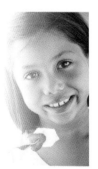

CHAPTER 4
Exploring Nutrition for Student Health   61

D. Gayle Povis

PART II   Components of Health-Related Fitness

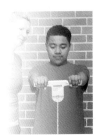
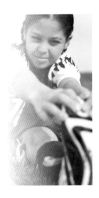
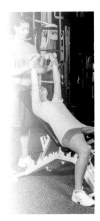

PART III Curriculum and Teaching Methods

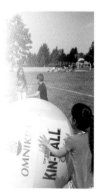

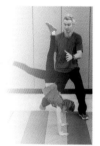

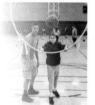

PART IV Foundations of Assessment in Health-Related Fitness and Physical Activity

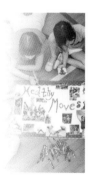

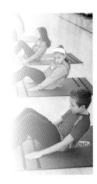

Preface

Physical educators around the country face a unique challenge. We live in a nation of cutting-edge medical advancement, yet members of the current generation of Americans are predicted to be the first in recent history with a shorter life expectancy than their parents. The challenge posed by this reality also gives physical educators a unique opportunity to enable positive changes, help reverse the health decline in U.S. society, and help improve individuals' health for generations to come. By helping students gain the necessary knowledge and skills to become physically literate individuals, as well as the confidence to do so, we prepare them to live healthier, less stressful, more productive lives.

Physical education has a clear role in preparing students for lifelong health. It is well documented that regular physical activity is linked with good health and improved cognitive function. Physical education—along with physical activity before, during, and after school—provides the best opportunities to reach most of the young population. But physical education and activity programs that prepare students for healthy lives must offer far more than a single-person effort or a mere "roll out the ball" program. Fortunately, many cooperative efforts are under way to provide the necessary education, professional development, and resources for promoting effective physical education and physical activity programs that lead to healthier lifestyles among young Americans. This powerful, unified effort to improve the health of current and future generations can be aided by every physical education teacher in every gymnasium and classroom and on every field. One tool that can help physical educators succeed in this effort is the Physical Best program, and *Physical Best: Physical Education for Lifelong Fitness and Health* is your guide to using it.

Who Should Use This Book?

For veteran teachers, *Physical Best* outlines strategies for emphasizing health-related fitness within an existing program; it also offers an opportunity to refresh and update one's content knowledge of health-related fitness and incorporate engaging health-related fitness activities based on the newest research. At the same time, new teachers will learn how to create an effective education program for health-related fitness by following examples from master teachers. For district coordinators, this book provides useful information for professional development and continued education in physical education. And for preservice teachers in teacher education programs, it provides an overview of current research, trends, and best practices for teaching health-related fitness.

Physical Best Content

This book was developed to provide a comprehensive guide to incorporating health-related fitness and lifetime physical activity into physical education programs. It provides examples of best practices, current research on core content, and numerous practical examples of how to integrate health-related fitness education into an existing physical education curriculum. Examples from this fourth edition include how to teach health-related fitness concepts through enjoyable physical activity and how to use health-related fitness assessment as an instrument for inspiration rather than a "tool for torture."

In the previous edition, the Physical Best resources included three books:

- *Physical Education for Lifelong Fitness: The Physical Best Teacher's Guide, Third Edition*
- *Physical Best Activity Guide: Elementary Level, Third Edition*
- *Physical Best Activity Guide: Middle and High School Levels, Third Edition*

With this edition, information from all three books has been condensed into one book, and the sample Physical Best activities—which had made up the bulk of the two *Physical Best Activity Guides*—are now presented in an online web resource. This change was made so that we could provide you a complete K-12 package in streamlined form.

Part I introduces you to the Physical Best program and health-related fitness by providing an in-depth look at behavior and motivation related to physical activity; it also examines basic training principles for health-related fitness. Because nutrition is an essential component of body composition, part I concludes with an overview of nutrition, including the foundations of a healthy diet, and provides resources for dietary tools.

Part II provides an overview of health-related fitness concepts. Specifically, this edition addresses cardiorespiratory endurance; muscular strength, endurance, and power; and flexibility and body composition—all as they relate to K-12 students. Because knowledge of health-related fitness continues to evolve rapidly, and some disagreement exists (even among exercise physiologists) about appropriate exercise protocols, this book provides guidance on controversial topics, along with recommendations for addressing them in a physical education program. Part II also provides teaching tips to help you address each component of health-related fitness in your physical education program.

Part III offers strategies for integrating health-related fitness education throughout the curriculum, as well as effective teaching methods that encourage inclusion of all students—in the gymnasium, on the field, and in the classroom.

Part IV introduces assessment and assessment strategies as they relate to effective teaching and health-related fitness. This part of the book covers appropriate collection and use of health-related fitness assessment results, as well as ways in which to assess concept knowledge, application of knowledge, and participation in physical activity. The associated web resource gives you access to assessment-related documents that can be downloaded for personal use.

The book concludes with a glossary and a reference list that you can use as a resource guide.

Part V is now available online through the web resource (access is provided with this text). It offers ready-to-use activities from master instructors to guide you in incorporating health-related fitness content into your teaching. These activities reflect current research and have been designed to align with SHAPE America's National Standards and Grade-Level Outcomes for K-12 Physical Education (2014). Activities are divided according to grade level: elementary and middle school and high school. Activities can be downloaded and printed as needed. In addition to useful reference documents, the web resource also provides ready-to-use worksheets and masters.

Instructors also have access to other online resources to help teach the content provided in the book: a presentation package, instructor guide, and test package. The presentation package presents PowerPoint slides of key concepts covered in each chapter. The instructor guide provides tools for teaching a course using *Physical Best, Fourth Edition,* as your textbook. The test package consists of multiple-choice and true-or-false test questions covering the content from all chapters.

How This Edition Was Developed

Good teaching is both an art and a science. The National Association for Sport and Physical Education (now SHAPE America—Society of Health and Physical Educators) developed the first edition of Physical Best by combining extensive research on the science of physical activity for children and young adults with the vast knowledge and experience of master physical education teachers from across the country. This fourth edition is designed to help preprofessionals and professionals in physical education stay current with content connected to health-related fitness education and teaching fitness to students in physical education and physical activity programs, from kindergarten through grade 12. See the acknowledgments for a list of experts and master teachers who helped create this edition of Physical Best.

Your Physical Best

As a physical educator, you do an important job—one that can literally shape the future health of the nation. I hope that you will find this book both informative and inspirational in your journey to being the best physical educator you can be.

Jackie Lynn Conkle, DHEd
Editor
Health and Physical Education Teacher
Peters Township School District
McMurray, Pennsylvania

Acknowledgments

Many physical education professionals contributed their time and expertise to this project. Content experts were sought to bring the newest research to this edition. Many researchers and educators shared their ideas and experiences, which are referenced throughout the book. I thank both the new contributors listed in each chapter and those who provided content for earlier editions, which served as the basis for the cutting-edge content provided in this edition. Significant roles in coordinating this revision were played by Thomas Lawson and Joe McGavin of SHAPE America and Ray Vallese and Scott Wikgren of Human Kinetics. I also wish to recognize and thank Chuck Corbin for his contributions to this and previous editions.

Special thanks to the activity editors for this edition, who supervised the content of the elementary and secondary activities included in the web resource for *Physical Best*:

Clayton Ellis, Mrachek Middle School, Aurora, Colorado

Joanna Faerber, Louisiana State University Laboratory School

The following people served as content experts for this fourth edition:

Suzan F. Ayers, Western Michigan University

Mary Jo Sariscsany, California State University, Northridge

Hannah Brewer, Slippery Rock University

Ethan Hull, Slippery Rock University

Randy Nichols, Slippery Rock University

Sean Bulger, West Virginia University

Brooke Towner, West Virginia University

D. Gayle Povis, University of Arizona

Jan Galen Bishop, Central Connecticut State University

Bette Jean Santos, Albemarle County (Virginia) Public Schools

Scott Going, University of Arizona

Melanie Hingle, University of Arizona

Elizabeth A. Burkhart, Wilson (Pennsylvania) High School, Penn State Berks

Philip C. Dlugolecki, Lansdale (Pennsylvania) Catholic High School

Patrick McHenry, Castle View (Colorado) High School

Bane McCracken, Marshall University (retired)

Betsy Gunther, Peters Township (Pennsylvania) High School (retired)

Keith Johannes, Santa Ana (California) Unified School District (retired)

Brian Culp, Kennesaw State University

David Lorenzi, Indiana University of Pennsylvania

Christina Sinclair, University of Northern Colorado

Lynn V. Johnson, Plymouth State University

Web Resource Contents

The web resource for *Physical Best, Fourth Edition,* includes 100 sample activities that show you how to put into action the health-related fitness principles detailed in the book. These teacher-tested activities can be used in your gym immediately or serve as templates you can use to create your own activities. In previous editions, these activities were presented in separate books: *Physical Best Activity Guide: Elementary Level* and *Physical Best Activity Guide: Middle and High School Levels.* But now the whole Physical Best package has been streamlined into one book and one web resource, which can be found at www.HumanKinetics.com/PhysicalBest.

The Physical Best activities have always been valued for their quality content: clear, step-by-step instructions for setting up and leading activities, practical teaching tips, modification ideas for inclusion, built-in assessments, home extensions, and ready-to-use posters and worksheets. In this edition, not only have the activities been completely updated to reflect current physical education and health education standards, they've also been reformatted to make searching for specific aspects of components of health-related fitness (such as flexibility) and fitness concepts (such as intensity and progression) faster and easier. This will help you pick the activity that best aligns with your lesson.

We've also made the activities easier to use than ever. You can access the activities your way—print them out or pull them up on your phone, tablet, or laptop. And you can use the activity menu to search for activities by standard, fitness component, fitness concept, or age level.

The Physical Best web resource also features forms and reproducibles that help you implement health-related fitness concepts into your curriculum, including sample assessments explained in the book that you may use in your own class as-is or customize to better fit your needs.

The following is a list of all the activities included in the web resource.

Elementary School Activities

- Activity Pyramid Circuit
- Aerobic Sports
- Animal Tag
- Around the Block
- Artery Avengers
- Beginning Yoga Poses
- Bowl a Snack
- Brown Bag Dinner
- Caterpillar Stretch
- Circulatory Scramble
- Clean the Beach
- Dash for Cash
- Disc Golf and Body Composition
- Fitness Four-Square
- Flexibility Activity Picture Chart
- Flexible Fun
- Give It Away
- Healthy Hearts
- Hoop It Up With Food
- Intermediate Yoga Poses
- Maintaining Balance
- Metabolism Medley
- Muscle Hustle
- Musical Sport Sequence
- Partner Pyramid Workout
- Push-Up Curl-Up Challenge
- Push-Up Dance
- Roll the Stretch
- Shuffle Activity
- Stretching Out Tag
- Stretch Marks the Spot
- Survivor Course

- Towel Stretching for Flexibility
- Treasure Island
- The Ultimate Game
- Up and Down With Jump Ropes
- You Can Bend

Middle and High School Activities

Aerobic Fitness:
- Cardio Benefit Hunt
- Cardiorespiratory Endurance Is FITT
- Chart Your Heart Rate
- Clean Out Your Arteries
- Continuous Relay
- Cross Training Trio
- FITT Log
- Four-Corner Heart-Healthy Warm-Up and Cool-Down
- Heartbeat Stations
- Know the Risks and Benefits
- Mini Triathlon
- The Ultimate Game (T.U.G.)
- Wanderer

Being a Good Health and Physical Activity Consumer:
- Evaluating Health Products
- Health and Fitness Quackery

Body Composition:
- Body Composition Survivor
- Build-a-Healthy-Body Ball
- Calorie-Balancing Act
- Cross-Training Triumph
- Frisbee Calorie Blaster
- One Thousand Repetitions

Combined Component:
- Component Countdown
- Deal a Healthy Body
- Fitness Adventure
- Fitness Bingo
- Fitness Unscramble
- Fortune Cookie Fitness
- Health-Related Fitness Warm-Up
- Jump Band Fitness

- Medicine Ball Circuit Training
- Monopoly Fitness
- Partner Racetrack Fitness
- Partner Racetrack Fitness Using Stability Balls
- Speed Circuit
- Sporting Fitness

Musculoskeletal Fitness:
- All-Star Stretches
- Flexibility FITT Log
- Flexibility Fling
- Flexibility Puzzles
- Get FITT
- Go for the Team Gold
- Introduction to Yoga
- Know Your Way Around the Weight Room
- Mission Push-Up Possible
- Muscle FITT Bingo
- Muscle Up
- Muscles for Money
- Muscles in Action
- Muscular Endurance and Strength FITT Log
- Muscular Fitness Scavenger Hunt
- Resistance Band Repetitions
- Rev-Up Roulette
- Safely Finding the 8 to 12 Rep Range
- Sport Spectacular
- Stretch Marks the Spot
- Type Cast
- Understanding Progression Through Functional Fitness
- Warm Up With Weights

Program Planning, Self-Management, and Goal Setting:
- Enrichment Activity: Fitness Trail
- "Exercise Your Rights!" School-Wide Special Event
- Fitness Olympics
- Goal Setting
- Learning Self-Management Skills

Foundations of Health-Related Fitness and Physical Activity

Part I introduces Physical Best, which is SHAPE America's approach to providing health-related fitness instruction, and shows how this approach encourages students to make positive changes for their health through fitness and nutritional choices. Chapter 1 examines the Physical Best philosophy and approach to give you a clear understanding of its purpose and usefulness in your teaching. Specifically, the chapter explains the comprehensive nature and unique qualities of the Physical Best instructional approach. Chapter 2 focuses on how and why children and adolescents choose to be physically active. It includes suggestions to help you motivate your students to become more physically active and makes connections between motivation and Physical Best instruction. Chapter 3 presents applications of the philosophical and behavioral concepts of the Physical Best instructional approach, including an overview of the basic training principles for key components of health-related fitness: cardiorespiratory endurance, muscular strength and endurance, and flexibility components. This first part ends with chapter 4, which covers nutrition and ways to guide your students to make positive nutritional choices for improved health.

CHAPTER 1

Introduction to Physical Best

Suzan F. Ayers and Mary Jo Sariscsany

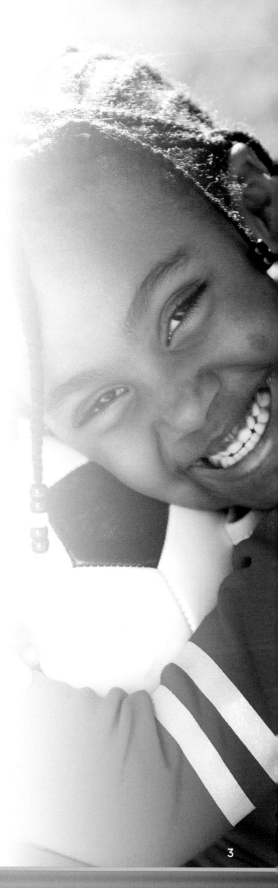

CHAPTER CONTENTS

Even as an increasing number of American adults recognize that physical activity is important to their health, physical education is being challenged in the nation's schools. In fact, the number of states requiring physical education in their public schools declined during the four-year period from 2012 to 2016 (SHAPE America, 2016). Moreover, 31 states allow other activities as substitutions for physical education credit, and 30 allow student exemptions from physical education class time or credit. In addition, 15 states allow school districts to apply for a waiver from state physical education requirements. Even worse, several states allow physical activity to be withheld or used as a punishment, although only 10 prohibit withholding physical activity as a punishment.

At the same time, physical education is more important than ever. It is still the best means available for schools to teach students the benefits of participating in regular physical activity. In addition, early physical education experiences play a key role in

Benefits of Physical Education and Physical Activity

In addition to knowing the risks of a sedentary lifestyle, students must also understand the many benefits of engaging in sufficient physical activity and remaining active for life. Research continues to affirm the benefits of physical activity, both for children's bodies and for their minds, including the following:

- Improved cardiorespiratory endurance and muscular fitness
- Favorable body composition
- Improvement in biomarkers for cardiovascular and metabolic health
- Reduced symptoms of anxiety and depression

Studies also continue to reveal new benefits, such as improved bone health and weight status for children of ages 3 to 5 and improved cognitive function for children of ages 6 to 13 (U.S. Department of Health and Human Services, 2008, 2018).

Recent research has also defined more clearly the link between school-based physical activity and academic achievement (Corbin et al., 2014). For example, a literature review published by the Centers for Disease Control and Prevention (2010b) identified policy implications of school-based physical activity, including physical education, and found "substantial evidence that physical activity can help improve . . . grades and standardized test scores" (p. 2). In addition, articles included in the review provided support for the positive effect exerted by physical activity on cognitive skills, attitudes, and academic behavior—all of which are precursors for academic success and harbingers of student success in school. The review also noted that increasing or maintaining physical education time has only a positive effect on students' academic performance. Taken together, this research highlights the need for well-conducted, standards-based physical education in K-12 schools.

Positive experiences with physical activity at a young age can help lay a foundation for being active regularly throughout one's life, according to the U.S. Department of Health and Human Services (USDHHS; 2018). The USDHHS recommends that young people (aged 6 to 17) participate in at least 60 minutes of physical activity per day; however, as of 2018, 30 percent of the U.S. population engages in *no* moderate or vigorous physical activity (USDHHS, 2008, 2018).

Physical activity exerts a positive influence not only on individual health but also on society as a whole, because a physically active population is able to be more productive. Physically active people also have healthier attitudes (USDHHS, 2018), which allows them to handle the larger problems associated with work or home in a more positive, reflective manner.

helping children develop fundamental locomotor and nonlocomotor skills required for participation in organized sports and activities in later years. Even though parents and guardians (or at least those who can afford it) have increasingly enrolled their students in physical activities outside of school, there remain few high-quality substitutes for the broad base of knowledge, skills, and attributes that students develop in a standards-based physical education program.

SHAPE America addresses this need for high-quality, standards-based physical education through the Physical Best approach to fitness education. This comprehensive program for health-related fitness education provides both conceptual information and a series of activities that can be included in physical education programs. Physical Best focuses on the benefits of physical activity (not just exercising), offers a variety of enjoyable activities, and helps students develop the necessary knowledge and skills to be confident and successful in a variety of movement activities across the life span. Thus the program aligns with the physical literacy approach that undergirds the National Standards for K-12 Physical Education (SHAPE America, 2014).

The provision of effective physical education has long been a priority for SHAPE America (Le Masurier & Corbin, 2006; National Association for Sport and Physical Education, 2004) and continues to be a concern of various national health organizations (Centers for Disease Control and Prevention [CDC], 2010a). SHAPE America's *National Standards & Grade-Level Outcomes for K-12 Physical Education* (2014) defines the primary goal of physical education as the development of *physically literate* individuals "who have the knowledge, skills, and confidence to enjoy a lifetime of healthful physical activity" (p. 1). This focus on physical literacy is holistic and supports children's development in the psychomotor, cognitive, and affective domains, thus addressing not just physical competence but also knowledge, attitudes, and psychological and social skills needed for lifelong participation in physical activity. As a result, the National Standards frame K-12 expectations as follows:

Standard 1. The physically literate individual demonstrates competency in a variety of motor skills and movement patterns.

Standard 2. The physically literate individual applies knowledge of concepts, principles, strategies and tactics related to movement and performance.

Standard 3. The physically literate individual demonstrates the knowledge and skills to achieve and maintain a health-enhancing level of physical activity and fitness.

Standard 4. The physically literate individual exhibits responsible personal and social behavior that respects self and others.

Standard 5. The physically literate individual recognizes the value of physical activity for health, enjoyment, challenge, self-expression and/or social interaction.

Standards-based physical education programs can help prepare children and adolescents to live physically active and healthy lives as part of becoming physically literate. This outcome is produced when teachers integrate skill- and health-related fitness instruction, because people can participate only in those activities for which they have developed a basic level of skill competence.

Physical educators are positioned both to help students become physically literate individuals and to help the community understand the relationship between physical activity and a healthy life. In turn, community support may increase when people understand how an effective physical education program can positively influence children and adolescents. To this end, physical educators can develop strong relationships with allied community health practitioners, physicians, and local government

Comprehensive School Physical Activity Programs (CSPAPs)

As noted by Corbin et al. (2014), the increased attention and visibility given to physical education by the medical and public health communities resulted in a prominent report by the Institute of Medicine (IOM) titled *Educating the Student Body: Taking Physical Activity and Physical Education to School* (2013). One of the key findings shared in this report is the role played by physical education and other school-based activity programs in enhancing student learning. One cooperative effort under way to promote physical activity and healthy lifestyles among youth involves the creation of Comprehensive School Physical Activity Programs (CSPAPs). This initiative, co-designed by SHAPE America and the Centers for Disease Control and Prevention in 2013, encourages the provision of high-quality physical education and a variety of physical activity opportunities—before, during, and after the school day—to foster participation in the nationally recommended 60-plus minutes of physical activity each day. This approach is intended to encourage student, community, faculty, and staff opportunities coordinated to help participants develop the necessary knowledge, skills, and confidence to be physically active for a lifetime (SHAPE America, 2015).

This approach to increasing quality movement opportunities has also been fostered by many other school-based relationships, including the NFL's Fuel Up to Play 60 (in partnership with the National Dairy Council) and the NFL Play 60 Challenge (in partnership with the American Heart Association). In addition, organizations such as Action for Healthy Kids and the Alliance for a Healthier Generation have established national training and support networks to help schools create a healthier environment. The visibility and accessibility of these and other programs has helped to build momentum for enhanced physical education programming in the United States.

officials, as guided by the CDC's Whole School, Whole Community, Whole Child (WSCC) model (Lewallen, Hunt, Potts-Datema, Zaza, & Giles, 2015). When we help people think of schools as contributing to the physical *and* cognitive well-being of children and adolescents, we can develop greater support. Physical education not only teaches children about a wide range of healthy habits but also provides them with opportunities to participate in health-enhancing physical activity.

What Is the Physical Best Instructional Approach?

In the early 1980s, SHAPE America recognized the need for a program that would help youth understand the importance of lifetime physical activity and fitness through regular participation in physical activity. The program would focus on educating all students from a health-related perspective regardless of their abilities. Thus, in 1987, Physical Best was developed as a comprehensive, health-related fitness education curriculum supplement for existing physical education programs. Physical Best helps both teachers and students meet the K-12 national physical education standards in order to help students achieve their individual physical best.

To reiterate, Physical Best was not designed to be used as a stand-alone curriculum. Rather, its materials can be used in conjunction with existing curricula and should be viewed as instructional materials, not as a curriculum framework.

To fully understand the mission of Physical Best, clarity on a few commonly used terms is needed. Specifically, *fitness*, *physical activity*, and *exercise* are frequently presented in the popular media as synonymous terms, when in fact they are not. In addition, the term *fitness* can be subdivided into *health-related fitness* and *skill-related fitness*. Long-established definitions of these terms (Caspersen, Powell, & Christenson, 1985) have been updated over the years and have served as the bedrock of health-related fitness instruction (Institute of Medicine, 2012, 2013):

- **Health-related fitness** is a measure of a person's ability to perform physical activities that require endurance, strength, or flexibility. This kind of fitness is achieved through a combination of regular exercise and inherent ability. The components of health-related physical fitness are cardiorespiratory endurance, muscular strength, muscular endurance, flexibility, body composition, and power as they relate specifically to health enhancement.

- **Skill-related fitness** is quite different than health-related fitness. Skill-related fitness often goes hand in hand with certain physical activities and is necessary for a person to accomplish or enhance a skill or task. Skill-related components include agility, balance, coordination, power, reaction time, and speed. An individual can still achieve and maintain a healthy lifestyle and lifelong participation in physical activity without possessing a high degree of skill-related components.

Health-related components and skill-related components are not mutually exclusive, but Physical Best focuses primarily on health-related fitness components (see figure 1.1).

In contrast, the terms *physical activity* and *exercise* have been defined by the U.S. Department of Health and Human Services (2008) as follows:

- **Physical activity** is strictly defined as any bodily movement produced by skeletal muscles that results in an expenditure of energy. It includes a broad range of occupational, leisure-time, and routine daily activities such as manual labor, gardening, walking, and performing household chores. Such activities may require light, moderate, or vigorous effort and can lead to improved health when performed regularly.

- **Exercise** is physical activity of a repetitive nature that is planned or structured to improve or maintain one or more of the health-related fitness components.

Here it may be helpful to briefly explain the relatively recent inclusion of power as a component of both skill-related and health-related fitness. As defined by the Institute of Medicine, **power** is "the peak force of a skeletal muscle multiplied by the velocity of the muscle contraction" (2012, p. S-7). The rationale for including power as a health-related fitness component has been outlined by Corbin et al. (2014, p. 27):

Among adults, improved strength, muscular endurance, and power are related to a variety of health benefits (e.g., lower mortality, lower risk of heart disease, better metabolic profiles, lower risk of osteoporosis) and reduce the chance of musculoskeletal disorders (American College of Sports Medicine, 2013). The appropriateness of resistance training for youth was questioned until recent years, but new guidelines from the National Strength and Conditioning Association (Faigenbaum et al., 2009) indicate that properly conducted programs are appropriate for youth. Although the associations of strength, muscular endurance, and power are not as strong among youth as among adults, the IOM report (Institute of Medicine, 2102) documents the relationship between these fitness components and health markers, especially bone health, among youth. . . . [In addition], the relationship between muscle power and health is more established among youth (Institute of Medicine, 2012) and older adults (American College of Sports Medicine, 2013) than it is among young adults.

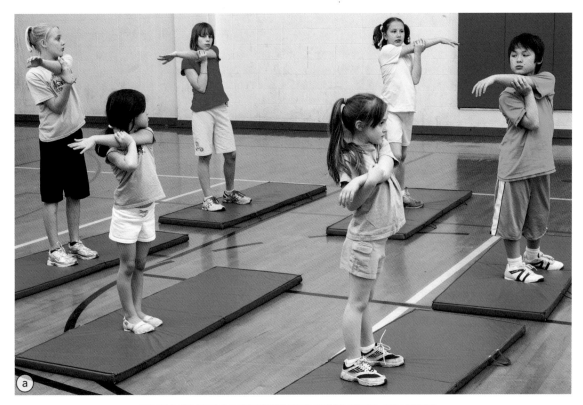

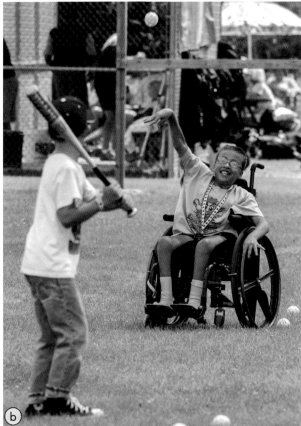

FIGURE 1.1   *(a)* Health-related fitness includes the components of cardiorespiratory endurance, muscular strength, muscular endurance, flexibility, body composition, and power. *(b)* Skill-related fitness includes the components of agility, balance, coordination, power, reaction time, and speed.

Health-Related Fitness Education

The Physical Best instructional approach recognizes the importance of assessment in health-related fitness education. Although individual fitness performance results should not be used as part of students' grades, they can and should be used to help students set personal fitness goals and to help teachers prepare and adjust curriculum. The Physical Best approach is characterized by eight key elements (see figure 1.2):

- *Fitness concepts.* The Physical Best approach educates students about fitness concepts and the role of regular exercise in preventing disease. These foci lay the foundation for understanding the relationship between physical activity and lifelong health benefits, as well as the health-related fitness components and the concepts necessary to develop and improve health-related fitness.

- *Preparing students.* Helping students prepare for assessments should include showing them pictures, videos, and examples of what the assessments will involve. This interaction, as well as communicating with administrators and parents about testing content and procedures, will help establish open lines of communication among stakeholders.

- *Practicing procedures.* Giving students multiple opportunities to practice will help them understand the protocols and feel comfortable and confident during assessments. It is also necessary to explain why fitness is important for overall health, as well as which health-related fitness component is measured by each

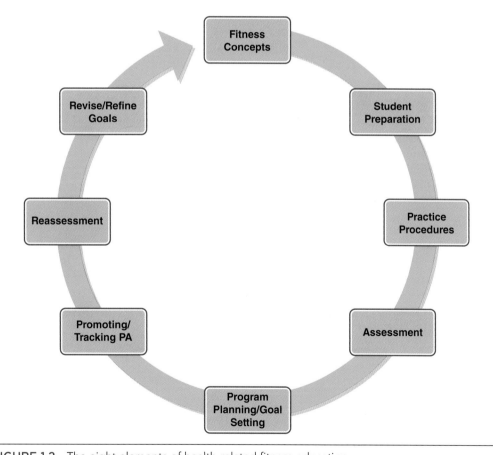

FIGURE 1.2 The eight elements of health-related fitness education.

Reprinted by permission from The Cooper Institute.

assessment. Ensuring students understand procedures—for example, what constitutes a performance error—helps clarify expectations.

- *Assessing health-related fitness.* Using the six recommended FitnessGram **assessments** to evaluate health-related fitness provides data for decision making. Details of how to conduct each assessment are provided in the *FitnessGram Administration Manual* (The Cooper Institute, 2017).

- *Program planning and goal setting.* Teachers can synthesize class- and school-level assessment results to help them make programmatic and instructional decisions that positively affect students' health-related fitness. For example, a teacher who analyzes school-level data might discover that a majority of students lack adequate flexibility as compared with the healthy values based on age and gender. In response, the teacher could address this need by adding a flexibility station to the warm-up routine in each class. On the individual level, helping students use personal results to set goals that are SMART (i.e., specific, measureable, attainable, realistic, and time-bound) can motivate them to achieve and maintain lifelong health-related fitness. Moreover, sharing assessment results with students and parents opens the door for families to consider ways to become and remain active together. Part of this family outreach is ensuring that all parties understand and can accurately interpret individual results. Once this understanding is established, helping students set goals will enable them to adjust their physical activity and health-related fitness pursuits across the life span.

- *Promoting and tracking physical activity.* Giving students opportunities to promote and track their physical activity helps them understand the relationships between regular physical activity and health-related fitness. When students are encouraged and given opportunities for physical activity—both within and beyond the classroom—they can develop healthful patterns of physical activity that will last a lifetime. Tools for tracking physical activity include programs such as PALA+ (Presidential Active Lifestyle Award) and ActivityGram. Other simple options include tracking one's steps and using pedometer or Fitbit data to set and adjust goals. The value of regularly tracking physical activity lies in the process of focusing attention on one's personal fitness regimen and the activities it includes (this focus relates to the process of revising and refining goals, noted a bit later in this list).

- *Reassessing student fitness.* Reassessing the health-related fitness components, in both standardized (e.g., FitnessGram) and less formal ways (e.g., comparing levels of effort required to walk up stairs or noting how clothes fit differently over time), can reinforce students' interest and desire to participate in regular physical activity and meet their goals. In addition, participation can also be incentivized by offering recognition for improved levels of health-related personal fitness.

- *Revising and refining goals.* The process of revising and refining goals is necessary to address what is and is not working. Consistently monitoring health-related fitness levels and making appropriate revisions and refinements in a physical activity plan demonstrate a personal commitment to personal wellness. Keeping an eye on personal fitness provides updated information that reflects progress toward individual goals. It also provides feedback about the effectiveness of changes and helps determine which activities are most effective and enjoyable. Teaching students to evaluate their own health-related fitness results, revise their goals, and set new goals is essential to a fulfilling life of regular participation in physical activity, which can foster health-related fitness.

What Makes Physical Best Unique?

The uniqueness of Physical Best lies in its comprehensiveness, which combines the latest scientific research with practical experience and activities from physical educators around the country. As noted at the beginning of this chapter, Physical Best is aligned with the National Standards for K-12 Physical Education (SHAPE America, 2014), and this approach is supported by the profession's definition of quality physical education:

> The goal of physical education is to develop physically literate individuals who have the knowledge, skills and confidence to enjoy a lifetime of healthful physical activity. (SHAPE America, 2014, p. 11)

The following list highlights some of the features of Physical Best that make it a valuable tool for physical educators and students alike:

- *Comprehensive conceptual framework.* Physical Best provides a framework that educators can use to teach conceptual information about health-related fitness and nutrition in the activity setting. In turn, the program provides students with information to help them understand and value the concepts of health-related fitness and its relationship to a healthy lifestyle; it also provides information about assessment, goal setting, and motivational strategies. In addition, Physical Best offers ideas and suggestions for integrated curricula (across subject areas and in the three learning domains—cognitive, affective, and psychomotor), as well as parent and community involvement.

- *Active participation.* The Physical Best activities, available in the web resource accompanying this book, are designed to involve all students and help them remain active most of the time. Teams are limited in size (two to four students per team) so that each student has numerous practice opportunities. In addition, student wait time can be limited by setting up multiple stations.

- *Individualized activities.* Activities are designed so that students can work at their own level of health-related fitness or activity. Physical Best also provides avenues for students to excel by moving beyond the minimum. The activities may provide various levels to achieve, different practice times, variety in the number of trials, choices of task difficulty, and so forth. In turn, individuals have the opportunity and freedom to choose activities that are interesting to them. They can also modify an activity to suit their needs, goals, and abilities without losing the activity's health-related benefits. In short, Physical Best emphasizes enjoyment in participation and encourages students to strive for personal success in a positive learning atmosphere.

- *Tools for lifelong activity.* Students gain the knowledge, skills, and self-motivation to engage regularly in one or more physical activities as an ongoing lifestyle choice.

- *Health-related physical activity.* Students are provided with safe and sequential activities that help maintain or improve the components of health-related fitness (cardiorespiratory endurance, muscular strength and endurance, flexibility, body composition, and power). Activities focus on personal improvement

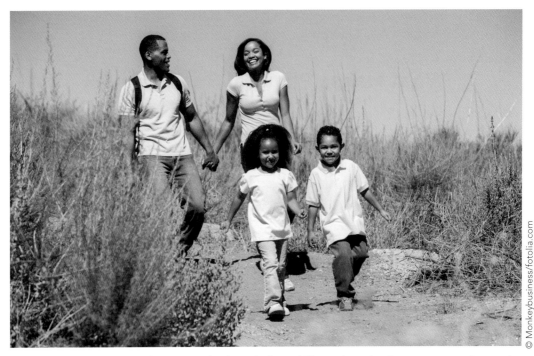

In physical education, students gain the knowledge, skills, and motivation to engage in regular physical activity as an ongoing life choice.

rather than attaining unrealistic standards. The program incorporates the latest health-related fitness testing (FitnessGram) and combines assessment and activities into a plan for individual improvement.

- *Adherence to standards.* Physical Best was developed to help teachers meet national standards for physical education, health education, and dance education (see chapter 9). It also supports the *Healthy People 2020* objectives and the 1999 *Surgeon General's Report on Physical Activity and Health* and its updates, and it is consistent with the 2018 *Physical Activity Guidelines for Americans.*

Rather than just teaching sports, physical educators are encouraged to teach the how and why of a physically active, healthy lifestyle. In Physical Best, these components are combined into a comprehensive K-12 education program for health-related fitness. The program uses a variety of resources, as well as professional development training, to facilitate success for both students and teachers.

Physical Best Activities

This textbook provides a foundation of knowledge in health-related fitness education. The accompanying web resource equips teachers to take the knowledge off the page and into the gym with ready-to-use activities for the elementary, middle school, and high school levels. The web resource is available by means of the key code bound into this book. Its table of contents can be found at the beginning of this book.

Physical Best Activities for the Elementary Level

The elementary-level activities are designed to help kindergarten through fifth-graders gain the knowledge, skills, appreciation, and confidence to lead healthy, physically active lives. The easy-to-use instructional activities have been developed and used successfully by physical educators across the United States. This collection includes competitive and noncompetitive activities, demanding and less demanding activities, and activities that allow for maximum time on task. Above all, the activities are designed to be educational and fun.

Physical Best Activities for the Middle School and High School Levels

The secondary-level activities are geared toward 6th- through 12th-grade students. The information presented enables deeper and richer understanding of the importance of daily physical activity. The activities include an additional section focused on personal health and health-related fitness planning. This section provides students with an introduction to the skills needed to be physically active for life after high school.

Related Resources

During a typical school year, many educators use more than one program, drawing on a variety of teaching resources and overlapping various approaches on a day-to-day basis. With this reality in mind, it may be reassuring to know that although Physical Best is designed to be used independently for teaching health-related fitness, it can also be used in conjunction with the following resources.

FitnessGram

FitnessGram (developed by the Cooper Institute) provides a comprehensive assessment for health-related fitness and activity, as well as a web-based reporting system. All elements of FitnessGram are designed to help teachers achieve the primary objective of health-related fitness programs for youth—namely, to help young people establish physical activity as a regular part of their daily lives. FitnessGram is the only nationally supported assessment tool for health-related fitness, and it can be used with minimal investment and access to online training (additional resources are available in the online version).

FitnessGram is based on the belief that extremely high levels of health-related fitness, though admirable, are not necessary in order to achieve key objectives associated with good health and improved function. Indeed, all children should have adequate levels of activity and health-related fitness. To this end, FitnessGram enables students and teachers to assess health-related fitness performance in a way that connects participation in physical activity with related outcomes, including good health, growth, and function.

The *FitnessGram Administration Manual* (The Cooper Institute, 2017) is published by and available through Human Kinetics, as are the materials for the Brockport Physical Fitness Test, which is a health-related fitness assessment for students with disabilities. For complete information about FitnessGram, FitnessGram software, and other resources, visit www.cooperinstitute.org/fitnessgram.

Fitness for Life

Fitness for Life is a comprehensive K-12 program that helps students take responsibility for their own activity and health-related fitness, thus preparing them to be physically active and healthy throughout their lives. This standards-based program has been carefully articulated with a pedagogically sound scope and sequence to enhance students' learning and progress. It is philosophically compatible with Physical Best and in pursuit of helping students develop lifelong physical activity habits. Research has shown that Fitness for Life is effective in promoting physically active behavior among students after they finish school.

Fitness for Life and Physical Best complement each another because Physical Best activities can be used before, during, and after a Fitness for Life course. Both programs are based on the HELP philosophy of promoting *H*ealth for *E*veryone with a focus on *L*ifetime activity of a *P*ersonal nature. For more information about Fitness for Life, visit www.fitnessforlife.org.

SHAPE America Resources

SHAPE America publishes many useful resources, which are available on its website and through its online store at www.shapeamerica.org. Given the ever-changing nature of online resources, this website is provided in lieu of listing publications that may not be current by the time this textbook is purchased.

Physical Best Certificate

Physical Best provides accurate, up-to-date information and training to help physical educators create a conceptual and integrated format for health-related fitness education. In addition to providing the program itself, SHAPE America offers the option of earning a certificate to indicate that educators have developed the knowledge, skills, and ability to provide effective health-related fitness instruction. The certificate was created specifically to recognize physical educators who remain up to date on the most effective strategies for helping students gain the necessary knowledge, skills, appreciation, and confidence to lead healthy, physically active lives. It focuses on application—that is, how to teach health-related fitness concepts using developmentally appropriate and age-appropriate activities and FitnessGram assessments.

To earn the Physical Best certificate through SHAPE America, the following steps are necessary:

- Attend a one-day Physical Best Health Fitness Specialist workshop or complete a semester-long college or university course that includes Physical Best content.
- Read this book and the latest version of the *FitnessGram Administration Manual*.
- Use these resources to complete an online open-book examination. Successful completion of the exam results in awarding of the Physical Best certificate.

Summary

Physical Best complements and supports existing physical education programs by teaching and applying health-related fitness concepts to promote lifelong physical activity. The program excels at providing this component of a well-rounded physical education curriculum by

- basing its philosophy and materials on current research and expert, field-tested input;
- teaching the benefits of lifelong physical activity;

- offering a national certificate as a Physical Best Health Fitness Specialist;
- focusing on the positive (e.g., students' strengths, enjoyable activities); and
- individualizing instruction so that all students can benefit and succeed.

The Physical Best instructional approach increases the odds that students will pursue healthy, physically active lifestyles after they leave quality physical education programs and move into adulthood.

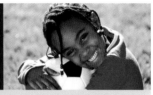

Discussion Questions

1. Describe the Physical Best mission and how it relates to providing quality physical education instruction.
2. How does the comprehensive nature of Physical Best help teachers provide quality instructional activities that foster learning?
3. Discuss the features of Physical Best that can help teachers incorporate the program into any lesson.
4. Give examples of how the information presented in this guide can be coordinated with the Physical Best activities provided in the web resource to provide active learning experiences.

CHAPTER 2

Creating Physical Activity Behaviors That Last a Lifetime

Hannah Brewer, Ethan Hull, and Randy Nichols

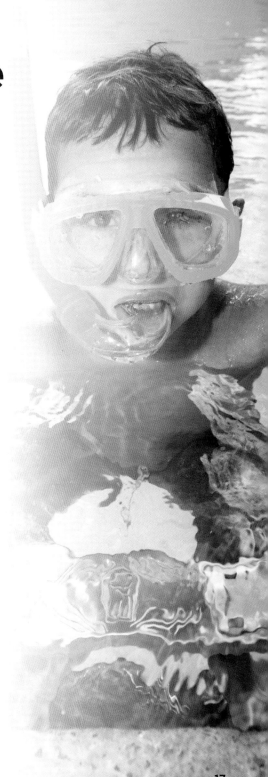

CHAPTER CONTENTS

Meeting physical activity guidelines can be challenging for children, adolescents, and adults alike. Lifelong habits of physical activity come naturally for some students, but most need to be taught how to be physically active; why physical activity is important; and how to value, appreciate, and become intrinsically motivated to engage in lifelong physical activity. In other words, effective physical education is vital for shaping healthy physical activity habits among children and adolescents. Beyond physical education, we must provide learning experiences that inspire children and adolescents to be physically active before, during, and after the school day. We can shape positive attitudes and embed physical activity into a student's day in a variety of ways, but evidence clearly indicates that effective physical education programs must also motivate students. To this end, Physical Best focuses on each child's preferences and capabilities in order to motivate all children to be physically active, not just during their school days but for a lifetime.

This chapter investigates how physical educators and physical activity specialists can motivate school-age children and adolescents to develop physical activity habits that last a lifetime. More specifically, the chapter addresses how the pursuit of this mission is facilitated by the Physical Best program. In 2016, SHAPE America (the Society of Health and Physical Educators) launched its 50 Million Strong by 2029 initiative with the goal of ensuring that all students are empowered to live healthy and active lives. With that goal in mind, some of us may need to approach teaching physical education differently from how we've taught it in the past. Our focus must shift from teaching students how to play a variety of games and sports to teaching them how to live a life of wellness and lifelong physical activity. With that need in mind, this chapter provides information about (1) physical activity and obesity trends among children, adolescents, and adults; (2) research on the success of interventions intended to increase physical activity; (3) current national initiatives promoting school wellness; (4) strategies for motivating school-age children and adolescents based on Physical Best recommendations; and (5) tips from current K-12 physical and health education teachers.

Physical Activity Trends

The importance of daily physical activity for improving and maintaining health is well known, especially among physical educators. Even so, population data show that large proportions of U.S. children, adolescents, and adults are overweight and inactive (Ogden, Carroll, Fryar, & Flegal, 2015; Ogden, Carroll, Kit, & Flegal, 2014; U.S. Department of Health and Human Services, 2008), and few Americans meet the recommendations for physical activity (Centers for Disease Control and Prevention, 2016b; U.S. Department of Health and Human Services, 2008). In 2008, the U.S. Department of Health and Human Services (2008) issued guidelines for physical activity and musculoskeletal health recommending that children and adolescents should be physically active for at least 60 minutes per day. Moreover, at least 30 minutes of that activity should occur during a physical education class (American Heart Association, 2015), and students should spend at least half of that 30 minutes in moderate- to vigorous-intensity physical activity (Institute of Medicine, 2013; SHAPE America, 2016a). Teachers should view these recommendations not as limits but as minimal starting points for children and adolescents.

According to the CDC, since the 1960s, obesity levels have risen among adolescents (aged 12 through 19 years). In contrast, since 2005, obesity rates appear to be decreasing in children of ages 2 through 5 years and leveling off in children of ages

6 through 11 years (figure 2.1). Nevertheless, over the past 50 years, obesity levels have nearly doubled in children of kindergarten age or younger, more than tripled in elementary-age children, and quadrupled in adolescents. Although obesity can be attributed to numerous factors, one of the most commonly cited reasons for weight gain is physical inactivity (Centers for Disease Control and Prevention, 2016a).

Although plenty of data support the preponderance of obesity, tracking physical activity levels is more difficult. As compared with obesity data, physical activity data are less reliable, require more effort to measure, and are more subject to recall bias. Still, nearly all of the physical activity data suggest that both school-age children and adolescents and adults are insufficiently active. Research shows that only about 25 percent of adolescents aged 12 to 15 years meet the recommendations for physical activity (PA) on all seven days of the week, whereas 49 percent meet the recommendations on five days per week, and 15 percent do not engage in *any* physical activity (Fakhouri et al., 2014).

The evidence is even worse for adults. Figure 2.2 shows the trend in adult obesity and adult PA levels from 1994 through 2014. Since the 1990s, the percentage of obese adults has risen from 23 percent to nearly 37 percent, and only 20 percent of adults engage in the recommended 30 minutes of daily PA on five days per week. Additional data from the Centers for Disease Control and Prevention (CDC) show that a large proportion of American adults (48 percent) do not meet the daily or weekly PA recommendations (National Center for Health Statistics, 2016).

Perhaps the only silver lining in figure 2.2 involves the small increase in adults who met the physical activity recommendations, which may seem counterintuitive. How can adults be more active *and* more obese? Keep in mind that measuring body weight is not the same as measuring physical activity levels. Still, if adults are slowly becoming more physically active, then that trend is worth supporting and nurturing. It may relate to the fact that adults are more susceptible to chronic diseases associated with physical inactivity and are starting to take ownership of their health due to the prospect of impending chronic disease.

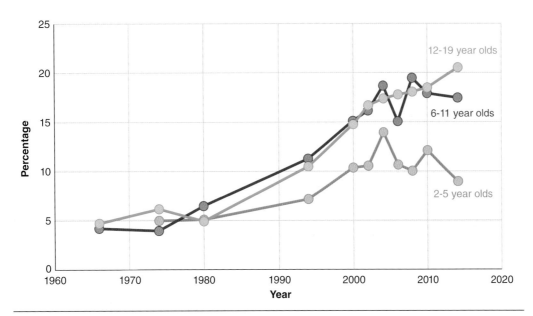

FIGURE 2.1   Obesity levels of children in the United States.

From Ogden et al. (2015); Ogden et al. (2014).

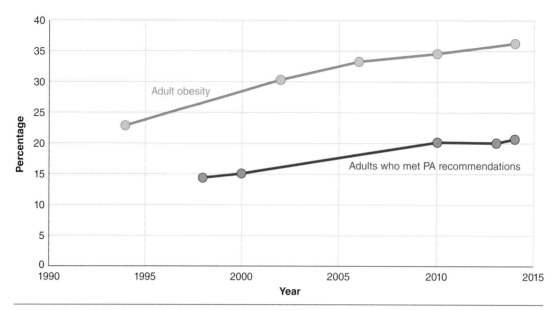

FIGURE 2.2   Percentage of adults who were obese and those who met physical activity recommendations, 1994-2014.

Based on National Center for Health Statistics (NCHS) (2016).

Of course, adults typically do not have the luxury of a daily physical education class to help them stay active, but many children do not have that opportunity, either. As shown in figure 2.3, the percentage of young people participating in daily physical education classes fell sharply during the early 1990s, then largely leveled off at about 30 percent. Meanwhile, even as television viewing decreased, 25 percent of adolescents still watch three hours or more of television per day, and more than 40 percent play video games for three hours or more per day—nearly double the rate from 2005. These trends reinforce the importance of motivating children and adolescents to be physically active beyond their school-based physical education classes.

Thus the public health problem is clear: School-age children and adolescents must be more active, and schools can serve as the primary vehicle for helping students create positive physical activity behaviors that are sustainable. Physical education is the only academic subject dedicated to motivating students to be physically active, yet most school districts (70 percent) don't have a policy for physical education time requirements (Committee on Physical Activity and Physical Education in the School Environment; Food and Nutrition Board, 2013a). According to CDC research, only about 25 percent of districts recommend that their schools meet the federal physical activity guidelines; moreover, only 4 percent of elementary schools, 2 percent of middle schools, and 2 percent of high schools are required by their district to meet the guideline of offering 30 minutes per day of moderate- to vigorous-intensity physical activity in physical education (Committee on Physical Activity and Physical Education in the School Environment; Food and Nutrition Board, 2013b). This reality means that, now more than ever, physical education teachers are responsible not only for producing effective lessons and programs to encourage physical activity but also for serving as physical activity advocates in their schools.

Given that physical education teachers shoulder so many responsibilities, they will benefit from knowing how to motivate students to be active both in the classroom and in the community. This chapter covers several school-based initiatives and explains how you can take an active role in promoting physical activity at your school. More

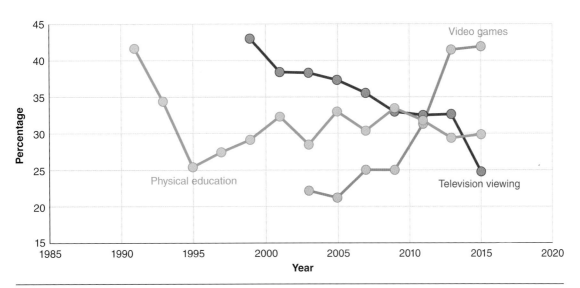

FIGURE 2.3   Percentage of U.S. adolescents (grades 9 through 12) who participated in physical education five days per week, played video or computer games for three hours or more per day, and watched three hours or more of television per day.

Based on Center for Disease Control and Prevention (2015), *Trends in the Prevalence of Physical Activity and Sedentary Behaviors National YRBSS: 1991-2015.* https://www.cdc.gov/healthyyouth/data/yrbs/pdf/trends/2015_us_physical_trend_yrbs.pdf

specifically, the next section of the chapter discusses physical activity behavior, which we must understand in order to motivate school-age children and adolescents to adopt positive physical activity habits that last a lifetime.

Physical Activity and Behavior Change

A person may adopt and sustain a behavior for any of many reasons, some of which may not be apparent to either an independent observer or the person making the decision. The factors that influence a person's internal and external motivation often change throughout the person's life, and what works today may not work tomorrow. Likewise, a physical education teacher may help students maximize movement during physical education, but that pattern may not transfer outside of school if the child lacks support or access to external physical activity programs. Given these various factors, it is worth stepping back to consider the role of a physical education teacher. Specifically, can teachers improve health status on a societal scale when most schools allocate only limited time to physical education? As one answer to that question, this chapter discusses how physical education teachers can help students develop self-determined motivation to be physically active for a lifetime.

The role of today's physical education teachers should be to advocate, teach, and promote a physically active lifestyle for all students. Who else has the knowledge, skill, and training to positively influence children to build a culture of health in schools? Children are more active and have higher health-related fitness levels when the physical education class is led by a physical education teacher than by another professional, according to Sallis, McKenzie, et al. (1997). Their landmark study suggests that physical education teachers are the optimal choice when creating physical activity opportunities in school. We can all remember when a teacher positively influenced us, but did that influence transfer into a lifelong habit related to the activity in question? If so, it is a type of opportunity that is worth re-creating, and such opportunities constitute a top priority in physical education.

To create lifelong learners who choose to engage in health-enhancing physical activities on a daily basis, you should be well versed in the theory and practice of motivation. Although it lies beyond the scope of this chapter, further reading in motivational interviewing and the theory of unified behavior can help you understand decision making and behavior change (Herman, Reinke, Frey, & Shepard, 2013). For now, the following section reviews concepts and motivational theories that have shown some success in promoting motivation for physical activity among school-age children and adolescents.

Social Support for Physical Activity

Social support is one of the primary modes through which a person establishes patterns of behavior. For children and adolescents, social support comes in three major forms: parental support (when the child is young), parental and peer support (as the child ages through middle school and high school), and teacher and coach support (throughout childhood).

Of these three factors, parental involvement has been shown to have the strongest connection with a child's PA level (Davison, Downs, & Birch, 2006; Prochaska, Rodgers, & Sallis, 2002; Sallis, Alcaraz, McKenzie, & Hovell, 1999; Trost et al., 2003). When parents support their children through encouragement, praise, teaching, transportation to a facility or other location for activity, and playing with their children, those children are significantly more active than are children of parents who support activity at a lower level. For this reason, programs should encourage parents to be active with their children before, during, or after school. This involvement increases children's motivation to be active and leads to increased physical activity by the parents as well.

Although parental involvement is strongly correlated with child PA levels, most physical activity programs have not attempted to involve parents, and those that have done so have struggled (Gentile et al., 2009; Luepker et al., 1996; Pate et al., 2003). Leaders of these programs have stated that efforts to involve parents are difficult, require considerable planning and organization, and should offer incentives for participation. Given this advice, the task of trying to start community, family, and school-based PA programs should not be attempted alone; instead, such efforts may benefit from a committee of dedicated planners, coordinators, staff members, and volunteers.

Engaging parents and families may be a key aspect of motivation. For example, one physical activity initiative, the Bienestar Health Program, demonstrated success in involving parents and improved children's health-related fitness levels (Trevino, Hernandez, Yin, Garcia, & Hernandez, 2005). Leaders of the program, which took place in a community with relatively low socioeconomic status, attributed the improvements in children's health-related fitness to increased levels of child self-efficacy and increased social support from parents and teachers. The innovative nature of the project created the expectation that parents would participate in games, presentations, and programs, and feedback from parents suggested that they found the experience both meaningful and fun. For instance, in one activity, children prepared a theater performance addressing diabetes, and parents were asked to play the roles of glucose, insulin, and cells (fat or muscle). Parents each wore a card around their neck and imitated the flow of glucose in both a healthy and an unhealthy state. As a result of its positive outcomes, the program continues to operate (Texas Education Agency, 2017), and its results suggest that focusing on children's needs and creating a supportive environment can enable sustainable and positive change.

Strategies for Engaging Families

Here are some specific strategies for enhancing motivation for physical activity through parent involvement.

Elementary

- *Communicate.* Create a school website for physical education and wellness and use it to provide ideas for family fun that includes physical activity. Routinely update the site to show the physical activities that children are engaging in at school. Consider also providing such updates via social media.

- *Support.* Create positive relationships with parents so that they feel valued as members of the school community and share in the school's vision of success. Provide support to help parents become involved to the point where they are not only encouraged but also expected to participate (Herman et al., 2013).

- *Engage.* Create at-home challenges, share them with students during class, and encourage students to get their parents or guardians involved at home. Ask children to initiate a specific physical activity at home—for example, a walking challenge, a TV commercial fitness challenge (family members perform various exercises during commercial breaks), or a simple dance performed to a popular children's song that they have learned in physical education.

- *Find opportunities to move.* Encourage children to work with their parents to create as many opportunities to move as possible throughout the day (Segar, 2015). Examples include parking far away from the grocery store, standing instead of sitting while completing homework, walking while waiting to pick up an older sibling at an after-school activity, and taking a "longcut" while walking to a neighbor's house or running errands.

- *Share resources.* Create a take-home kit of various physical activity equipment (e.g., jump rope, set of cups for stacking, flying disc, plastic bat and ball). Allow children to take the kit home and engage their family in physical activity, then share with the class about the activity they did at home.

- *Make health-related fitness a part of education.* Take every opportunity to include physical activity in schoolwide events, including those that involve parents and families. Can band and choral concerts include a physical activity component, such as dancing? Can physical activity also be incorporated into book fairs, indoor carnivals, reading clubs, and before- and after-school programs?

Secondary

- *Communicate.* Create a school website for physical education and wellness and use it to provide ideas for family fun that includes physical activity. Routinely update the site to show the physical activities that children are engaging in at school. Consider also providing such updates via social media.

- *Advocate.* Ask students to analyze and reflect on their family's physical activity habits. They can then help their family become more active by creating a SMART plan—that is, a plan focused on a goal that is specific, measurable, attainable, realistic, and time sensitive. This approach gives students ownership of PA recommendations for themselves and their family members and allows them to advocate for physical activity within their home.

- *Find opportunities to move.* Encourage students to find as many opportunities to move as possible throughout the day (Segar, 2015). Middle school and high school students may do so either individually or with their family. Encourage them to create an in-home challenge where they compete with a sibling or parent to identify the most creative opportunity to move that day.

- *Share resources.* Create a list of simple workouts that can be done at home with minimal or no equipment and post them on the website. Include both individual workouts and ones that can be done with a peer or buddy. These ideas may encourage secondary students to ask a parent, sibling, or guardian to participate in an at-home workout with them.

- *Make students the experts.* Host an evening or weekend event focused on health-related fitness where students teach and lead a variety of physical activities for parents and teachers. Examples include Zumba, Drums Alive, yoga, team handball, and walking groups.

Thus physical education teachers may find that incorporating similar strategies for parental involvement in activities that are deemed meaningful and enjoyable will help them create a successful physical activity program for the school community. Of course, each school community is unique in its social and built environments, and the resulting constraints and opportunities should be factored into any physical activity project carried out at the school. Creating an environment that supports daily PA requires both time and a committed staff that shares a viable vision and framework for the project.

Efforts to encourage PA behavior change in an organized fashion may benefit from a solid grounding in theory, perhaps even in multiple theories (Reis et al., 2016). Fortunately, people's motivations for change have been studied extensively in terms of stages of readiness and awareness (Cardinal, 2000; Carron, Hausenblas, & Estabrooks, 2003; Prochaska, Norcross, & DiClemente, 1994).

Stages of Change

The predominant change theory—the transtheoretical model (TTM), or stages-of-change model—is used in public health to understand and describe an individual's level of readiness to change (McKenzie, Neiger, & Thackeray, 2017). Understanding the **stages of change** can help wellness professionals (and individuals seeking to change) understand the process one goes through to become ready to change an unhealthy behavior or adopt a healthier behavior. More specifically, TTM posits that all individuals go through the following series of stages when beginning a physically active lifestyle:

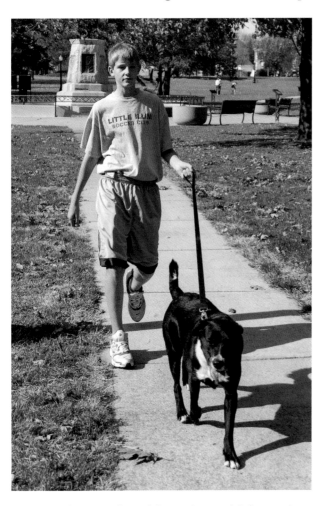

The transtheoretical model may be useful for working with mature middle school and high school students who are ready to make changes toward a more active lifestyle.

- *Precontemplation.* In this stage, the person has no intention of changing and is not motivated to do so.
- *Contemplation.* This stage is marked by thinking about change but not being motivated to take immediate action. In this stage, the individual hopes to make a change within the next six months.
- *Preparation.* This stage involves some activity or preparation to take action in the near future.
- *Action.* In this stage, the individual is making specific, overt, positive changes in lifestyle (and within the past six months).
- *Maintenance.* In this stage, the individual has made a positive change and is actively maintaining the new healthy lifestyle.

In order to move from any of the first three stages to the action stage (for example, to engaging in regular physical activity), the person must have knowledge, support, tools, and intrinsic desire to want to change. Thus, for inactive students, you must find ways not only to provide the needed tools and supports but also to foster intrinsic desire within the student to adopt lifelong physical activity behaviors (that is, to reach the maintenance stage).

Perhaps more important, you can help students create healthy behaviors while they are young so that they do not have to make such changes in their adult years. Among at-risk populations, only a minority (usually less than 20 percent) of individuals are prepared to take action at any given time (McKenzie et al., 2017). Therefore, changing unhealthy behaviors in relation to physical activity is more challenging than helping students develop positive physical activity patterns while they are young and their behaviors are more malleable. As a result, the transtheoretical model may be useful for middle school and high school teachers, who are working with more mature students, or students who are already choosing a sedentary lifestyle.

Social Cognitive Theory

Most programs that have been implemented in schools to improve physical activity behavior and motivation do not appear to be purposefully based on a theoretical framework. Among those that are, social cognitive theory (SCT) appears to be the most common choice (Dobbins, Husson, DeCorby, & LaRocca, 2013). According to Bandura (1986), SCT holds that behavior is affected by personal, behavioral, and environmental influences. Bandura's articulation of SCT suggests that each of these three factors affect the other two and that a behavior becomes more likely when an individual develops competency, increases self-efficacy, and enhances self-motivation through goal setting. To elaborate, competency is the ability to perform a task, self-efficacy is the belief that one can be effective at accomplishing the task, and goal setting creates a positive idea about what one wants to achieve. In a physical education setting, students' competency should increase with skill building and practice, their self-efficacy should increase when they succeed at applying practiced skills, and goal setting should stimulate their **intrinsic motivation** (internal desire to perform a particular task) to achieve and improve. These are all important facets of motivation.

In turn, Physical Best may help students develop self-efficacy and a personal commitment to their own health by focusing on health-related fitness concepts and attitudes in an inclusive and enjoyable manner. Specifically, physical education teachers can use the following strategies: skill building and practice, goal setting to improve health-related fitness and wellness, and opportunities for parents and other family members to provide social support that reinforces a pattern of daily PA.

The next section discusses recent initiatives to promote physical activity among children and adolescents and considers ways in which schools can help students develop the motivation needed to sustain positive physical activity behaviors.

Current Initiatives Promoting School Wellness

Recently, several local, state, and national initiatives have been developed to improve health and increase physical activity levels among school-age children and adolescents. From Michelle Obama's Let's Move! campaign to the Surgeon General's Step it Up! challenge, the message is clear: Today's children and adolescents need to move more, and we are seeking innovative ways to motivate them to be physically active. One common theme among several national initiatives is the notion that health-enhancing physical activity can be simple: Walking, dancing, standing instead of sitting, and simply playing are among some of the most recent initiatives designed to improve the health and well-being of school-age children and adolescents (Batch-elder & Matusitz, 2014). Accordingly, we can frame physical activity not in terms of a course that emphasizes performance or skill but as a positive, enjoyable activity that can be experienced by anyone. When we lead or allow students to view physical activity as complicated, strenuous, or enjoyed only by "athletes," we run the risk of failing to empower *all* children to lead healthy and active lives (SHAPE America, 2016a). According to Davies et al. (2015), "The key to reversing the growing trend of inactivity among today's youth begins with adjusting the attitude and environment surrounding physical education" (p. 9).

This view is consistent with the approach taken by Physical Best as it focuses on guidelines for health and personal improvement rather than on meeting unrealistic performance-based standards, which may be viewed as overly strenuous or compli-cated. In this and other ways, the studies and initiatives mentioned in the preceding paragraph are critical for understanding the role that physical education teachers play in inspiring children and adolescents to be physically active, both during physical education class and throughout the day.

The next section reinforces how physical activity and physical education are con-nected to students' overall well-being. More specifically, it defines the Whole School, Whole Community, Whole Child (WSCC) approach, which takes into account several concepts that are important for motivation, including parental support, peer support, and teacher support.

Whole School, Whole Community, Whole Child

The WSCC model (see figure 2.4) serves as a blueprint for improving health among school-age children and adolescents by establishing a positive and inclusive school climate. A supportive school climate includes physical education and physical activity, as well as other concepts of healthy living, such as nutrition and social and emotional wellness (Birch & Videto, 2015). This approach was developed to provide positive supports for students not only within the school but also at home and throughout the community. This approach may be especially important for shaping positive physi-cal activity behaviors because parental support is one of the strongest predictors of obtaining sufficient physical activity levels among children and adolescents (Davison et al., 2006; Prochaska et al., 2002; Sallis, Alcaraz, et al., 1999; Trost et al., 2003). The WSCC model includes 10 interrelated components that are essential for improving students' academic performance by ensuring that they are physically, socially, and emotionally well (Lewallen, Hunt, Potts-Datema, Zaza, & Giles, 2015).

The 10 WSCC components are as follows:

- Physical education and physical activity
- Health education
- Health services
- Counseling, psychological, and social services
- Social and emotional climate
- Physical environment
- Employee wellness
- Family engagement
- Community involvement
- Nutrition environment and services

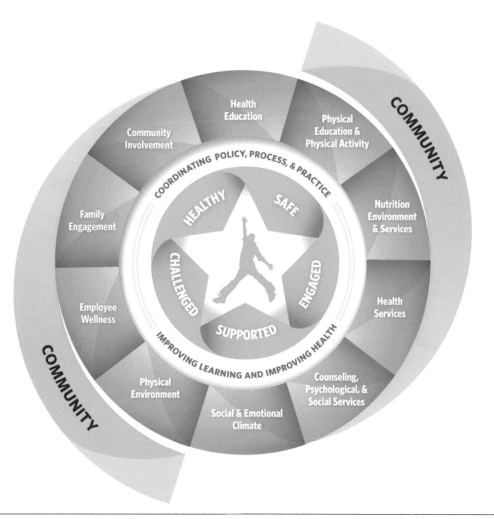

FIGURE 2.4   Whole School, Whole Community, Whole Child model.

Reprinted from ASCD, *Whole School, Whole Community, Whole Child: A Collaborative Approach to Learning and Health* (Alexandria, VA: ASCD, 2014).

Here, we focus on the role of physical and health education teachers in ensuring that the WSCC model is implemented in their schools. We also discuss how quality physical education programs can be enhanced through a whole-school approach.

SHAPE America recommends that physical education teachers take an active role in coordinating and implementing the WSCC model (SHAPE America, 2016b). Although they will spend most of their efforts in planning and implementing effective physical education, they should also serve as the wellness champion for their school (Centers for Disease Control and Prevention, 2013). This role includes pioneering wellness beyond their traditional classes and encouraging all stakeholders in the WSCC model to work together to increase physical activity throughout the school. This collaborative approach is critical for increasing students' motivation for lifelong physical activity. The cohesiveness of the 10-component WSCC model is what helps students to not only feel that physical activity, physical education, and their own health are important but also that they have opportunities to engage in physical activity and other health-enhancing behaviors before, during, and after school.

A whole-school approach to promoting physical activity allows students to apply the skills they learn in physical education throughout their everyday lives. Such experiences encourage students to be physically active in their community at large. When Jayne Greenberg (2011) implemented Let's Move! Miami, a successful branch of the Let's Move! campaign, she reported, "Schools cannot do it alone. All you have to do is ask for support, and community members are front and center. After all, it is their children that we are educating, and what parent or caregiver does not want the best for their kids?" (p. 6).

Thus the WSCC approach provides supports for the goals of healthful living and lifelong physical activity pursued by Physical Best. The next section explains how the WSCC model, including collaboration between families and the community, connects with three key elements of motivation.

Motivation

Motivating students to participate in regular physical activity requires a continued and consistent emphasis on providing them with a variety of daily physical activity experiences. As a result, physical activity cannot be confined within the walls of the gymnasium; if it is, students' motivation for physical activity will wane between physical education classes. Findings from Weiss (2000) suggested that children and adolescents maintain or increase their participation in physical activity when given opportunities to enhance their perceptions of competence, social support, and enjoyment. Similarly, when Cox, Smith, and Williams (2008) examined motivation-related variables in middle school physical education and leisure-time physical activity behaviors, their findings suggested that in order for students to experience self-determined motivation, they must feel competent, autonomous, and connected—or able to relate—both to the physical activity and to those around them. Self-determined motivation was defined as intrinsic desire to be physically active and was measured by participation in leisure-time physical activities.

Among these three elements essential for self-determined motivation—competence, autonomy, and connection—feeling competent was associated with students' confidence in their ability to perform the physical activity. Confidence can be achieved through effective physical education programs that address SHAPE America's National Standards and Grade-Level Outcomes and use Physical Best. Physical education programs have traditionally taught, and continue to teach, skills for physical activity, which is an essential piece of the motivation puzzle. Yet the physical educator's role cannot stop there: Confidence is also enhanced through before- and after-school physical activity programs, as well as other offerings within a Comprehensive School Physical Activity Program (CSPAP) model. The role of CSPAP in enhancing motivation for lifelong physical activity among students is defined later in this chapter; for now, suffice it to say that CSPAP provides a clear strategy for helping all students, not just athletes, attain the confidence needed to engage in health-enhancing levels of physical activity.

Other strategies for improving confidence include the following:

- *Refrain from assigning grades based on skill level.* Instead, teach students to set their own goals for personal health and fitness and to record whether or not they meet those goals. You can then grade students' ability to set personal goals and establish a plan to attain them. It is appropriate to grade students' improvement or ability to reach their goals and their reflections on the experience, but it is not appropriate to grade their actual fitness scores because there are many factors contributing to these scores, many of which are outside students' control. This strategy supports Physical Best recommendations, which focus not on skill but on improvement.

- *Add a variety of activities to the curriculum.* Add health-related fitness and **circuit training** stations to lessons that align with Physical Best strategies and allow students to choose the intensity at which they work.

In addition to confidence, autonomy is a key element in developing self-determined motivation for physical activity. One proven strategy for improving autonomy is to give students choices within the physical education curriculum (Carlson, 1995; Davies et al., 2015). Adolescents want to feel some level of control or ownership of their physical activity experiences; therefore, allowing them to choose which activities they will participate in almost automatically enhances their motivation. This concept may appear simple, but it is often overlooked in physical education and physical activity programs. Examples of how to implement it include giving students opportunities to set their own goals, develop a personal health-related fitness plan, choose a type of activity in which to participate, and choose the intensity at which to perform.

To further reinforce the importance of choice, think about your own daily physical activity habits. How would you feel if someone told you that you had to take a one-hour indoor cycling class on a day that your body was telling you that you would benefit from a yoga class? Or, how would you feel if you were told that you had to complete a 40-minute, high-intensity interval workout in the gym when it was 70 degrees and sunny and you were looking forward to taking an hour-long walk with your dog? In this regard, children and adolescents are no different from adults. They need to learn how to listen to their own bodily signals about physical activity and

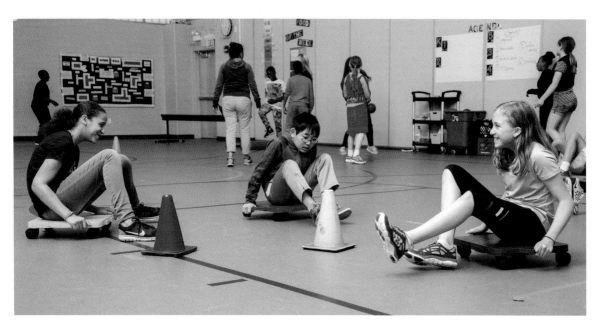

Station activities allow students to work at their chosen intensity and develop confidence.

choose to be active in ways that feel good to them (Segar, 2015). The following strategies can help improve students' autonomy through choice and taking ownership for their own health.

- In physical education, ask students to reflect daily on how they feel before, during, and after physical activity. Doing so allows them to identify which types of physical activity help them feel good and which types they do not enjoy (and why). This self-reflection helps students get in tune with their bodies and find physical activities that work for them and will motivate them to stay active for a lifetime.

- When teaching a specific skill (e.g., ball handling), give students choices regarding types of equipment to use. When throwing and catching, allow elementary students to choose between activity balls of different sizes and weights; other options include beach balls, rubber rings, and even beanbags or stuffed animals. Whatever they choose, the skill is the same (ball handling), and giving students choices may enable them to better succeed at catching, thereby increasing their confidence. This concept can be paralleled at the secondary level by allowing students to choose how to improve, say, their cardiorespiratory endurance. This goal could be achieved in any of various ways, such as riding a stationary bike, doing a high-intensity interval workout (HIIT), participating in a group exercise class, running on a treadmill or outdoor trail, and playing a team sport.

- At the beginning of the school year (or at various times throughout the year), ask students how they prefer to move. Specifically, ask them to identify physical activities that they enjoy, and why. Incorporate these movements and activities into your curriculum. Remember: The sports or activities you favor are not necessarily the ones your students are passionate about.

Providing choice in physical education is known to increase participation rates (Weiss, 2000). Therefore, teachers are encouraged to ask students what activities they enjoy most and incorporate students' preferences into curricular offerings for physical education. Weiss (2000) reported that students feel more empowered when given the opportunity to choose how to be physically active; moreover, ownership is positively correlated with the motivation to pursue a lifetime of physical activity. At the secondary level, it is appropriate to allow students to choose from a variety of physical education elective courses—for example, aquatics, personal physical fitness, team sports, dance, and group exercise.

The third element of self-determined motivation—feeling connected—may involve both connection to the physical activity itself and social connection to peers during the activity (Cox et al., 2008). We can help students feel connected through intentional team-building activities, teaching them about the cultures associated with various physical activities, and giving them opportunities to support each other socially during physical activity. We can create a positive physical activity culture among peers at school through wellness clubs; intramural activities; team challenges; and opportunities to be active before, during, and after school. Focusing on the social element of physical activity helps build sustainable physical activity behaviors (Segar, 2015). For example, think about adults who are physically active for a lifetime. These individuals often have a walking buddy, a friend to play tennis with, or a group of acquaintances they look forward to catching up with at their weekly Zumba class. These positive and supportive relationships can also be established in schools to help students see that physical activity can be an enjoyable and social part of their lives.

Here are a few specific strategies for increasing motivation through social activities that support physical activity:

- At the elementary school level, identify motivation buddies who are responsible for encouraging each other during physical education. Motivation buddies do not define groups for activities or games; instead, they provide a guaranteed network of support for each student. For example, a motivation buddy might give a peer a high five before or after an activity, comment on something that the buddy did well in class that day, or encourage the buddy to be physically active on the playground. In order to help all children feel included in physical education, Tingstrom (2015) asserts that we must "expect all students to be supportive of one another" (p. 12). She recommends identifying students who are naturally supportive and pairing them with students who may need extra support to be physically active.

- At the middle school level, the sport education model, developed by Daryl Siedentop (2009), may help increase social support for physical activity. In this model, students participate as members of teams in seasons that last longer than the usual physical education unit. This approach allows students to participate in a sport experience while developing camaraderie through team uniforms, names, and motivational support for their team. Thus students are able to feel as though they are part of something special while also enhancing their skill development in sport.

- At the high school level, consider using ideas from a new and increasingly popular activity among adults of all ages and fitness abilities—namely, obstacle course racing (Mullins, 2012). Races such as the Tough Mudder, Warrior Dash, and Spartan Race series include physical challenges requiring strength and endurance while promoting camaraderie and teamwork. You can create obstacle-style or adventure challenges in secondary physical education classes that are based not on individual success or competition but on peer support and group completion of the course. Be sure to add a fun element to these activities (Kulik, Brewer, Windish, & Carlson, 2017).

Another way to add a social element that helps students provide peer support for physical activity is to use specialized apps and websites. Table 2.1 describes some options that can foster a sense of community and connectedness through the common theme of physical activity.

Findings about motivation for physical activity among children and adolescents nearly parallel recent research on sustainable physical activity patterns among adults (Segar, 2015), and several strategies can be used in schools to enhance competence, autonomy, and feelings of connectedness during physical activity. Focusing on these three outcomes will inspire the self-determined motivation necessary for school-age children and adolescents to engage in lifelong physical activity behaviors. Michelle Segar, behavior expert and author of *No Sweat* (2015), reports that enjoyment of physical activity is the strongest predictor for maintaining a health-enhancing level of physical activity throughout the life span. In other words, physical activity must be enjoyable in order to be sustainable. In accordance with this finding, Physical Best prioritizes enjoyment and learning over skill, an approach that may be especially important in creating sustainable physical activity habits among children and adolescents, because experiences in childhood and during K-12 physical education programs can shape individuals' views about physical activity for a lifetime.

TABLE 2.1   Technology That Enables Social Support for Physical Activity

App or website	Description	Social element	Grade level
Endomondo	Tracks bike rides, runs, and other outdoor activities.	Allows users to add friends, who can encourage physical activity habits and engage in friendly competition.	Secondary
Strava	Started as a cycling and running app but now tracks almost any type of physical activity, including paddle boarding, yoga, and high-intensity interval training (HIIT); tracks heart rate, speed, distance, and duration of activity; stores physical activity data for years and allows users to map running or cycling routes.	Allows users to follow other users, give kudos to followers, and comment on activity; also allows users to upload pictures.	Secondary
MapMy	Tracks routes and progress, including distance, pace, calories burned, and more.	Allows users to post a diet log, running routes, and accomplishments to social media.	Secondary and upper elementary
Nike + GPS	Tracks runs, including mileage, pace, and time.	Cheers every time someone likes or comments on a user's status update.	Secondary and upper elementary

Technology Box was created by Certified Google Innovator and Professor of Physical and Health Education at Slippery Rock University, Dr. Joanne Leight.

These views can be positive or negative, depending on each student's unique experience. Take, for example, a student who remembers being "placed" in the goal during a middle-level physical education class and feeling as though she is the reason her team lost because she let three balls float into the net. This experience may cause the student to hold negative views of physical activity as she transitions into adulthood. The negative mental image generated through this specific experience may also affect her view of other physical activity behaviors or even lead her to avoid all types of physical activity—even ones completely unassociated with soccer. Indeed, most adults who hold a negative perception of physical activity can identify one or more specific events in their past that shaped these negative views (Segar, 2015).

Thus, physical activity experiences in school can exert a powerful influence on future behavior, which means that physical education teachers must strive to create positive physical activity experiences for students. Yes, this approach could mean, for example, that students spend less time in their target heart rate zone while the teacher uses class time to create a learning community that promotes confidence, autonomy, and positive feelings of connectedness to the activity and to peers. However, the time devoted to influencing students' perceptions of physical activity will be well spent toward achieving the greater goal of lifetime physical activity. In addition, Physical Best activities (available in the web resource associated with this book) give teachers opportunities to teach through activities that are enjoyable for students and individualized for preferences and health-related fitness levels.

The next section discusses how students' motivation for physical activity—based on confidence, autonomy, and connection—can be enhanced by Comprehensive School Physical Activity Programs (CSPAPs).

Comprehensive
School Physical Activity Programs

In support of the Whole Child model, and encompassing several components that enhance students' motivation for physical activity, SHAPE America recommends that schools use the Comprehensive School Physical Activity Program (CSPAP) approach. CSPAP provides a national framework for physical education and physical activity in schools and pursues the goal of enhancing physical activity opportunities and involving the whole school community (SHAPE America, 2016b). Led by a certified health and physical education teacher, also referred to as a Physical Activity Leader (PAL), a CSPAP is a sequential K-12 curriculum that helps students develop the competence, autonomy, and connectedness necessary to live healthy and active lives.

The CSPAP approach consists of five key components that serve the common goal of ensuring that school-age children and adolescents meet the recommended 60 minutes of physical activity per day. These components include physical education, physical activity before and after school, physical activity during school, staff involvement, and family and community engagement. The cohesiveness of these five components helps students build competence in their physical activity behaviors. First, competence is built through the multiplicity of the CSPAP model. Students learn skills for movement and skills for healthy living during physical education classes and are then given opportunities throughout the rest of the day to practice these skills and engage in health-enhancing physical activity. In this way, the CSPAP model helps equip students for lifelong physical activity by enabling them to experience physical activity in multiple areas of life (Centers for Disease Control and Prevention, 2013). Thus, although physical education is the main ingredient in a successful CSPAP program, all five components must be included in order to shape positive, lifelong physical activity behaviors.

Physical Education

Effective physical education programs are vital to both health promotion and disease prevention among children and adolescents (Birch & Videto, 2015). Although physical education teachers would appreciate more time for physical education in schools, the reality is that we need to focus on preparing physically literate individuals in whatever amount of time is given to us for physical education. To that end, we need to use students' time in physical education not only to give them opportunities to be active but also to help them become physically literate members of society. Physical literacy has been defined as including the necessary skills to engage in a variety of lifelong physical activities, knowledge of the benefits of physical activity, opportunities to engage in daily physical activity, physical fitness, and valuing of physical activity and its contribution to a healthy lifestyle (SHAPE America, 2014). Understanding physical literacy is important for understanding why motivation and promotion of physical activity outside of traditional physical education classes are essential for helping children and adolescents develop positive physical activity habits that last a lifetime.

Physical Activity During School

Physical activity during school demonstrates that all persons at the school, not just health and physical education teachers, value movement and the health benefits that accompany regular physical activity. Whether this approach consists of activity breaks led by classroom teachers or takes place on a schoolwide level (e.g., everyone using

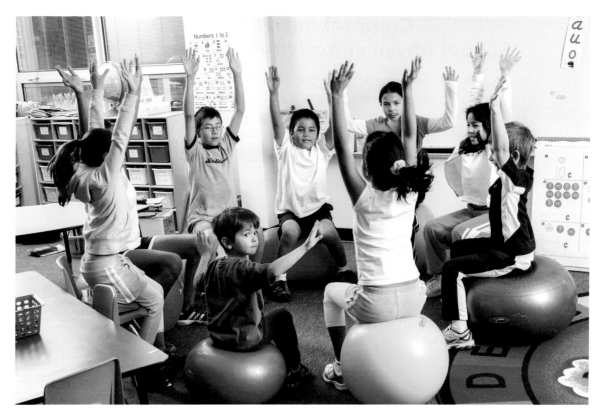

Incorporating physical activity during the school day helps create a culture of wellness at the school.

a standing desk or taking a walking break between classes), incorporating physical activity during the school day goes much further toward creating a culture of wellness among all students, faculty, and staff than does confining physical activity to the gymnasium. Creating this culture of wellness also builds on the autonomy and connectedness that are essential for instilling intrinsic motivation in students. Consider the following suggestions for ways to integrate physical activity into various parts of the school day:

- *Physical activity as a reward.* Classroom teachers can use physical activity, even something as simple as extra recess, as a reward for the entire class. Doing so helps children achieve the recommended 60 minutes of physical activity per day and develop a positive mind-set regarding physical activity—that is, viewing it not as a chore but as a gift (Segar, 2015).

- *Starting the day with movement.* To begin the day (or class), classroom teachers can lead simple warm-up activities, such as jogging in place, jumping jacks, cross-jacks, arm circles, and stretches. Another idea is for physical education teachers to lead the entire school in a one-minute physical activity to begin the day as part of morning announcements. Another option is for physical education teachers to create simple "brain boosts" for the school district and post them on the school website for classroom teachers to use when their students need a moment to recharge during the school day.

- *Classroom yoga.* Classroom teachers can lead students through a series of yoga stretches and poses in the classroom. Some of these movements can be performed in a very small space—for example, diaphragmatic breathing, mountain pose, and tree pose. Here are two detailed examples of classroom yoga for the elementary level (Ebert, 2012):

1. Desk Puppy
    - Stand behind your desk with your chair pushed in. Place the palms of your hands on the middle of your desk.
    - Take a step back and bend forward so that your head comes down between your arms.
    - Check your alignment. Your arms and legs should be straight. Your back is flat with your hips pressing backward and your tailbone reaching up. Your heels are on the floor.
    - Let your head hang and relax between your arms. Feel the stretch in your shoulders, arms, hamstrings, and calves. Release into the stretch a little more with each exhalation. (Encourage students to hear their exhales ["ahhh"]).
    - When you are finished, step forward and roll your spine back up to standing. Shake out your limbs as needed.
2. Open Heart
    - Begin in Sitting Mountain pose and reach back to hold onto the sides of your chair. Mountain pose is a position used to improve posture. For Sitting Mountain, find a comfortable seated position on the chair. Lift and spread your toes and the balls of your feet, then lay them back onto the floor with your big toes touching. Press gently into your toes and the balls of your feet, feeling the earth beneath you.
    - Inhale as you roll your shoulders back and lean forward, opening your chest toward the sky.
    - Hold this pose for three to five full breaths, imagining that each exhalation sends love from your heart to the rest of the school.
    - Slowly exhale and return to Sitting Mountain pose. Repeat.

- *Brain boosts.* Types of brain boosts include physical movement, thinking, and crossing the midline of the body. Examples of "brain boosts" or "brain busts" (formerly referred to as "brain breaks") can be found on a variety of websites. One such site is PECentral (www.pecentral.org/brainboosts.html).
- *Walking.* Provide opportunities for students to walk throughout the day. For example, at the secondary level, all students and teachers could participate in a scheduled three-minute walk for health-related fitness between classes, before the bell rings and they begin walking to their next class. Another option is the Daily Mile, which is making waves in schools across Europe. In this option, every class and every student who is able has an opportunity to run or walk a full mile at some point during each day. Those who are unable may work on a personal goal of physical activity minutes.

As this discussion illustrates, schools can use various approaches to promote physical activity throughout the school day. Moreover, students who see teachers, staff members, and administrators engaging in regular physical activity alongside physical education teachers come to understand that physical activity is for everyone (Kulinna et al., 2016). Additional strategies for integrating physical activity into the school day include ensuring recess opportunities for all grade levels and providing chances for voluntary physical activity at lunchtime in the gymnasium, fitness room, or outdoor areas. As shown in table 2.2, teachers of all disciplines can also promote physical activity during school by means of specialized apps and websites.

Promoting physical activity during school requires strong coordination between physical education teachers and other personnel who work with school-age children and adolescents. These key individuals include classroom teachers, administrators, parents and other family members, and the community at large. In addition to encouraging physical activity during school, the CSPAP approach connects students to events and organizations in the community that provide opportunities for physical activity before and after school. These activities can be held both on school grounds and in the larger community. In either case, they are integral to helping students apply the knowledge and skills they learn in physical education consistently throughout their daily lives.

The next section discusses how integrating physical activity into before- and after-school programs can enhance motivation for lifelong physical activity among children and adolescents.

Physical Activity Before and After School

Physical activity before and after school helps build competence by letting students choose what type of movement or activity to participate in and providing them with opportunities for practice and autonomy. Choice is known to enhance autonomy in physical activity behaviors among children and adolescents (Sanders et al., 2016); in addition, providing students with more choices of physical activity motivates them

TABLE 2.2   Technology for Promoting Physical Activity

App or website	Description	Application	Grade level
FitQuote	Provides daily fitness motivation (in the form of affirmations, push notifications, images, and reminders) to help users achieve goals related to fitness, workouts, walking, running, cycling, and more.	Can be used either by students or by teachers (to role-model by sharing with students how you are using the app to achieve your goals); can help users remember to get up and *move* throughout the school day.	Elementary and secondary
GoNoodle	Turns movement into a game and makes it easy to be active; offers hundreds of videos that get students of all ages running, dancing, stretching, jumping, and practicing mindful movements.	Can be used by teachers of all disciplines for brain breaks during class.	Elementary and secondary (Who doesn't want to dance in the middle of the school day?!)
Sworkit	Named for the slogan "simply work it"; allows users to choose and follow along with a workout based on time (e.g., 5 to 60 minutes) and type (e.g., strength, cardio, yoga, stretching).	Can be used easily by teachers of all disciplines, as well as staff members, parents, and community members; can help individuals who are not certified in physical education feel comfortable leading an activity break during the day.	Elementary and secondary

Technology Box was created by Certified Google Innovator and Professor of Physical and Health Education at Slippery Rock University, Dr. Joanne Leight.

to engage based on their personal preferences. Recommendations for increasing physical activity and fostering autonomy among school-age children and adolescents include walking or biking to school, voluntary physical activity clubs and intramural programs, informal recreation or play on school grounds, and integration of physical activity into homework during after-school programs. We can also enhance students' ability to achieve the recommended 60 minutes of daily physical activity by engaging with external constituents, such as YMCAs, parks and recreation programs, and faith-based organizations that provide opportunities for physical activity (Centers for Disease Control and Prevention, 2013).

Staff Involvement

To get students moving during the school day, the school staff must participate in, model, and promote physical activity during school and in their free time. You can make this easier by providing suggestions and activities for staff to engage with students in physical activity, leading wellness staff–student initiatives, and seeking interested staff members to lead opportunities. For example, you can make equipment available and invite teachers to bring their students to use it or provide in-service training to colleagues to familiarize them with quick and easy ways to incorporate physical activity in the classroom. (A classroom teacher may ask students to "show" the answer to a multiple-choice question by using their bodies to respond. To indicate choice A, the students may perform jumping jacks; to indicate choice B, they may perform spine twists; and so on.)

You can also take the lead in wellness initiatives. Organize faculty versus student volleyball matches or staff step challenges, and allow staff and students to sign up for yoga during study periods. Reach out to other staff members to participate in fitness activities before or after school; you might find some physical activity enthusiasts who can take the lead on starting a student running club, lead a staff Zumba class, or use their expertise to further spread your message. For example, a technology education teacher might base a student project on creating health-related fitness videos or promote physical activity opportunities in the school or community. You need supportive staff members (hopefully including some administrators as well) to role model physical activity for your students.

Family and Community Engagement

The last component of CSPAP involves engaging families and the community. The positive influence of schools can be perpetuated when the students' families and community support healthy actions. Educate parents regarding health-related fitness through newsletters and your physical education website. Invite them to your school and allow them to learn along with your students through family fitness events. Ask parents to volunteer in your classes as appropriate. Seek out community leaders who will support your efforts to improve or maintain health-related fitness in your students. Perhaps a local business will provide donations for equipment purchases or send volunteer speakers to inform students about what is available in their communities and motivate students as well. Be proactive in seeking and maintaining family and community relationships; it can benefit your students through support outside of school and by showing them the opportunities that exist to be active. You can learn more about CSPAP integration in the book *Comprehensive School Physical Activity Programs: Putting Evidence-Based Research Into Practice* (Carson & Webster, 2020).

Goal Setting

Goal setting helps students understand their potential and take personal responsibility for their health and fitness. Including goal setting in physical education is an effective way to encourage students to maintain healthy behaviors or adopt better habits of physical activity. Using goals created from students' personal assessments establishes ownership and fosters their pride in the process. They can then establish a pathway for achieving their goals by writing an action plan. The types of behaviors (goals) that students need to establish in order to improve their health-related fitness can be determined through preassessment. Thus, as in other areas of life, goal setting can be a valuable process in physical education.

The positive relationship between motivation and self-determination, or autonomy, is important in physical activity settings. The theory rests on the assumption that people who have input or choices regarding their activities and goals are more vested in the time and energy (effort) required to accomplish those goals. On the other hand, when goals are externally controlled, people tend to lack commitment and are more likely to withdraw or expend less effort. Goal setting can be divided into two distinct areas: establishing a desired outcome and working to achieve it. For students' goals to be motivational—and for students to incorporate goals into their physical activity behaviors—teachers should encourage them to set goals for learning new tasks, practicing drills and skills, and participating in physical activity and health-related fitness assessments.

We recommend using healthy fitness zones (HFZs) as the standards or goals that students strive to attain in order to live healthy lives (see chapter 13). To help students begin the goal-setting process, establish a time when they can assess their health-related fitness. This assessment will provide a baseline to help each student decide which areas of health-related fitness to work on through the goal-setting activity. For the assessment, ask students to compare their results with the HFZ charts and identify their personal strengths and areas needing work. Then use FitnessGram resources, which are designed for individualized goal setting and self-assessment and can help students identify their current status in each area of health-related fitness and where they would like to be.

Goal Striving

Goal striving is the effort that a person makes toward attaining a goal. To enhance motivation, consider focusing less on goal attainment and more on goal striving (and the overt actions that students take toward reaching their goals). Goal setting can be a simple part of physical education class that enables beneficial outcomes in students' ability to take ownership for their health and understand why it is important to engage in a variety of health-enhancing physical activities. Goal setting promotes self-regulation and awareness of one's physical health status. These capacities are especially important in today's society, in which only half of children and adolescents meet the recommendations for daily PA on five days per week and only one in four do so on all seven days of the week (Fakhouri et al., 2014). Young children can set simple goals, such as being physically active outside for 30 minutes after school or riding a bike on two days per week.

After students have set their first goal and worked to attain it, ask them to state what they did to support their goal striving. Then ask them to think about how they feel when participating in physical activities (Segar, 2015) and how these activities affect their personal health-related fitness. Next, ask students to establish a revised goal based on their experience with and reflections on their first attempt. Reinforce the goal-setting process by drawing attention to goal striving, checking in with students, and asking whether they have met their goals. If they have not, ask them to identify the barriers that got in the way. Then ask them to identify strategies to help them attain their goals on the next try. You might also ask students whether they think their goals were too difficult, which can help them refine and set more realistic goals.

This introduction to the goal-setting process teaches students the importance of decision making and self-assessment. It also shows them that their everyday habits and choices exert a big influence on their physical activity level and overall health.

Older students should write their goals, identify potential barriers, and hold themselves accountable for meeting their goals. Reflection and critical thinking are important steps in goal setting; they also enhance learning. For secondary students, it may be useful to use the SMART goal template (specific, measurable, attainable, realistic, and time framed), which is often used in public health settings and in community and commercial physical activities. Here are some guiding questions for setting SMART goals:

1. Is it specific? (Who? What? Where? When? Why?)

2. Is it measurable? (How will I measure progress? How many? How much?)

3. Is it attainable? (Can this really happen? Is it attainable with enough effort? What steps are involved?)

4. Is it realistic? (Do I possess or can I acquire the knowledge, skills, and abilities that are necessary to reach this goal?)

5. Is it time framed? (Can I set fixed deadlines? What are the deadlines?)

Figure 2.5 shows a worksheet you can give students to help them write SMART goals. It is available in the web resource.

Pursuing goals based on personal choice (i.e., exercising autonomy) motivates students to work toward achieving them. In contrast, pursuing goals because of external regulation leads to decreases in effort and motivation over time. Effort also tends to decrease when more challenging goals are imposed on individuals (e.g., students) by external agents (e.g., teachers). These patterns demonstrate the importance of giving students ownership of the goal-setting process, allowing them to establish their own goals (big or small), and prompting them to reflect on the process and modify their goals when necessary.

Although we recommend using the healthy fitness zones, student autonomy can be undermined if the focus of the goals becomes solely to achieve scores in the zones. Healthy fitness zones do delineate fitness levels required for good health (for more information, see chapter 13). However, although they present desirable targets for health-enhancing levels of muscular strength,

SMART Goal Template

	Questions to Ask Yourself
SMART criteria	What is your basic goal?
1. Is it specific?	Who? What? Where? When? Why?
2. Is it measurable?	How will I measure progress? (How many? How much?)
3. Is it attainable?	Can this really happen? Attainable with enough effort? What steps are involved?
4. Is it realistic?	What knowledge, skills, and abilities are necessary to reach this goal?
5. Is it time-bound?	Can I set fixed deadlines? What are the deadlines?

From I. Conkle, *Physical Best. Physical Education for Lifelong Fitness and Health*, 4th ed. (Champaign, IL: Human Kinetics/SHAPE America, 2020).

FIGURE 2.5 SMART goals worksheet.

Goal-Setting Steps

1. *Establish a baseline.* The baseline is an accounting of the current health-related fitness level or the behaviors needing change. Thus, in setting goals to enhance personal health-related fitness, the first step is to assess one's current level of health-related fitness.

2. *Define the desired outcome.* If a student determines in the initial assessment that he or she needs to improve flexibility in the right shoulder, the student can use the FitnessGram healthy fitness zone charts as a guide in setting the desired outcome. That outcome might be that the student can touch fingertips when reaching with the right hand down over the shoulder and with the left hand up behind the back from the waist.

3. *List the necessary activities and strategies for attaining the desired outcome.* Students can use the FITT guidelines to ensure specificity in setting their activities: frequency (e.g., how many times per day or week a stretch will be performed), intensity (e.g., whether the stretch will be performed by the person alone or with partner assistance), time (e.g., how long the stretch will be held), and type (e.g., the types of stretching that will enhance shoulder flexibility).

4. *Identify a time line for reassessing and attaining the goal.* The time line is often included at the beginning of the goal, as in the following example: "At the end of six weeks, I will be able to touch fingertips when performing the right shoulder flexibility assessment."

5. *Commit to attaining the goal.* The best way to make this commitment is to use peer support. (You also can provide support in your role as teacher.) Assign students "goal buddies" to encourage them to work toward their goals. Ask students to check in daily with their goal buddies to provide and receive encouragement. They can do so in person or by phone, e-mail, text, or social media.

6. *Reassess and reinforce.* Reassessment should occur not only at the end of the period but also (at least) on a weekly basis. Reinforcement can be given daily by both the goal setter and the goal partner after each reassessment period. For students who need **extrinsic motivation**, reinforcement might come in the form of tokens (e.g., stickers) that can be exchanged at the end of the goal period for something of value—for instance, free time, choice of activities, points toward a grade, or even a day off.

muscular endurance, body composition, and flexibility, they should not become the sole focus of goal setting. More specifically, teachers must be careful not to overemphasize achievement of HFZ targets as their desired goal for students. Rather, they should teach students about health-related fitness—that the scores in the zones are related to health and well-being, that they differ by age and gender, and that a variety of factors affect personal health.

When students independently choose an HFZ target as their goal, the goal is more autonomous. Some students may even wish to set goals above the zone, and others may set goals that progressively move them toward the zone. Although the outcome of student choice and the teacher's desired outcomes may be the same for many students, the *process* is the critical focus of goal-setting exercises. Applying a personal approach helps students select their own goals, and facilitating discussions about personal health can help students see the connection between the healthy fitness zones and physical and psychological well-being. In short, teachers should provide students with meaningful reasons to use HFZs in goal setting, including the fact that achieving HFZ targets will help them enjoy what matters most to them in life—even if health-related fitness itself is not their passion.

Goal setting often takes practice, both for students and for teachers. However, when it is introduced early and included as part of a comprehensive physical education curriculum, students of all ages can learn the process. This approach helps children and adolescents establish meaningful personal goals for themselves and use those goals to enhance their own motivation to be physically active.

Summary

The fields of public health and exercise science have long been researching the process of behavior change. Several well-researched models and theories exist to describe the path that individuals take toward changing unhealthy behaviors or adopting healthier ones. As indicated by the stages-of-change theory, behavior change is a difficult process (Prochaska et al., 2002). As a result, we recommend that instead of expecting children and adolescents to change unhealthy physical activity habits when they reach adulthood, physical education teachers help them create behaviors of healthy living while they are still developing. School is a central location where teachers help students develop skills in math, literacy, science, the arts, and other areas. Most children do not come to school to *change* their skills; instead, they come to *develop* them. Similarly, childhood and adolescence are the most effective times for teaching students valuable life skills, including physical activity habits that can last a lifetime. You can foster skills of healthy living while your students are still forming their views and personal preferences regarding physical activity. Helping students shape healthy behaviors proves to be a complex phenomenon, but Physical Best can help you with this process.

Because our goal is to motivate students to engage in sustainable physical activity patterns for a lifetime, we as physical education teachers must view our area of influence not as the gymnasium or playing field alone but as the entire school. To help bring life to the motivational strategies discussed in this chapter, use the questions listed in the next section to discuss and review chapter content. Also, see the web resource for tips from current teachers who discuss strategies that they have used to motivate students to engage in physical activity (figure 2.6). Many of the strategies that practicing teachers have identified as "what works" to motivate children and adolescents to be active are consistent with the Physical Best recommendations and current research on motivation and sustainable physical activity behaviors.

Chapter 3 addresses basic training principles. Because confidence is enhanced partially through knowledge, teaching students basic training principles (overload, progression, specificity, regularity, and individuality) contributes to their motivation for lifelong physical activity by increasing their knowledge of how the body responds to physical activity.

Teacher Tips for Motivating Students

What strategies and techniques have you used to motivate students in physical education?

1. Exposure to a variety of activities and opportunity for choice in activity preference (autonomy) during 11th and 12th grade. At the beginning of the school year, we provided students with an explanation of lifelong wellness [see the Lifetime Wellness Definition form in the web resource] and gave students a survey to see what activities they were interested in doing [see the Lifetime Wellness Activity Interest Survey in the web resource]. We used the results of this survey to base our selections off of for class [see the Lifetime Wellness Class Schedule in the web resource]. This seemed to improve interest and participation rates because students felt a sense of ownership of their health and physical activity choices.
—Chris Mooney, Slippery Rock Area School District, Slippery Rock, Pennsylvania: Secondary Health and Physical Education

2. Empowering student choice, voice, and responsibility have led to nearly every student participating every day. When students feel like their input is valued, they are more likely to be part of a wellness community. Fostering wellness is about building relationships with all students, not just the kids who love sports. Relationships lead to communities, and communities are able to support change.
—Brett Slezak, Allegheny Valley School District, Cheswick, Pennsylvania: Secondary Health and Physical Education

3. Our students take surveys at the beginning of the year to list what their own priorities are in life. This year, the generalized results of the survey suggested that students valued family, friends, athletics, grades, work, their personal health, and religion. Through physical education class, we follow up with that survey by teaching them that being active both now and as an adult will have a positive impact on those priorities and improve their daily lives.
—Shawn Bean and Andrea Barrett, Cranberry Area School District, Seneca, Pennsylvania: Secondary Health and Physical Education

4. Individualizing goals for each and every student along with seeking and listening to the student's voice. For example, during the indoor winter cardio unit, I presented guided choices for students after a discussion and stories from Dr. Segar's book No Sweat. Students were asked: "What are your goals for this unit? Check one."

From J. Conkle, *Physical Best: Physical Education for Lifelong Fitness and Health*, 4th ed. (Champaign, IL: Human Kinetics/SHAPE America, 2020).

FIGURE 2.6 See the web resource for tips on motivating students to be physically active.

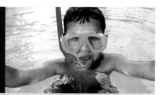

Discussion Questions

1. Why are so many children and adolescents not meeting recommended physical activity guidelines despite the clear benefits of regular physical activity?

2. Think about a time when you really enjoyed physical activity. What elements of this experience made it enjoyable?

3. Think about a time when you were *unmotivated* to be physically active. What elements of this experience made you avoid physical activity?

4. How can you, as a teacher, motivate students to adopt healthy behaviors for a lifetime?

5. How can students benefit immediately from goal setting? How might they benefit from it in the future?

6. Explain how to use healthy fitness zones effectively in the goal-setting process.

7. Explain how confidence, autonomy, and connectedness increase motivation. How can you foster these three characteristics in your students?

8. Physical Best focuses on each student's individual preferences and capabilities. How does this approach enhance the motivation and encourage desirable physical activity behaviors?

9. How can the Physical Best approach and the Whole School, Whole Community, Whole Child model be implemented together to support health, well-being, and physical activity in schools?

10. Explain the transtheoretical model, including why behavior change is a difficult process. Comment on how health and physical education teachers can motivate students to create healthy lifestyle behaviors that are sustainable for a lifetime.

Basic Training Principles

Sean Bulger and Brooke Towner

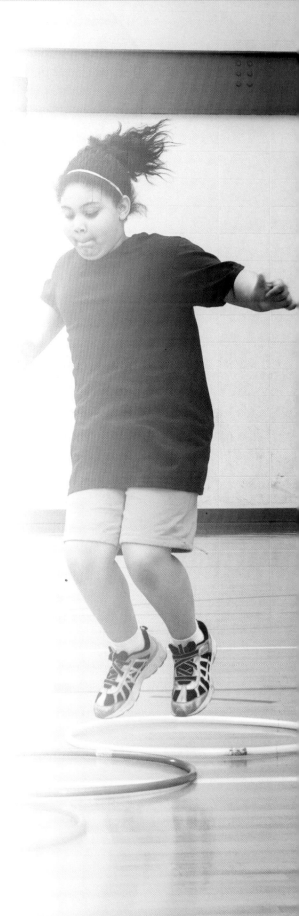

Habitual physical activity is one behavior known to help protect against a variety of chronic diseases in adults, including cardiovascular disease, hypertension, obesity, type 2 diabetes mellitus, and osteoporosis (Rowland, 2016). Although the link between physical activity and health is less well established among children and adolescents, many of the chronic diseases affecting older adults are thought to be the product of lifelong processes. As a result, the promotion of physical activity among youth has gained considerable support as a recommended strategy for reducing disease risk and improving public health. Moreover, leading professional and governmental organizations have indicated that this effort can be significantly aided by school-based programs (American Heart Association, 2006; SHAPE America, 2015; U.S. Department of Health and Human Services, 2018).

By teaching youth about basic training principles and FITT guidelines (frequency, intensity, time, and type), you can provide them with the conceptual foundation for designing safe and effective physical activity programs for themselves. Basic training principles consist of the scientific concepts that underlie program design, whereas the FITT guidelines address key decisions for physical activity and health-related fitness. Even if you are already familiar with this information, this chapter provides a quick reference to make it easier to teach.

Understanding the Basic Training Principles

The basic training principles—overload, progression, specificity, regularity, and individuality—indicate how the body responds to the physiological stress of physical activity across the components of health-related fitness: cardiorespiratory endurance, muscular strength, muscular endurance, flexibility, body composition, and power. The principles are applied to bring about desired physiological changes through manipulation of the frequency, intensity, time, and type (FITT) of physical activity performed. The physiological changes that occur in response to regular physical activity or exercise are called **training adaptations**. Although the basic training principles serve as the foundation for all physical activity programs, the magnitude of training adaptations in children is limited because children do not respond to training as adults do.

When applying the basic training principles to learning activities, you should individualize the lesson to meet the needs of students at all levels of ability, including athletes, students who are inactive, students with disabilities, and students who are unmotivated. It is unrealistic to expect all students to set the same personal goals, take interest in the same physical activities, or achieve the same level of health-related fitness. To the contrary, each student will respond individually to the activities involved in a given physical education lesson, and adherence to the basic principles of training provides a basis for a more personalized approach. For example, rather than requiring all children to run around the track during a physical education lesson, you might give students a choice between walking, jogging, or doing a mixture of the two. If this approach is used across multiple lessons, it can account for all of the basic training principles and allow students to participate at a level that is consistent with their individual interests and needs.

The **overload principle** states that a body system (cardiorespiratory, muscular, or skeletal) must be stressed beyond what it is accustomed to in order to bring about a desired training adaptation. Thus overload is considered a positive stressor when applied through careful manipulation of frequency, intensity, or time (Brooks, Fahey, & Baldwin, 2005). The overload principle should not be confused with **overtraining**, which is a condition caused by training too much or too intensely and not providing sufficient recovery time (Roy, 2015). Signs and symptoms of overtraining include the following:

Signs
- Prolonged decreases in performance (over two months or longer)
- Chronic injuries
- Elevated heart rate

Symptoms
- Persistent sore muscles
- Fatigue
- Depression
- Disruption in sleep habits
- Loss of appetite
- Increased susceptibility to infection

The **progression principle** holds that an overload must be increased gradually in order to remain efficient and safe (see figure 3.1, *a* and *b*). If too much overload is applied too soon, the risk increases for injury from overtraining or overuse, either of which may discourage or prevent a person from participating in physical activity. Conversely, failure to progress in terms of frequency, intensity, or time may result in diminished training adaptations over an extended period. Therefore, you should emphasize that becoming more physically active and improving health-related fitness is a gradual and ongoing process.

The **specificity principle** states that physical activities produce training adaptations by stressing a particular body part or system and do little to affect other body parts or systems (Brooks et al., 2005). For example, in order to develop muscular strength or muscular endurance in the knee extensors, a person must perform resistance-training exercises (e.g., leg press, knee extension) that stress the quadriceps muscle group. Similarly, a student interested in increasing hamstring flexibility must include several stretches targeting that muscle group—for example, the back-saver sit-and-reach stretch. This stretch differs from the back-saver sit-and-reach assessment that is used to evaluate flexibility. The stretch should be performed on each leg for two or three repetitions and held for 15 to 60 seconds in order to specifically target hamstring flexibility. When training for cardiorespiratory endurance, a distance runner would employ a training program involving runs of longer duration and lesser intensity as compared with the program of a sprinter. These differences in exercise intensity and time reflect the specific metabolic demands of the desired outcomes.

At the same time, training techniques can be used to address multiple body systems and multiple health-related components of fitness. For example, a student who wants to improve both cardiorespiratory endurance and muscular endurance could use circuit training that combines strength training and aerobic exercises in brief, intermittent bouts. Another option is **functional training**, which is designed to increase muscular strength while emphasizing flexibility, balance, and coordination of

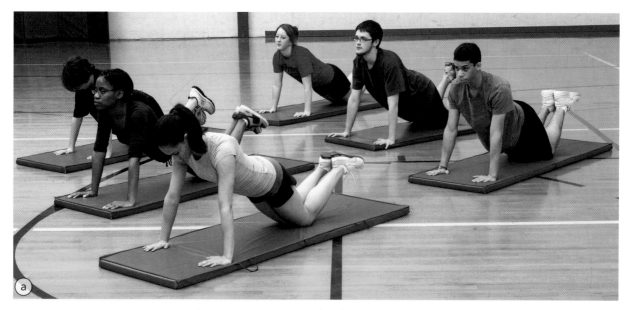

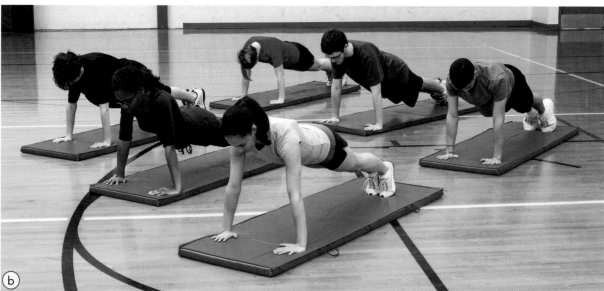

FIGURE 3.1   Students demonstrate progression through increasing intensity by moving from (a) a modified push-up to (b) a regular push-up.

movements in multiple planes. In this way, any physical activity program or training technique should reflect the desired training outcomes or adaptations.

The **regularity principle** holds that physical activity must be performed on a regular basis in order to be effective. In other words, any health-related fitness gains achieved through physical activity will be lost if the person does not continue to be active. To put it bluntly, use it or lose it! Applied over the long run, this basic training principle reinforces the importance of physical activity across the life span. Specifically, any improvements that a student makes in health-related fitness performance during an active childhood or adolescence will be lost if the person becomes inactive as an adult. For this reason, physical education programs should promote regular involvement in physical activity before, during, and after the school day. Physical education is a place to learn *how* to be physically active and to participate in fun learning opportunities, but it is not the only place to *be* physically active. With this need in mind, Physical Best educates and develops students who understand how to be active in order to produce health benefits and enjoy what they are doing; as a result, they are more likely to continue with a physically active lifestyle beyond their school years.

The **individuality principle** takes into account that people enter into physical activity programs with individual biological potentials for change, personal goals and interests, current activity patterns, health-related fitness levels, psychosocial characteristics, and environmental determinants. As a result, if we give children plenty of opportunities to make choices about the FITT guidelines in physical education, we help them develop physical activity patterns that may extend across the life span. In its most complex form, this kind of student choice could involve an elective physical education program at the high school level, in which students select from lifetime leisure pursuits such as rock climbing, tennis, golf, and weight training. In its simplest form, the choice could occur during a tag game at the elementary level, in which the students select from a list of alternatives (ranging from simpler to more complex) to perform when tagged—for example, line jumps, cone jumps, and rope jumps.

These basic training principles provide the foundation for engaging in lifelong physical activity. The time that students spend in physical education is not enough. They must also understand the principles and be able to apply them in order to find fun and enjoyable ways to be physically active and maintain health-enhancing levels of fitness over the long run.

Applying the Basic Training Principles

Exercise prescription is the process of designing an individualized physical activity program to improve health, health-related fitness, and sport performance (Garber et al., 2011). When your students develop exercise prescriptions, help them make key decisions regarding the FITT guidelines (frequency, intensity, time, and type) and an appropriate rate of progression. These decisions need to take into account a variety of issues, including the participant's health status, current activity level, exercise history, personal preferences, and goals.

FITT Guidelines

The **FITT guidelines** address how to apply the basic training principles during program design (see table 3.1). Whether the program is intended for a high school student enrolled in a personal wellness course or for an elementary student joining an after-school club for health-related fitness, the physical educator needs to facilitate responsible decision making. The particulars will vary based on several factors, including the program's goals and desired outcomes, the physical activity setting or context, the developmental readiness of participants, and the instructor's qualifications. Specific FITT guidelines for each area of health-related fitness are discussed in later chapters of this book.

TABLE 3.1   Sample Applications of FITT Guidelines

Fitness component	FITT guidelines
Cardiorespiratory endurance	F—most days of the week I—60%-90% of maximal heart rate T—60 min T—walking, jogging, biking, swimming, rowing
Muscular fitness	F—2-3 days per week with rest days between I—weight that allows for 8-12 reps per set T—1 set of 8-10 lifts with 1-2 min rest (~20 min total) T—free weights and resistance machines
Flexibility	F—at least 3 days per week (preferably more) I—stretching to mild discomfort, backing off slightly, then holding T—holding each stretch for 10-30 seconds (repeating 4-5 times) T—static stretching that targets major muscles and tendons

Frequency

Frequency consists of *how often* a person performs the targeted physical activity. For each component of health-related fitness, the beneficial and safe frequency will vary. Cardiorespiratory endurance activities and flexibility activities can be performed all or most days. Most experts believe that muscular strength and endurance activities should be limited to three nonconsecutive days per week unless different muscle groups are exercised on alternating days.

Intensity

Intensity consists of *how hard* a person exercises and is therefore one of the most critical elements of program design. Appropriate exercise intensity depends on multiple factors, including the participant's developmental readiness, personal goals, and current levels of physical activity and health-related fitness. For example, a participant whose goal is to improve sport performance must exercise at a higher intensity than someone whose goal is to achieve general health benefits. Furthermore, a student who is already physically active on a regular basis is better prepared to tolerate high exercise intensities than as compared with a person who has been sedentary. When working with students who have lower levels of physical activity or health-related fitness, use activities of lower intensity to provide a more enjoyable experience and to minimize any potential discomfort or soreness.

Time

Time, or **duration,** consists of *how long* the activity is performed. As with other aspects of the FITT guidelines, it varies depending on the targeted component of health-related fitness. In addition, it is inversely related to intensity. Primary-grade children will have more difficulty than older children in understanding this concept and will be less able than older children and adolescents to complete intense physical activities in a single bout.

Type

Type consists of the mode, or *what kind*, of activity a person chooses to perform for each component of health-related fitness (see figure 3.2). For example, an individual can improve cardiorespiratory endurance by walking, riding a bike, skating,

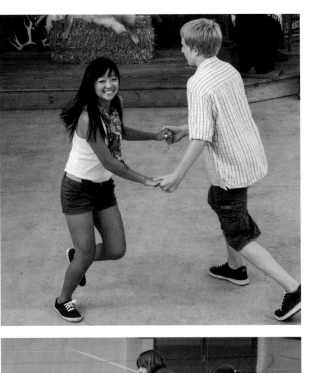
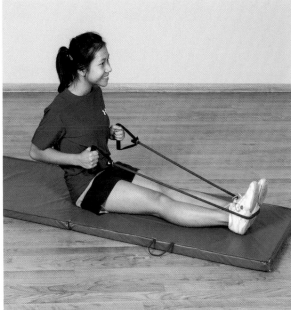
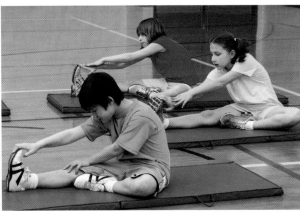
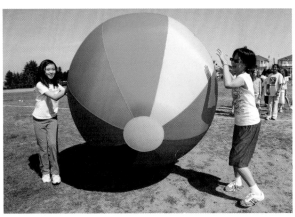

FIGURE 3.2   All of these activities improve students' health-related fitness. Best of all, students have fun doing them!

stair-climbing, or engaging in any number of other physical activities that elevate one's heart rate for an extended period. Muscular fitness, on the other hand, is developed by contracting a muscle or a muscle group against external resistance, which may be provided by, for example, free weights, variable resistance machines, elastic tubing, body weight, a medicine ball, or a partner. And flexibility can be enhanced by repeatedly stretching a muscle beyond its normal resting length in any of several training modes, including static and dynamic stretches.

Physical educators should encourage students to select activities that they enjoy and that target their personal goals for health, health-related fitness, or sport performance. In addition, instructors of elementary and middle school students should provide a variety of activities to prepare students for responsible decision making at the high school level and beyond.

FITT Age Differences

Physical activity guidelines provided by the U.S. Department of Health and Human Services (2018) for children and adolescents can help teachers understand the over-

Activity Tracking

Websites and mobile apps that track physical activity can be used to reinforce the importance of the basic training principles. Students can use these resources to log their physical activity before, during, and after school or to build personalized physical activity programs that adhere to the training principles. For a list of examples, see tables 2.1 and 2.2 in chapter 2.

Heart rate monitors can give you and your students useful feedback about the intensity of moderate and vigorous activities; for example, they can measure a student's heart rate during exercise, during recovery, and at rest. Another useful category of devices includes pedometers, activity monitors, and accelerometers, which can be used to measure activity levels both inside and outside of physical education. This type of technology is simple to use and increasingly cost-effective, and its outputs (such as number of steps or distance covered) are easy to understand.

Utilizing available technology can help students better understand and apply the basic training principles and FITT guidelines. In a fun and interactive way, students can measure and assess personal physical activity levels, set goals and monitor goal attainment, and even collaborate and compete with others as a form of motivation.

all needs of these demographic groups. The department's guidelines indicate that children and teenagers from age 6 through 17 should accumulate 60 minutes or more of daily physical activity. They should also engage in a variety of enjoyable and developmentally appropriate activities that address the following outcomes:

1. *Cardiorespiratory endurance.* Most of the 60 minutes or more per day should consist of either moderate or vigorous aerobic activity; in addition, vigorous physical activity should be included on at least three days per week.

2. *Muscle strengthening.* As part of their 60 minutes or more of daily physical activity, children and adolescents should include muscle-strengthening activity on at least three days per week.

3. *Bone strengthening.* As part of their 60 minutes or more of daily physical activity, children and adolescents should include bone-strengthening physical activity on at least three days per week.

To help teachers determine what activities are considered moderate, vigorous, or age appropriate, the following definitions are provided by the National Association for Sport and Physical Education (2004). **Developmentally appropriate physical activity** involves "activity of a frequency, intensity, duration, and type that leads to optimal child growth and development and contributes to the development of future physically active lifestyles" (p. 8). **Moderate physical activity** is defined as "activity of an intensity equal to brisk walking . . . and can be performed for relatively long periods of time without fatigue" (p. 7). The authors suggest brisk walking, bike riding, some household chores, low-intensity games (e.g., disc golf, four-square), and yard games (e.g., ladder golf). **Vigorous physical activity** is defined as "movement that expends more energy or is performed at a higher intensity than brisk walking. Some forms of vigorous activity, such as running, can be done for relatively long periods of time, while others may be so vigorous (e.g., sprinting) that frequent rests are necessary" (p. 8).

When applying basic training principles and FITT guidelines to program design, remember that youth respond differently from adults and that the traditional idea of exercise prescription should not be rigorously applied to younger children. Instead, use instructional approaches that focus on the process of engaging in enjoyable activity rather than the product of becoming physically fit through structured forms of exercise training (National Association for Sport and Physical Education, 2004). For various reasons, children exhibit different physiological responses to structured exercise than adults do; the reasons may include a range of factors, such as lower anaerobic fitness, limited aerobic trainability, less movement economy, different thermoregulatory reactions, and more intermittent patterns of activity (Rowland, 2016).

As a result, the lifetime activity model, which emphasizes the accumulation of physical activity in a less structured manner, enables appropriate application of the FITT guidelines for most children (National Association for Sport and Physical Education, 2004). In this model, a child is encouraged to accumulate at least one hour, and up to several hours, of play each day through a range of lifestyle activities, active aerobics, active sports, flexibility exercises, and muscular exercises—all of which minimize extended periods of sedentary living. As age and year in school increase, you can introduce students to more structured and adultlike exercise programs based on goals and interests. The Physical Activity Pyramid is an effective tool for teaching students how to weigh each component of health-related fitness while incorporating sufficient variation in their personal physical activity programs (Corbin, 2014). Figure 3.3 shows the pyramid for children, and figure 3.4 shows the pyramid for teenagers.

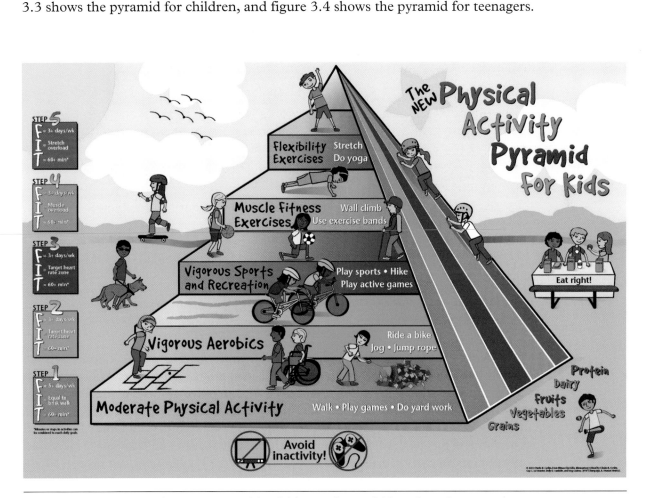

FIGURE 3.3   The Physical Activity Pyramid for children is also available in the web resource.

Reprinted, by permission, from D. Lambdin et al., *Fitness for Life: Elementary School Classroom Guide Kindergarten Classroom Guide* (Champaign, IL: Human Kinetics, 2010), 11.

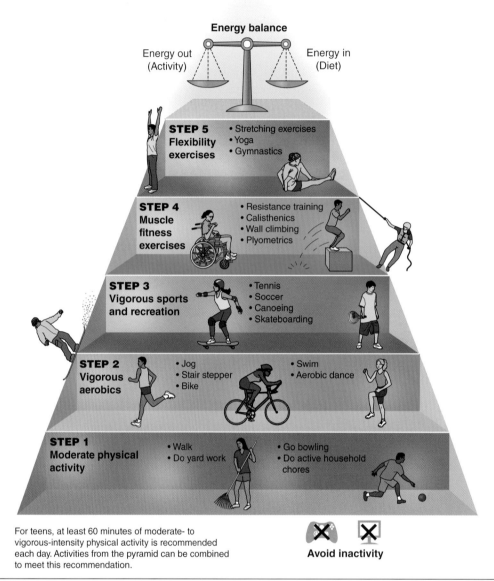

FIGURE 3.4   The Physical Activity Pyramid for teenagers is also available in the web resource.
© Charles Corbin

Although the FITT guidelines remain applicable when using the lifetime activity model for program design, they are applied in a less structured manner, which is thought to be suitable for younger children and inactive adults. At the elementary level, remove the stringent three-day-per-week training requirement, place less emphasis on minimum intensity levels, remove the time limits frequently suggested as minimums for the development of health-related fitness, and emphasize increased daily physical activity. Certainly, the adult-model FITT guidelines can be presented, but the emphasis should be on increasing physical activity.

To prevent students from losing interest, and to keep them from losing the desire to become more physically fit, you can help each student explore a variety of recreational activities and ways to vary their physical activity choices. Encourage students to participate in school athletic programs and in before- and after-school programs for activity and health-related fitness. You can also role-model active behavior for students through such measures as taking the stairs, parking away from the building, and taking classes outside to walk the longest distance to the activity area. The importance of these types of activities must be explained to students in ways that relate directly to them. For example, discuss how improved cardiorespiratory endurance will enable them to play longer without getting tired. Explain how improved muscular fitness will help them perform their daily chores, such as taking out the trash, or how extra strength can help them better navigate playground bars and equipment. Just like other components of health-related fitness, improvements in muscular strength can increase feelings of overall well-being and enhance performance in activities that students find enjoyable. You can also serve as a liaison between students and the community by pointing out recreational programs, such as sport leagues, health clubs, and park district activities.

If a child, a parent, and a physical educator agree that a more structured, adultlike exercise prescription is needed in order to enhance a child's health-related fitness or sport performance, then the program must adhere to the basic training principles. In addition, the FITT guidelines must be applied based on the individual's stage of maturation rather than on chronological age (Bompa, 2000). We must also consider when a child is ready to begin a resistance training program. According to the prevailing recommendation, if a child is ready—based on maturation—to participate in sport activities, then the child is ready for some resistance training (Faigenbaum et al., 2009). The basic training principles and FITT guidelines can help us minimize the risk of injury and appropriately design lessons. As a rule, teachers and coaches of younger children should focus on age-appropriate activities that give all participants an equal opportunity to play, make friends, and improve their social skills while enhancing their health-related fitness. In the Elementary section of the web resource, each activity indicates which of the FITT guidelines is being applied during that specific activity so that you can highlight its importance with your students to help them make the mental connection to their learning activity. For example, Treasure Island focuses on time, while Aerobic Sports focuses on type of exercise. At the middle and high school levels, students are closer to adulthood and respond to training and conditioning more like adults do. At this point, you can begin transitioning to more structured physical activity programs by helping students apply the FITT guidelines in a more prescriptive manner. From the web resource, you might use Aerobic Fitness Is FITT to teach your students about intensity or Continuous Relay to teach the importance of time and intensity.

Components of a Physical Activity Session

Every physical activity session should follow a systematic method that includes a warm-up, a main physical activity, and a cool-down. This approach helps to ensure participants' safety by preparing their bodies for the demands of physical activity and then gradually reducing the workload at the end of the session. Warming up and cooling down properly may also prevent injuries (see figure 3.5) and aid in postexercise recovery, respectively. As for the main physical activity, it should be conducted in a way that helps students feel and understand, through participation, the importance of being physically active.

Injury Prevention Strategies

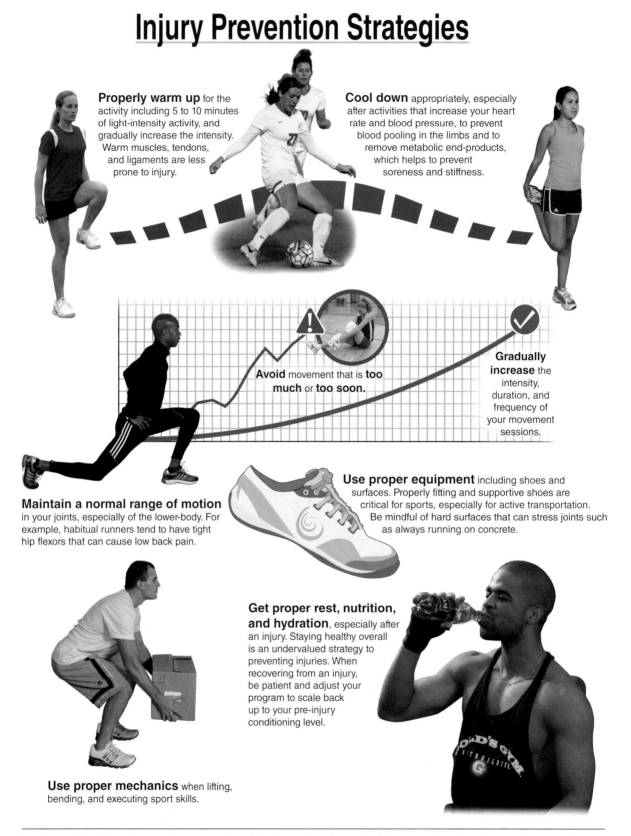

Properly warm up for the activity including 5 to 10 minutes of light-intensity activity, and gradually increase the intensity. Warm muscles, tendons, and ligaments are less prone to injury.

Cool down appropriately, especially after activities that increase your heart rate and blood pressure, to prevent blood pooling in the limbs and to remove metabolic end-products, which helps to prevent soreness and stiffness.

Avoid movement that is **too much** or **too soon.**

Gradually increase the intensity, duration, and frequency of your movement sessions.

Maintain a normal range of motion in your joints, especially of the lower-body. For example, habitual runners tend to have tight hip flexors that can cause low back pain.

Use proper equipment including shoes and surfaces. Properly fitting and supportive shoes are critical for sports, especially for active transportation. Be mindful of hard surfaces that can stress joints such as always running on concrete.

Get proper rest, nutrition, and hydration, especially after an injury. Staying healthy overall is an undervalued strategy to preventing injuries. When recovering from an injury, be patient and adjust your program to scale back up to your pre-injury conditioning level.

Use proper mechanics when lifting, bending, and executing sport skills.

FIGURE 3.5   Properly warming up and cooling down is an important injury prevention strategy.

Warm-Up

A **warm-up** is a low-intensity activity done before a full effort and should be organized to meet the goals of the main physical activity. The primary purpose of the warm-up is to prepare the participant for the moderate to vigorous physical activity that will occur during the session. For example, a person intending to engage in a vigorous physical activity, such as a game of full-court basketball, needs to complete a more thorough warm-up than does a person simply going out for a brisk walk.

The structured warm-up, in this case focused on basketball, incorporates a general warm-up followed by a specific warm-up that includes sport-related stretches and movement patterns performed with increasing intensity. The general segment of the warm-up can include activities such as walking, jogging, swimming, and cycling to prepare the cardiorespiratory and musculoskeletal systems for both the sport-specific segment of the warm-up and the main physical activity that follows. The specific warm-up may include a combination of static and dynamic stretches. Dynamic stretching uses movement to gradually increase the range and intensity of motion. A specific warm-up that uses dynamic stretching might include walking or light jogging, arm circles, lunges that progress to walking lunges or lunges with a torso twist, and squats performed to half depth or squats to a calf raise. The specific warm-up is more efficient if the activities target the primary muscles that will be used to perform the main physical activity; stretches that put unnecessary stress on the joints, such as the hurdler stretch, should be avoided. This type of structured warm-up routine offers the following benefits:

- Increases blood flow to the working muscles.
- Increases circulatory parameters and blood flow to the heart.
- Raises body temperature and aids temperature regulation.
- May reduce the risk of muscular injury and soreness.

In many instances, however, structured warm-up routines can be difficult to incorporate into physical education classes. For instance, in a 40-minute elementary physical education class, allocating 10 to 15 minutes to an extended warm-up may not be the best use of instructional time. It is also inadvisable to commit large chunks of lesson time to less active types of exercise, such as static stretching. As an alternative approach, Physical Best activities can be used throughout the year as warm-up activities to help students understand, in age-appropriate ways, that warming up prepares the body for the main activity by gradually increasing heart rate and blood flow to muscle and other tissues. A more specific warm-up could incorporate, for instance, dynamic movements that target the prime movers acting on the shoulder joint, including jumping jacks, arm swings in multiple planes of movement, and pull-up and push-up variations to prepare the arms for throwing activities.

Although gentle stretching and walking (or slow jogging) for about five minutes are common and safe warm-up activities, you should vary student warm-ups to prevent boredom and carelessness in the routine. For younger children, plan and lead warm-ups that provide instant activity as students arrive at the lesson site in order to prevent management problems (Graham, Elliott, & Palmer, 2016). An instant activity section in a lesson could include challenge activities such as jumping back and forth across a line (or turning a jump rope) as many times as possible, completing a short circuit-training course, or engaging in a dribbling activity. Instant activities may also work for older students by providing an opportunity for them to socialize while

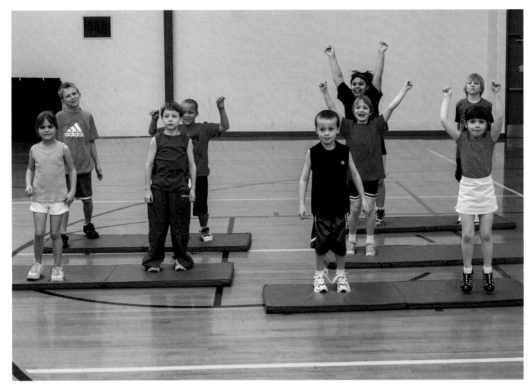

A warm-up should precede moderate to vigorous physical activity.

warming up. For older students, you can also post the warm-up in the locker rooms or at the lesson site and let students be responsible for carrying it out independently.

Main Physical Activity

The main physical activity provides the core of the physical education lesson and is intended to improve or maintain one or more of the health-related fitness components. The frequency, intensity, time, and type of physical activity depend on the goals of the lesson, the length of the class period, and the current levels of health-related fitness among the students. Whether you are teaching kindergarteners or high school seniors, explain the purpose of the lesson and how the day's activity will help students reach class or personal goals.

Like adults, children will express and act on preferences within the many physical activities available. When possible, therefore, provide a wide variety of activities and allow a broad range of personal choice in your program. Ensure, however, that students understand the need to address each component of health-related fitness and monitor the intensity of the activity performed. When developing lessons, plan to provide students with easy ways to measure moderate to vigorous physical activity (MVPA)—for example, by using heart rate monitors or rating of perceived exertion (ways to monitor MVPA are discussed in greater detail in chapter 5). In short, emphasize the importance of total health-related fitness and the need to engage in an activity for each component of health-related fitness. For instance, one student may elect to swim laps while another goes cross-country skiing, and both are addressing cardiorespiratory endurance but still need to work on flexibility, muscular strength and endurance (for muscle groups not addressed by the chosen activities), and body composition.

Cool-Down

A proper **cool-down** includes a period of light activity following exercise that allows the body to slow down and return to resting parameters. Students must understand that the body needs this gradual recovery in order to reduce muscle stiffness and soreness; remove lactic acid; and prevent light-headedness, dizziness, or even fainting. Teach students to resist the urge to sit or lie down after physical activity; instead, they should gradually slow down their activity by walking or jogging slowly for three to five minutes or until their heart rate returns to near resting level. Continued light activity facilitates recovery by "milking" blood in the veins back toward the heart. In contrast, abruptly stopping exercise facilitates pooling of blood in the extremities and decreases the return flow of blood to the heart, and subsequently to the brain, which leaves the person susceptible to fainting. Stretching exercises should also be performed during the cool-down, when muscles are warmest and most pliable, thus providing maximum benefit toward improving flexibility. For examples of stretching exercises and activities, refer to chapter 7 of this book and to the Physical Best activities in the flexibility section of the web resource. The cool-down also provides an opportunity for you to bring closure to the lesson by reviewing key concepts and facilitating students' self-evaluation in relation to personalized goals for the workout.

Social Support and Safety Guidelines

In addition to using the basic training principles, the FITT guidelines, and the three major components of a physical activity session in a developmentally appropriate manner, you must be careful to provide your students with a teaching and learning environment that is both socially supportive and safe. As introduced in chapter 2, the Association for Supervision and Curriculum Development (2014) recommends taking a whole-child approach to the long-term development of children and suggests five keys for developing each child: health, safety, engagement, support, and academic challenge. If these features are absent, a physical education program is not likely to influence physical activity or other health-related behaviors in a positive manner.

You can adopt the whole-child approach through Physical Best. First, teach your students in an environment that supports *health*. Physical Best activities focus on health-related fitness to teach students the basic information they need in order to make good health choices, measure their own health-related fitness, plan for improving or maintaining health-related fitness, and continue participating outside of physical education. Second, ensure students' *safety* in your class: Be knowledgeable about exercise principles and teaching strategies that are developmentally appropriate, construct a supportive emotional environment (for more, see chapter 11), and understand your students' individual health needs and conditions. Notice that this text highlights safety guidelines in many chapters. Third, Physical Best activities are meant to teach health-related fitness concepts while helping students to be active. This type of *engagement* enhances student learning, motivation, and enjoyment and makes the best use of precious class time. In addition, Physical Best activities provide many opportunities for you to encourage individuals and help ensure success for each child, which fosters improved self-esteem and perceived competence in a safe and *supportive* instructional environment. Finally, Physical Best activities can be individualized to ensure that each student is *challenged* both intellectually and physically. Push your students to expand their physical activity pursuits and motivate them to become their own physical best!

Providing Social Support

Children do not choose to exercise or remain physically active for the associated health benefits, but they are more likely to be physically active if they perceive their physical abilities to be high (National Association for Sport and Physical Education, 2004). Therefore, we must take care to help children experience some measure of success when they are introduced to new physical activities. With this in mind, activities that are initially very intense or difficult may prove discouraging and lead children to opt out of further participation. In addition, in order to promote continued engagement in physical activity beyond the school setting, we should incorporate forms of physical activity that carry cultural and geographical relevance for students and their families (Braga, Elliott, Jones, & Bulger, 2015). Toward this end, it is important to consider students' voices and interests when developing the curriculum.

Your role as a primary source of social support is also paramount. Physical Best emphasizes the development of long-term learning and activity habits by calling attention to health-related fitness as a lifelong process rather than a product of isolated training and conditioning. The literature demonstrates that, in the right circumstances, physical education and sport in schools can help students develop a lifestyle that includes physical activity and health-related fitness, fundamental movement skills, social responsibility, self-esteem and pro-school attitudes, and perhaps cognitive development and academic achievement (Bailey, 2006). These positive outcomes do not, however, result directly from participation in regular physical activity, and we must be careful to acknowledge that "the effects are likely to be mediated by the nature of the interactions between students and their teachers, parents, and coaches who work with them" (Bailey, 2006, p. 397). In short, these important learning outcomes are most likely to be realized if the physical education environment is positive and characterized by high levels of student engagement, enjoyment, diversity, and social support from knowledgeable practitioners and well-informed parents.

You are in a position to influence both student behavior and the environment before, during, and after school in order to promote lifelong physical activity. This influence can take many forms. For instance, you can set up opportunities to increase successful practice and self-efficacy, use cooperative learning to shape group behavior, and correctly administer rewards to enhance students' motivation to engage in physical activity both in and beyond the physical education setting. As a place where youth spend considerable time, the school must provide students with access to a variety of opportunities to be physically active. These opportunities should facilitate students' progress in accumulating the recommended amounts of physical activity each day and in developing the behavioral skills and capabilities needed to remain active into adulthood.

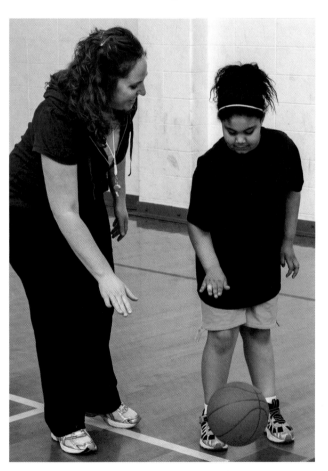

Your support can help students develop a lifestyle that values physical activity.

One way to pursue these goals is to implement a Comprehensive School Physical Activity Program (CSPAP), which is a multi-component approach including the following parts: (1) quality physical education during school activity, before- and after-school programs, staff involvement, and family and community engagement (Centers for Disease Control and Prevention, 2013; SHAPE America, 2015). A fully developed CSPAP supplements physical education by providing students with regular activity time throughout the entire school day, including recess, activity breaks, movement-based classroom lessons, and intramural clubs. It also promotes physical activity outside of the regular school day by involving school administrators and staff persons, parents, and community stakeholders in program planning, implementation, management, and evaluation.

Establishing a Safe Environment

Because physical activity participation involves some inherent dangers, we must take care to establish a teaching and learning environment that minimizes the risk of injury. This responsibility includes regular inspection and maintenance of all facilities and equipment. Preventive maintenance is of particular importance in high-risk areas marked by the potential for catastrophic injury (e.g., swimming pool, weight room, climbing wall, playground equipment). In addition, all physical education programs should implement meaningful preinstructional planning, effective teaching methods, and qualified supervision. For more information about facility safety and security in school, sport, and physical activity settings, visit the Athletic Business website (www.athleticbusiness.com); for information about risk management and shared-use agreements, visit the ChangeLabSolutions website (www.changelabsolutions.org/su-healthy-communities).

In addition to planning, management, and teaching, we must also consider various administrative factors. For instance, we must determine acceptable student-to-teacher ratios and make use of physical activity waivers and health history forms for students. We should also post a written emergency response plan, practice it on a routine basis, and maintain first aid and CPR certification. For more information about these issues, visit the website of the American Red Cross (www.redcross.org). You can also teach your students to become accountable for their own safety. Indeed, students seeking any level of health-related fitness must be encouraged to listen to their bodies and slow down if they feel overtired or suffer from soreness that is intense or lasts more than a day or so.

Common causes of injury include weakness, lack of flexibility, biomechanical problems, improper footwear, and doing too much too fast. Teach students to use proper pacing—beginning at low intensity and progressing slowly to longer, more intense activities. These concepts can be difficult to communicate, especially when working with younger children who still gauge success solely in terms of winners and losers in competition. Beginners frequently ignore early warning signs of overtraining and fail to recognize that they are overdoing it until it is too late to prevent injury or avoid undue fatigue. Regarding flexibility and muscular strength and endurance, students must understand that concentrating on only a few muscle groups while neglecting others can make an individual more susceptible to injury. For example, working only on pushing movements, such as the bench press and shoulder press, during resistance training can lead to muscle imbalances that increase the risk of harm. Instead, encourage students to take a whole-body approach to physical activity and health-related fitness.

Summary

Remember, we are talking about health-related physical activity—not Olympic training! Regardless of students' age, they should be presented with reasonable choices for how intensively they will work during a given physical activity session based on their personal goals. Health-related fitness is a journey, not a destination, and we want to help students develop positive lifelong habits for health-related physical activity. Moreover, students must understand the principles of training and the FITT guidelines so that, ultimately, they can choose to increase their levels of performance and health-related fitness as they desire—and know how to do so safely. The goal is to progress toward self-assessment and self-delivery of health-related fitness activities. Self-assessment and self-delivery can be carried over to a wide range of healthy lifestyle habits, including best nutrition practices, which are discussed in the next chapter.

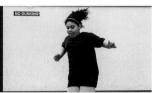

Discussion Questions

1. How can the basic training principles be used to inform development of unit plans and lesson plans in physical education?

2. Select one training principle and give examples of how it can be applied when working with students in elementary school, middle school, and high school.

3. Explain the FITT guidelines and describe how students can use them to reach training goals.

4. Why is it important to consider age-related differences when applying the FITT guidelines in school-based settings?

5. Describe each of the CSPAP components and provide real-world examples from your school.

6. How should a physical activity session be structured in order to achieve different training goals—improved health, health-related fitness, and sport performance? Remember to account for the warm-up, the main physical activity, and the cool-down.

7. Describe how you would explain the importance of warming up and cooling down to students in elementary school, middle school, and high school.

8. Select a Physical Best activity from the web resource and describe how it applies the training principles.

9. Explain the importance of facilitating a supportive and safe learning environment; illustrate your key points with examples from your own teaching.

10. Create a list of physical education reminders for students and staff.

CHAPTER 4

Exploring Nutrition for Student Health

D. Gayle Povis

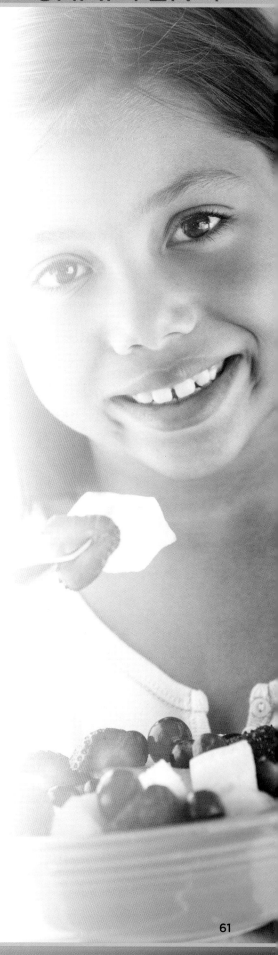

CHAPTER CONTENTS

Physical education teachers have a unique opportunity to help students develop healthy habits for life. Students look to physical education teachers as body experts, so it's natural to extend your teaching to help students choose nutritious foods for fuel. This chapter provides basic but thorough information about nutrients in foods to enhance your content knowledge and enable you to help students make wise choices. This information aligns with *2015-2020 Dietary Guidelines for Americans* (U.S. Department of Health and Human Services and U.S. Department of Agriculture, 2015a), which is based on hundreds of research studies that have been peer-reviewed for accuracy and reliability. This chapter also provides helpful suggestions and useful examples of practical ways in which to incorporate this information into your current program.

Helping students comprehend what constitutes a nutritious diet and then demonstrate that comprehension by the food choices they make is one of the goals set forth in the National Health Education Standards (NHES; Joint Committee on National Health Education Standards, 2007). Therefore, your efforts will help students attain not only just the physical education standards but also the NHES. The nutrition concepts found in this chapter can be taught through engaging physical activities that are described in the web resource. When you combine nutrition concepts with physical activity in a single lesson, you truly help your students become their Physical Best.

Healthy Students Do Better in School

You can play a critical role in helping students establish healthy behaviors by creating a culture in which physical activity is frequent and healthful food choices are the norm. Students spend up to 2,000 hours at school each year—nearly half of their waking hours—and as much as two-thirds of their food consumption occurs at school. The Institute of Medicine (IOM; 2012), which advises the U.S. population on ways to improve health, supports making schools the "heart of health" as a focal point for preventing childhood obesity and learning health-enhancing behaviors that lead to healthy lives. As you know, health and physical education teachers are responsible for carrying out such wellness activities in schools. IOM recommendations for a healthy school environment include the following (IOM, 2012):

- "All students in grades K-12 have adequate opportunities to engage in 60 minutes of physical activity per school day. This 60-minute goal includes access to and participation in quality physical education" (p. 329).
- All foods and beverages sold or provided in schools should meet strong nutrition standards.
- Schools should implement and monitor "sequential food literacy and nutrition science education, spanning grades K-12, based on the food and nutrition recommendations in the Dietary Guidelines for Americans" (p. 332).

The Institute of Medicine (2012) further notes that establishing a healthy school environment benefits educators and students in the following ways:

- "Physical activity and a nutritious diet are associated with" improvements in learning ability, behavior, and academic performance (p. 333).
- The benefits that students realize from practicing proper nutrition and physical activity are a prerequisite to optimal learning and are mutually reinforcing. Foods provide the nutrients needed for proper brain development, and physical

activity enhances learning, ability to focus, and mood. Brain research with children shows that improved nutrition and physical activity directly affect learning.

- "Physically active and well-nourished students are . . . less likely to miss school for health reasons" (p. 333).
- Improvements in physical activity and nutrition at school give students of all backgrounds the opportunity to lead healthier, more productive lives.
- Children who have early experiences with healthy foods are more likely to prefer and eat those foods later in life and to develop eating patterns that promote healthy growth and weight.
- Food and nutrition education can improve students' nutrition knowledge and eating habits, which may positively affect body weight.

Developing a healthy lifestyle early in life is critical because habits established in one's youth are typically carried into adulthood. Thus, physical educators have the opportunity to influence the future health of our nation by teaching students about physical activity and foods that promote a healthy mind and body and then guiding them to make healthy lifestyle choices on a regular basis. For teachers seeking to realize this opportunity, Physical Best is an excellent resource.

Physical activity and health educators are also encouraged to promote and participate in implementing their district's local school wellness policy, which sets standards for physical activity and nutrition education. Every school district is required to develop such a policy, assess its own compliance with policy at least every three years, and modify the policy as needed.

Road Map to Healthy Eating

The *2015-2020 Dietary Guidelines for Americans* (U.S. Department of Health and Human Services, 2015a) provides evidence-based recommendations for healthy eating patterns for all people of age two or older. Recognizing that everyone has a variety of eating habits, the guidelines are intended to help people make slight shifts in their eating patterns over time in order to consume healthier foods overall. **Eating patterns** consist of the combination of foods and beverages that a person consumes and the person's usual intake over time. In order to establish good eating patterns, students need to be educated about which foods contribute to good health, why, and how they can be identified. Students also need to understand the ramifications of good health versus poor health in order to be motivated to make smart food choices.

The Dietary Guidelines for Americans are updated every five years. One cornerstone of the current (2015-2020) guidelines is MyPlate, a graphic representation of the recommended proportions of various food groups for a typical meal (see figure 4.1). To help people put these guidelines into practice, many governmental agencies work together to provide education and recommendations. These agencies provide free educational materials with coordinated messages that are available

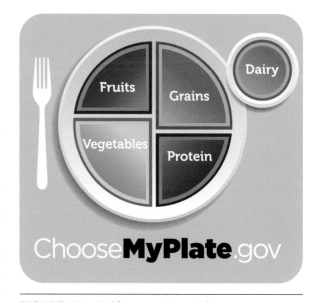

FIGURE 4.1 MyPlate nutrition guide.
USDA's Center for Nutrition Policy and Promotion.

A Healthy Eating Pattern

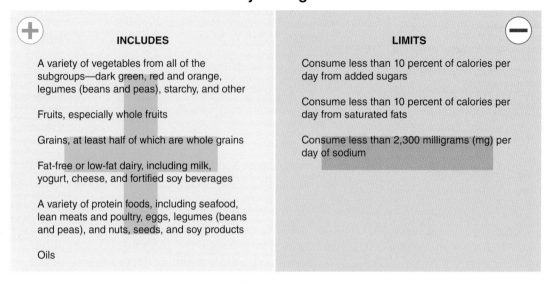

INCLUDES

A variety of vegetables from all of the subgroups—dark green, red and orange, legumes (beans and peas), starchy, and other

Fruits, especially whole fruits

Grains, at least half of which are whole grains

Fat-free or low-fat dairy, including milk, yogurt, cheese, and fortified soy beverages

A variety of protein foods, including seafood, lean meats and poultry, eggs, legumes (beans and peas), and nuts, seeds, and soy products

Oils

LIMITS

Consume less than 10 percent of calories per day from added sugars

Consume less than 10 percent of calories per day from saturated fats

Consume less than 2,300 milligrams (mg) per day of sodium

FIGURE 4.2   Summary of key recommendations from *2015-2020 Dietary Guidelines for Americans.*

online. For instance, the U.S. Department of Agriculture (USDA) offers an interactive website for MyPlate (https://www.choosemyplate.gov) and free printable materials (https://www.choosemyplate.gov/printable-materials).

In addition to MyPlate, the Dietary Guidelines for Americans offer recommendations. Key recommendations from the 2015-2020 guidelines are summarized in figure 4.2; the full guidelines provide much more depth.

The MyPlate graphic can be shared with students as an easy guide to making healthful choices from all food groups. Basic principles include the following:

- Fill half of the plate with fruits and vegetables—a little more of vegetables than of fruit.

- Just over a quarter of the plate should consist of complex carbohydrate, such as whole-grain foods (whole grains should account for at least half of the grain one eats).

- Just under a quarter of the plate should consist of lean animal protein or plant-sourced protein. Because protein is a concentrated food, large amounts are not necessary.

- Include a dairy or other calcium-rich food with each meal; choose dairy products that are nonfat or 1 percent fat.

Encourage students to choose healthful foods from each food group in order to meet their nutrient and calorie needs. Each food group provides a different set of nutrients, and the foods within each group provide similar but not identical nutrients. As shown in table 4.1, each food supplies higher amounts of certain nutrients and smaller amounts of others. For instance, an orange is packed with vitamin C, but an apple is not. Therefore, students should be encouraged to eat a wide variety of foods from within each food group in order to obtain all nutrients needed by their growing bodies.

The Dietary Guidelines for Americans recommend making slight shifts over time to include a variety of whole, unprocessed foods from each food group, as well as oils.

TABLE 4.1 Main Nutrients in Food Sources

Food source	Key nutrients	Tips for healthy choices
Fruits Fruits may be fresh, canned, frozen, or dried and may be whole, cut up, or pureed. Any fruit or 100% fruit juice counts as part of the fruit group.	Fruits provide carbohydrate, potassium, dietary fiber, vitamin C, and folate (folic acid). Most fruits are naturally low in fat, sodium, and calories. None have cholesterol.	The majority of fruit should come from whole fruits, including fresh, canned, frozen, and dried forms, rather than from juice. When juice is consumed, it should consist of 100% fruit juice. To limit intake of added sugar, fruit canned in 100% fruit juice is encouraged over fruit canned in syrup.
Vegetables Any vegetable or 100% vegetable juice counts as a member of the vegetable group. Vegetables may be raw or cooked; fresh, frozen, canned, or dried; and whole, cut up, or mashed. Based on their nutrient content, vegetables are organized into 5 subgroups: dark green, starchy, red and orange, beans and peas, and other vegetables.	Vegetables are low in calories and serve as important sources of many nutrients, including potassium, dietary fiber, folate (folic acid), vitamin A, vitamin C, and carbohydrate. Most vegetables are naturally low in fat, sodium, and calories. None have cholesterol.	Eat a variety of vegetables from each subgroup. Dark green and deep orange or yellow veggies are rich in vitamin A; eat them at least several times per week. Avoid adding fat (e.g., butter, oil, or cheese); bake or steam them instead of frying. When choosing frozen vegetables, select ones without creamy sauces to avoid excessive sodium, fat, and calories. When choosing canned vegetables, select ones labeled as "reduced sodium," "low sodium," or "no salt added."
Grains Any food made from wheat, rice, oat, cornmeal, barley, or another cereal grain is considered a grain product. Examples include bread, pasta, oatmeal, breakfast cereal, tortillas, rice, and grits. Grains are divided into two subgroups: whole grains and refined grains.	Grains serve as important sources of complex carbohydrate and many other nutrients, including dietary fiber, several B vitamins (thiamin, riboflavin, niacin, and folate), and minerals (iron, magnesium, and selenium).	Select whole grains most often, or at least half the time, to get fiber and nutrients that are otherwise removed during processing. Limit grain-based foods with added fat and sugar, such as cookies, cakes, and pastries. Also limit the amount of fat and sugar you add when preparing grain foods.
Protein Protein can be obtained from all foods made from meat, poultry, seafood, beans and peas, eggs, processed soy products, nuts, and seeds. Eat at least 8 ounces (225 g) of cooked seafood per week.	Foods in this group contain protein, B vitamins (niacin, thiamin, riboflavin, and B_6), vitamin E, iron, zinc, and magnesium.	Eat a variety of foods from the protein group each week. Experiment with main dishes made with beans or peas, nuts, soy, and seafood. Choose lean or low-fat cuts of meat, such as round or sirloin, and ground beef that is at least 90% lean. Trim or drain fat from meat and remove poultry skin. Eat eggs in moderation. Eat plant protein often. Try beans and peas (kidney, pinto, black, or white beans; split peas; chickpeas; hummus), soy products (tofu, tempeh, veggie burgers), nuts, and seeds.

(continued)

Table 4.1 *(continued)*

Food source	Key nutrients	Tips for healthy choices
Dairy This group includes all fluid milk products and foods made from milk that retain their calcium content (this definition excludes foods such as cream cheese, cream, and butter). Most dairy choices should be fat free or low in fat. The group also includes calcium-fortified milk substitutes, such as soy, almond, and rice milk.	Dairy foods provide a rich source of calcium, potassium, and protein. Most are also fortified with vitamin D.	Include milk or calcium-fortified milk substitutes as a beverage at meals. Choose fat-free or low-fat milk and milk products. If using whole milk, switch gradually to fat-free milk to reduce intake of saturated fat and calories. Calcium choices for those who do not consume dairy products include calcium-fortified juices, cereals, and breads, as well as calcium-fortified soy, rice, and almond milk. Choose reduced-fat cheeses (made from 2% milk or "part-skim" cheese). Look for reduced-fat or low-fat yogurt and frozen desserts. Limit full-fat cheeses and ice cream.
Oils Oils come from many different plants and from fish. Oils do *not* constitute a food group, but they do provide essential fatty acids and vitamin E. Examples in this group include vegetable oils, nuts, seeds, olives and avocados, and some seafood.	Oils contain high percentages of monounsaturated and polyunsaturated fats, some of which the body cannot make and therefore must be consumed. These oils are called "essential fatty acids." Oils also contain vitamin E.	Choose oils that are liquid at room temperature, such as canola, olive, corn, peanut, safflower, and soybean. Choose soft margarines that contain liquid vegetable oil and no hydrogenated or trans fat. Eat nuts and seeds in moderation. Consume oily fish several times per week. Replace saturated fats with oils whenever possible.

Reprinted from U.S. Department of Health and Human Services and U.S. Department of Agriculture. *2015–2020 Dietary Guidelines for Americans,* 8th ed. (Washington, DC: U.S. Department of Agriculture, 2015). http://health.gov/dietaryguidelines/2015/guidelines/

MyPlate Relay

Here's a fun way to get students of many ages thinking about food choices that align with MyPlate. Beforehand, collect a wide array of pictures of foods from each food group. One easy way to do so is to visit the National Dairy Council's website (www. NationalDairyCouncil.org), search for "food models," and print the resulting food pictures and nutrition labels. Scatter the food pictures on the ground or on a table near a large MyPlate poster or drawing at one end of the activity area. Divide the class into two teams with the food pictures located between them. To play the relay, students run, hop, or skip to a food picture and then place it in the corresponding part of the poster. Students then run back and tag the next person in line, who does the same thing. The goal is to be the first team to get a balanced meal (that is, one appropriate food in each food group). Repeat the activity using additional food pictures. The relay can be done three times—once each for breakfast, lunch, and dinner.

This healthy eating pattern supplies a person with the vitamins, minerals, carbohydrate, protein, essential fat, and nutrients needed by the body. (**Essential nutrients** cannot be made by the body and therefore must be obtained from food.)

People sometimes get stuck in a routine and eat the same foods day after day; therefore, students may need to be encouraged to eat a variety of foods. Doing so not only provides more nutrients but also keeps food interesting. Encourage students to be adventurous and try new foods. To help them meet this goal, offer them samples in small sizes or set up taste tests with fruits and vegetables in the cafeteria or classroom.

Carbohydrate, Protein, and Fat (Macronutrients)

Carbohydrate, protein, and fat make up the bulk of all of the foods listed in table 4.1. Known as **macronutrients** (i.e., large nutrients), they provide the energy that our bodies need in order to live, think, and move. They do so by providing calories in the following amounts:

Carbohydrate: 4 calories per gram

Protein: 4 calories per gram

Fat: 9 calories per gram

Carbohydrates

Carbohydrate, often referred to as "carbs," is the body's main source of fuel, or energy. This energy is provided by two categories of carbohydrate—complex and simple. **Complex carbohydrate** consists mostly of starch and fiber and comes from vegetables, fruits, and whole grains. **Simple carbohydrate** includes both naturally occurring sugars (such as those found in fruit and lactose) and added sugars (which include sweeteners such as white sugar and corn syrup). Because people tend to eat too much simple carbohydrate, we need to encourage students to shift toward eating more complex carbohydrate. Furthermore, the Dietary Guidelines for Americans recommend that no more than 10 percent of a day's calories come from added sugar; therefore, students should choose high-sugar foods only occasionally.

Whole Grains

As sources of complex carbohydrate, grains provide plenty of fuel for kids to move, think, grow, and be healthy. Whole grains provide more vitamins, minerals, and fiber than are found in processed (refined) grains. When whole grains are eaten in sufficient quantities, their fiber and nutrients provide health benefits that may include a reduction in the risk of cardiovascular disease.

A whole grain, such as a wheat kernel, contains all edible portions of the grain—bran, germ, and endosperm (see figure 4.3). In other words, when all three parts are present, the food is a whole grain. These three edible components contain the following nutrients:

Whole grain

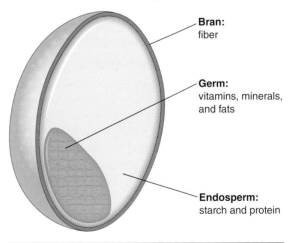

Bran:
fiber

Germ:
vitamins, minerals, and fats

Endosperm:
starch and protein

FIGURE 4.3 Components of a whole grain.

The Truth About Grains and Carbohydrate

Grains serve as a rich source of carbohydrate, which, despite the occasional popularity of "low-carb" diets, is the main fuel on which the body runs. During digestion, carbohydrate is broken down into glucose and either used for fuel right away or stored in the muscles and liver. The body needs glucose for all of its operations, such as breathing, muscle action, heart function, brain function, and formation of new tissue. When carbohydrate is in short supply, the body scrambles to break down fat reserves and turn them into a class of compounds known as *ketones*. The body can burn ketones for energy, though not efficiently, through the process of ketosis. At first thought, breaking down fat reserves might sound like a good thing, but as the body uses ketones instead of glucose for energy, side effects can occur, including headache, nausea, abdominal pain, fatigue, confusion, dizziness, aches, bad breath, and shortness of breath. Therefore, it is healthier for students to provide the body with the carbohydrate it needs. Long-term studies (Sacks et al., 2009) find that consuming a diet higher in protein and low in carbohydrate for weight loss results in insignificant differences in weight after one year as compared with eating a diet with a normal balance of protein and carbohydrate.

Carbohydrate is found in the following foods:

- Grains
- Fruits
- Vegetables
- Dairy products
- Nuts and seeds
- Legumes: beans (e.g., pinto, black, garbanzo), split peas, lentils, soybeans
- Sweeteners, such as white sugar, brown sugar, turbinado or raw sugar, molasses, honey, high-fructose corn syrup

Foods that contain *no* carbohydrate include the following:

- Animal sources of protein: meat, poultry, pork, fish, eggs
- Fats and oils

You can find out more about carbohydrate at the Mayo Clinic's website: https://www.mayoclinic.org/healthy-lifestyle/nutrition-and-healthy-eating/in-depth/carbohydrates/art-20045705

- The **bran** contains fiber.
- The **endosperm** contains mostly starch (carbohydrate) and protein.
- The **germ** contains vitamins, minerals, and a tiny amount of fat.

When grains are processed, or refined, the bran and the germ are removed, along with many vitamins and trace minerals. This removal leaves only the starchy endosperm. In the United States, as required by law, processed grains are enriched to return the thiamine, riboflavin, niacin, folic acid, and iron that were removed during processing. The refined grain is then referred to as "enriched."

The Dietary Guidelines and MyPlate recommendations urge everyone to eat whole grains for at least half of the grains. This goal can be met either by eating a few foods that are 100 percent whole grain or by eating more types of foods that are partially whole grain.

Whole grains can be consumed either in the form of a single food (e.g., brown rice, popcorn, oatmeal, 100 percent whole-wheat bread) or as one of multiple ingredient in a food (e.g., cereal, bread, crackers). Examples of whole-grain ingredients include buckwheat, bulgur, millet, oatmeal, quinoa, rolled oats, brown or wild rice, teff, whole-grain barley, whole rye, and whole wheat.

Teach kids to read the ingredient list on food labels to determine how much, if any, whole grain is contained. Look for the word *whole* in front of the name of a grain. The whole-grain ingredient should be the first one listed. For example, if the first ingredient is listed as "wheat" or "enriched wheat flour," then it is not whole wheat. Look for "whole wheat" or "whole oats" or "brown rice" and so on. A misleading label may say "100 percent multi-grain," which merely means that the product consists of more than one grain, none of which may be whole.

Gluten Sensitivity and Celiac Disease

Gluten is a protein found in certain grains. It can cause devastating health problems for people who have celiac disease by damaging the lining of the small intestine, which makes it difficult for them to absorb nutrients. If people with severe celiac disease consume gluten, they are at risk for nutritional deficiencies and health problems that stem from malnourishment. Ranging from slight to severe, this condition is estimated to affect one in every 141 people in the United States (Rubio-Tapia, Ludvigsson, Brantner, Murray, & Everhart, 2012), most of whom are never diagnosed with the disease. For more information about celiac disease, review the information page provided by the National Institute of Diabetes and Digestive and Kidney Diseases at https://www.niddk.nih.gov/health-information/digestive-diseases/celiac-disease.

Gluten can also cause problems for people with gluten sensitivity, which differs from celiac disease and affects more people. People with gluten sensitivity suffer adverse reactions after eating gluten, including gas, abdominal bloating, diarrhea (in adults), constipation and vomiting (in children), headaches, and fatigue. Such symptoms need to be evaluated by a health care provider.

The type of gluten that is harmful to celiac patients and people who are gluten sensitive is found in wheat, rye, barley, and other grains that contains any of these due to crossbreeding—for example, triticale (a cross of wheat and rye). Oats may also contain gluten from contamination in the field or during processing. Even pure, uncontaminated oats naturally contain a protein that causes an adverse reaction in a very small number of celiac patients.

Gluten is also contained in spelt and kamut, which are older species of wheat known as "ancient grains." In fact, gluten is found in wheat by any name, including bulgur, semolina, durum flour, and graham flour. It is *not* contained in rice, corn, buckwheat, teff, quinoa, millet, or amaranth.

Gluten appears not only in grain foods but also in many processed foods, such as soups, gravies, salad dressings, sauces, and even candy. Therefore, in order to completely avoid gluten, one must carefully read labels. You can find a listing of organizations that offer reliable information about health issues related to gluten, support groups, and more on the website of the National Institute of Diabetes and Digestive and Kidney Diseases at https://www.niddk.nih.gov/health-information/digestive-diseases/celiac-disease-organizations. These organizations may be useful for students who wonder if gluten poses a health issue for them.

Since 2015, food manufacturers are bound by Federal Drug Administration (FDA) regulations that apply to labeling food as gluten free. Details can be found on the

FDA website by doing a web search for "FDA gluten-free labeling of foods" or simply visiting www.fda.gov/Food/GuidanceRegulation/GuidanceDocumentsRegulatoryInformation/Allergens/ucm362510.htm.

Protein

Protein is made of amino acids, which are used by the body to grow, maintain, and repair itself. The body can make some amino acids from compounds that it stores, but others, referred to as *essential*, cannot be made by the body and therefore must be obtained from food.

Help students understand that there are two categories of proteins—those that come from animal-based foods and those that come from plant-based foods. Both types help grow healthy bodies; in fact, some of your students may be vegetarian. In addition, consuming plant-based proteins either occasionally or more often helps to prevent chronic conditions such as cardiovascular disease. The Dietary Guidelines for Americans recommend an eating pattern that includes a variety of protein-rich foods, such as seafood, lean meats, and poultry; eggs; legumes (beans and peas); and nuts, seeds, and soy products such as tofu. Most Americans get plenty of protein and in fact eat more than the recommended amount.

Fats and Oils

People often use the word **fat** to refer to a variety of solid fats and liquid oils; however, each type of fat affects health in its own way. Liquid oils contain essential nutrients needed by the body and are heart healthy. Specifically, they provide the following benefits:

- Help absorb and transport fat-soluble vitamins (A, D, E, and K).
- Form the cell membranes that surround every cell in the body; cell membranes contain a thin layer of fat that helps protect the cell's internal environment.
- Create regulatory compounds, such as prostaglandins, that regulate body processes including inflammation and blood pressure, as well as other compounds that regulate blood clotting, immune function, and more.

It's good to eat a small amount of healthy oils each day. This category includes omega-3, a type of essential fat. Foods that contain these healthy fats include nuts, nut butters, flax seed, avocados, olives, vegetable oils (especially canola and olive oils), and fatty fish (such as salmon, anchovies, herring, shad, sardines, Pacific oysters, trout, and Atlantic and Pacific mackerel—but avoid king mackerel, which is high in mercury) (U.S. Department of Health and Human Services and U.S. Department of Agriculture, 2015a, chapter 1). If students want to know more about which fish to eat or avoid, they can visit the website of the U.S. Environmental Protection Agency at https://www.epa.gov/choose-fish-and-shellfish-wisely/fish-and-shellfish-advisories-and-safe-eating-guidelines. One caveat: In order to avoid consuming too many calories, choose healthy oils to *replace* solid fats; for instance, fish or nuts can replace meat as a protein source.

In contrast, **saturated fat** and **trans fat** are considered solid fats and need to be limited or avoided for good heart health. The Dietary Guidelines recommend limiting solid fats and consuming recommended amounts of healthful oils for all people over the age of two. (Children who are younger than two need full-fat foods rather than reduced-fat ones to support proper brain and nerve development.)

Foods that are high in saturated fat come mostly from animal products, such as meat, poultry, pork, lard, tallow, butter, solid vegetable shortening, whole milk, and dairy products made from whole milk. Saturated fat also abounds in plant products from warm places, such as coconut, palm, and palm kernel oil. However, coconut oil, although saturated, contains a type of saturated fat referred to as "medium-chain triglycerides" (MCTs) and is considered healthful.

Trans fats are formed during food processing when hydrogen is forced onto the chemical bonds of **unsaturated fats**. This process keeps the fat from going rancid, thus lengthening shelf life. Trans fats formed during processing also enhance flavor and texture. These trans fats formed during processing are sometimes referred to as *synthetic trans fats* because they differ from the naturally occurring trans fats found in milk and some meats. It is the synthetic trans fats that pose a health concern.

The presence of trans fats is indicated by the terms *hydrogenated* and *partially hydrogenated* on food labels. This type of fat has not been very common in the U.S. food supply since 2006, when manufacturers were first required to list it separately on the nutrition facts label found on food products. In 2015, the U.S. Food and Drug Administration took further action to reduce the amount of synthetic trans fats in foods by requiring manufacturers to eliminate them within three years unless they are granted an exemption.

Make students aware of trans fats and how to avoid them by limiting intake of the following food items:

- Vegetable shortening
- Foods made with shortening, such as bakery pastries and refrigerated dough products (e.g., biscuits, cinnamon rolls)
- Processed foods made with hydrogenated or partially hydrogenated oils
  - Some crackers, cookies, cakes, frozen pies, and other grain foods
  - Some snack foods (such as microwave popcorn)
  - Frozen pizza
  - Stick margarines
  - Coffee creamers
  - Ready-to-use frostings
  - Fried foods from some restaurants (those who have not switched to frying oils free of trans fat)

The different types of fats, also called fatty acids, have different chemical structures and are categorized as being either saturated, monounsaturated, or polyunsaturated. All fats contain a mixture of these different kinds of fatty acids, as shown in figure 4.4; sharing this chart can help students understand the difference between healthful and less healthful fats. If a fat contains a high percentage of saturated fat, then it is referred to as a saturated fat even though not all of its fats are saturated. Similarly, fats that are high in monounsaturated and polyunsaturated fats are referred to as unsaturated. For another overview of the differences between the types of fat, see the fact sheet provided by Harvard Medical School at the following URL: www.health. harvard.edu/staying-healthy/the-truth-about-fats-bad-and-good.

Why limit foods that are high in solid fat?

- Solid fat (both saturated fat and trans fats) are turned into cholesterol in the body. Too much cholesterol in the bloodstream can result in artery damage and inflammation, plaque formation in the arteries, and, eventually, clogged arteries and heart disease. Sometimes plaques burst open, creating blood clots that can block arteries. If oxygen-rich blood is blocked from reaching an area of the heart, a heart attack can result; if blood is blocked from reaching the brain, a stroke can result. These scenarios may resonate with your students, because at least some of them will have a family member or family friend who has suffered a heart attack or stroke. The Dietary Guidelines for Americans state that a strong body of evidence supports limiting solid fat since it is linked to increased amounts of total cholesterol and "bad" LDL cholesterol, both of which are risk factors for heart disease (U.S. Department of Health and Human Services and U.S. Department of Agriculture, 2015a, chapter 1).

• High blood pressure is a common complication of heart disease. When blood pressure is high, the heart must work harder to push blood through partially blocked arteries.

• Coronary heart disease is the type most closely associated with diet. By limiting the intake of solid fats, we can diminish the risk of high blood pressure, heart attack, and stroke.

The Dietary Guidelines for Americans recommend obtaining no more than 10 percent of calories from saturated fat (U.S. Department of Health and Human Services

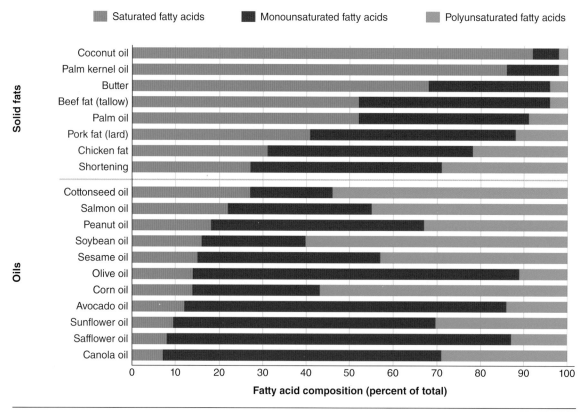

FIGURE 4.4   Fatty acid profiles of common fats and oils. * Coconut, palm kernel, and palm oil are called oils because they come from plants. However, they are solid or semi-solid at room temperature due to their high content of short-chain saturated fatty acids. They are considered solid fats for nutritional purposes. ** Shortening may be made from partially hydrogenated vegetable oil, which contains trans fatty acids.

Reprinted from U.S. Department of Health and Human Services and U.S. Department of Agriculture. *2015–2020 Dietary Guidelines for Americans,* 8th ed. (Washington, DC: U.S. Department of Agriculture, 2015). http://health.gov/dietaryguidelines/2015/guidelines/

and U.S. Department of Agriculture, 2015a). For a person who eats 2,000 calories per day, that means no more than 22 grams (about 5 1/2 teaspoons). Since solid fats are so abundant in the typical American diet, they contribute substantially to excess calorie intake, which can also result in weight gain. Experts recommend shifting from solid fats to oils and limiting solid fat by following these recommendations; share them with your students:

- Choose lean meats; remove all visible fat, as well as poultry skin.
- Replace animal-based foods with plant-based foods often.
- Replace solid fats with plant oils whenever possible.
- Read labels to choose foods low in saturated fat.

Help students learn the differences between types of fat and focus on eating fruits, vegetables, whole grains, lean meats, fatty fish, nuts, and healthful oils—which will automatically decrease solid fat intake while still supplying healthful oils. Students need to understand that consuming some fat, especially in the form of liquid oils, is necessary for human health and helps keep the heart and blood vessels healthy while performing the other favorable functions of fat. Although the emphasis is on keeping solid fats in check, remind students that too much *total* dietary fat can also contribute to health problems, including the following:

- *Overweight and obesity.* Because fat contains more than twice as many calories per gram as do protein and carbohydrate, eating too much fat may lead to weight gain. Being overweight can raise the risk of developing heart disease, type 2 diabetes, stroke, and certain cancers.
- *Type 2 diabetes.* As the rate of childhood obesity climbs, so does the number of children diagnosed with type 2 diabetes. In this condition, the body is no longer as sensitive to insulin as it used to be. To help the body regain its sensitivity to insulin, adults can lose weight. Children, however, are rarely put on weight-loss plans (only under a physician's orders); instead, the goal is to stop weight gain while the child increases in height. In addition, both children and adults can help themselves regain insulin sensitivity by increasing their level of physical activity.
- *Certain cancers.* High fat intake is associated with breast, prostate, colon, and other cancers.

Cholesterol

Cholesterol is a type of fat that comes from two sources—food and the human body. Foods that contain dietary cholesterol are animal based, such as meats, poultry, eggs, dairy products, and shellfish. Cholesterol is not found in plants.

The human body makes all the cholesterol it needs, mostly from saturated fat. A little of the body's cholesterol also comes from the cholesterol in foods. The body needs the cholesterol it makes for various purposes; for example, cholesterol is used to make substances, such as hormones and bile, and serves as a major component of every cell membrane in the body.

Dietary cholesterol (cholesterol obtained from food) should not be confused with serum cholesterol. Commonly called *blood cholesterol*, serum cholesterol is checked by a blood test. It is categorized either as HDL ("good") cholesterol, which helps clear the arteries, or as LDL and VLDL ("bad") cholesterol, which line the artery walls and obstruct blood flow.

Many foods that are high in saturated fat are also high in cholesterol. Therefore, teaching students to limit their intake of saturated fat will reduce their cholesterol intake as well.

Energy From Food Fuels Activity

Food and beverages provide the body with energy in the form of calories. The body uses those calories to fuel body functions and physical activity. People can control how many calories they consume in what they eat and drink, as well as how many calories they burn for physical activity. Because calories are used to measure energy, caloric balance is also called energy balance.

The body uses calories in three ways:

- *Metabolism.* The body uses calories to provide energy for growth, development, and maintenance of body tissues. Calories also fuel organ functions, such as heartbeat, breathing, growth, tissue repair, blood production, brain activity, and heat production. Some 60 percent to 75 percent of the calories converted by the body every day are used for metabolism, and we cannot influence the number of calories spent on these basic functions—with two exceptions. First, metabolic rate is influenced by the amount of one's muscle tissue. Muscle burns more calories, even at rest, than fat tissue does; as a result, the more muscle one has, the more calories one spends on metabolism. Thus, a muscular person has a slightly higher, or faster, metabolism than does a person with a higher percentage of body fat. Second, metabolism increases for an hour or two after a period of physical activity; therefore, frequent activity helps boost one's metabolic rate.

- *Food digestion.* About 10 percent of daily calorie usage fuels the process of breaking down food, digesting it, absorbing it, and transporting the nutrients to where they are needed in the body. The number of calories spent on digestion cannot be changed.

- *Physical activity.* Whether it's walking to school, playing at recess, or doing chores around the house or yard, physical activity uses 15 percent to 30 percent of calories consumed. People *can* alter how many calories they use in physical activity—the more activity, and the longer and more intense it is, the more calories are burned.

Anytime a person eats more calories than are used in a day, the body stores the extra calories as fat. It doesn't matter which foods have contributed the extra calories. However, fat in food contains more than twice as many calories per gram as do carbohydrate and protein. Thus, when fat is added to food, the food becomes much higher in calories, or more calorie dense. Fatty foods often taste good, which makes it easy to eat too much of them, in which case people end up eating more calories than are necessary to meet the body's needs. The point to emphasize with students is that regardless of which foods one eats, if one consumes more calories than one burns, then the body stores the extra calories as fat.

Energy Balance and Healthy Weight

Teach students that their food intake needs to be in line with their activity level in order for their body to maintain an appropriate weight. Increasing or decreasing food intake or activity level causes body weight to change. The concept is summarized nicely in the following simple equations from the National Heart, Lung, and Blood Institute (2013):

The same amount of energy in (calories consumed) and energy out (calories burned) over time = weight stays the same.

More energy in than out over time = weight gain.

More energy out than in over time = weight loss.

People who are sedentary most of the time—sitting or standing—need fewer calories than those who are more active. Therefore, in order to maintain weight, sedentary people need to eat foods in amounts at the low end of the recommended ranges. People who are more active—for example, doing 30 to 60 minutes per day of moderate physical activity—will need to eat in the middle of the recommended ranges. And people who are very physically active will need to eat at the high end of the ranges. For instance, if the recommendation is to eat 5 to 8 ounces of grains per day, then a sedentary person would eat 5 ounces, a more active person would aim for 6 ounces, and an athlete would eat even more.

To help with calorie balance, as well as health-related fitness, the *2018 Physical Activity Guidelines for Americans* (U.S. Department of Health and Human Services, 2018) recommend that children and adolescents engage in 60 minutes or more of physical activity per day. As much as possible, this time should include cardiorespiratory, muscle-strengthening, and bone-strengthening activities, which are covered in chapters 5 and 8.

Poor Practice: Physical Activity as Punishment for Poor Food Choices

Sometimes teachers and parents, in their enthusiasm to help kids be more active and maintain a healthy weight, negatively relate calories to physical activity. In other words, they use physical activity as a punishment rather than helping kids experience it as a fun thing to do. For instance, a teacher might misguidedly say something such as, "If you eat a donut, then you need to exercise 45 minutes longer to burn off the calories." Is this how kids should view physical activity? Not if they are to make it an enjoyable, normal part of their life! Think about it: How motivating is it if one is active only because it burns calories, makes up for eating something, or allows more calories to be consumed? If this is one's only motivation, it will be very hard to continue being active.

However, if kids learn to be active for the sake of playing, moving joyfully, feeling good, getting energized, and having fun, then they are more likely to keep moving. But if kids feel that they need to exercise for extended periods of time because they had some chips, then they may form a dangerous relationship between food and activity. They may also consider physical activity to be a punishment, which of course does not motivate them to engage in a healthy lifestyle.

Effective physical education, on the other hand, provides students with opportunities to learn to enjoy physical activity and become physically literate individuals. Physical educators should give lessons that help students develop knowledge related to being active and staying fit, appreciate and enjoy physical activity, and learn and practice skills that allow them to be active outside of class. One way to help students experience these types of lessons is through Physical Best activities, which equip students with knowledge and help them appreciate physical activity through active learning opportunities. Make a point to help students understand that food is fuel and that better fuel in the tank means they can perform and enjoy physical activities longer and more efficiently. In short, eating nutritious food helps them enjoy being active.

How Many Calories for Healthy Kids?

The total number of calories that a child needs each day depends on age, gender, and amount of physical activity. With that in mind, table 4.2 provides estimated calorie amounts needed to maintain caloric balance for various gender and age groups at three different levels of physical activity. The estimates are rounded to the nearest 200 calories, and a given child's calorie needs may be higher or lower than these averages. It can also be useful to consider food amounts, as shown in table 4.3.

These calorie amounts are provided to give you a general idea of children's caloric needs. It is not appropriate to recommend specific calorie levels for children. Do *not* give a calorie "prescription" to students—doing so can put too much focus on calories and lead to eating disorders. Be very careful not to make comments about any child's weight.

Instead of focusing on calories, teach kids to focus on eating recommended amounts of foods each day—several appropriately sized servings—from each food group. The amount of food recommended by the Dietary Guidelines from each food group provides the vitamins and minerals needed for good health. Students can get individualized calorie and meal plan recommendations from the MyPlate website by entering their age, height, weight, and activity level at https://www.choosemyplate.gov/MyPlatePlan. As the site explains, "The MyPlate Plan shows your food group targets—what and how much to eat within your calorie allowance. Your food plan is personalized, based on your age, sex, height, weight, and physical activity level." The page is also available in Spanish.

Listen to the Body

Students need to learn to recognize and follow the cues that their bodies send them. The body provides cues, or signals, to help maintain energy balance by announcing hunger, satiety, or fullness. No one needs to "clean their plate" if their body has had enough. Ignoring fullness cues leads one to eat more food than is needed to sustain the body, and continually overriding such cues may cause the body to stop sending them. To help students tune into their body's signals, encourage them to be thoughtful

TABLE 4.2   Recommended Calorie Intake by Age and Activity Level

	Age (yr)	ACTIVITY LEVEL		
		Sedentary[a]	Moderately active[b]	Active[c]
Girls	4-8	1,200-1,400	1,400-1,600	1,400-1,800
	9-13	1,400-1,600	1,600-2,000	1,800-2,200
	14-18	1,800	2,000	2,400
Boys	4-8	1,200-1,400	1,400-1,600	1,600-2,000
	9-13	1,600-2,000	1,800-2,200	2,000-2,600
	14-18	2,000-2,400	2,400-2,800	2,800-3,200

[a]*Sedentary* refers to a lifestyle that includes only the light physical activity associated with typical day-to-day life.

[b]*Moderately active* refers to a lifestyle that includes physical activity equivalent to walking about 1.5 to 3 miles (2.4 to 4.8 km) per day at 3 to 4 miles (4.8 to 6.4 km) per hour, in addition to the light physical activity associated with typical day-to-day life.

[c]*Active* refers to a lifestyle that includes physical activity equivalent to walking more than 3 miles per day at 3 to 4 miles per hour, in addition to the light physical activity associated with typical day-to-day life.

Reprinted from U.S. Department of Health and Human Services and U.S. Department of Agriculture. *2015–2020 Dietary Guidelines for Americans,* 8th ed. (Washington, DC: U.S. Department of Agriculture, 2015). http://health.gov/dietaryguidelines/2015/guidelines/

TABLE 4.3   Recommended Amounts[a] of Food for Moderately Active[b] Girls and Boys

	Vegetables	Fruit	Grains	Dairy	Protein	Oils[c]
BOYS						
5 yr, 1,400 cal	1-1/2 cup-eq	1-1/2 cup-eq	5 oz-eq	2-1/2 cup-eq	4 oz-eq	17 g
6-8 yr, 1,600 cal	2 cup-eq	1-1/2 cup-eq	5 oz-eq	3 cup-eq	5 oz-eq	22 g
9-10 yr, 1,800 cal	2-1/2 cup-eq	1-1/2 cup-eq	6 oz-eq	3 cup-eq	5 oz-eq	24 g
11 yr, 2,000 cal	2-1/2 cup-eq	2 cup-eq	6 oz-eq	3 cup-eq	5-1/2 oz-eq	27 g
12-13 yr, 2,200 cal	3 cup-eq	2 cup-eq	7 oz-eq	3 cup-eq	6 oz-eq	29 g
14 yr, 2,400 cal	3 cup-eq	2 cup-eq	8 oz-eq	3 cup-eq	6-1/2 oz-eq	31 g
15 yr, 2,600 cal	3-1/2 cup-eq	2 cup-eq	9 oz-eq	3 cup-eq	6-1/2 oz-eq	34 g
16-18 yr, 2,800 cal	3-1/2 cup-eq	2-1/2 cup-eq	10 oz-eq	3 cup-eq	7 oz-eq	36 g
GIRLS						
5-6 yr, 1,400 cal	1-1/2 cup-eq	1-1/2 cup-eq	5 oz-eq	2-1/2 cup-eq	4 oz-eq	17 g
7-9 yr, 1,600 cal	2 cup-eq	1-1/2 cup-eq	5 oz-eq	3 cup-eq	5 oz-eq	22 g
10-11 yr, 1,800 cal	2-1/2 cup-eq	1-1/2 cup-eq	6 oz-eq	3 cup-eq	5 oz-eq	24 g
12-18 yr, 2,000 cal	2-1/2 cup-eq	2 cup-eq	6 oz-eq	3 cup-eq	5-1/2 oz-eq	27 g

[a]Food group amounts are shown in cup- or ounce-equivalents (cup-eq, oz eq). Quantity equivalents for each food group are as follows:
- Fruits and vegetables: 1 cup-equivalent = 1 cup raw or cooked vegetable or fruit; ½ cup dried vegetable or fruit; 1 cup vegetable or fruit juice; 2 cups leafy salad greens.
- Grains: 1 ounce-equivalent = one 1-ounce slice bread; 1-ounce uncooked pasta or rice; ½ cup cooked rice, pasta, or cereal; 1 tortilla (6 in. or 15 cm diameter); 1 pancake (5 in. or 13 cm diameter); 1-ounce ready-to-eat cereal (about 1 cup cereal flakes).
- Protein foods: 1 ounce-equivalent = 1-ounce lean meat, poultry, seafood; 1 egg; 1 tablespoon peanut butter; ½ ounce nuts or seeds. Also, ¼ cup cooked beans or peas may be counted as 1 ounce-equivalent.
- Dairy: 1 cup-equivalent = 1 cup milk or calcium-fortified soy, almond, or rice beverage; 1 cup yogurt; 1½ ounces natural cheese (e.g., cheddar); 2 ounces of processed cheese (e.g., American).

[b]*Moderately active* refers to a lifestyle that includes physical activity equivalent to walking about 1.5 to 3 miles (2.4 to 4.8 km) per day at 3 to 4 miles (4.8 to 6.4 km) per hour, in addition to the activities of independent living.

[c]Oils do not constitute a food group, but they are included here to ensure that adequate amounts of heart-healthy oils are consumed. Healthy oils are extracted from plants and include canola, corn, olive, peanut, safflower, soybean, and sunflower oils. Oils are also naturally present in nuts, seeds, seafood, olives, and avocados.

Reprinted from U.S. Department of Health and Human Services and U.S. Department of Agriculture. *2015–2020 Dietary Guidelines for Americans,* 8th ed. (Washington, DC: U.S. Department of Agriculture, 2015). http://health.gov/dietaryguidelines/2015/guidelines/

before eating. They can ask, "Am I hungry?" If the answer is no, they can wait a while to eat. Similarly, before cleaning their plate or having seconds, they can ask, "Am I satisfied?" If the answer is yes, they can stop eating. We do not have to feel "full" or "stuffed" in order to be done with a meal or snack.

Students on the Move: Athletes

Students involved in athletic endeavors have higher calorie needs than do nonathletic students. However, they still need to make smart food choices in order to provide their active bodies with premium fuel. Protein in normal amounts will suffice—protein builds a matrix inside muscles. Carbohydrate, on the other hand, needs to be supplied in somewhat larger amounts than normal, and within two hours of vigorous activity, in order to replenish glycogen stores in the protein matrix of muscle (American Dietetic Association, 2009). Carbohydrate stored in the protein matrix as glycogen enables strength and endurance. Fat is recommended in normal amounts, and athletes typically need extra water because of loss due to perspiration.

Making Sense of Food Labels

Teaching students how to read food labels will help them make smart choices throughout their lives. Labels are full of information—much more than just the name and picture of the food in the package. Specifically, food labels include the following information:

- *Product brand and name.* Look for clues in the name of the product. For example, if it says "frosted," then the product is going to have more sugar than an unfrosted version of the same food. If it says "nonfat," then it may be heart healthy, but more facts are needed in order to say for sure.
- *Location of company.*
- *Nutrition facts.* Notice the nutrients, and how much of each, is contained in a serving of the food. This portion of the label is the most crucial for students to understand.
- *Amount in the package.* Expressed in weight, measure, or numeric count.
- *Ingredient list.* Ingredients appear in the list in order of their prominence in the product in terms of weight. The first item on the list is the main ingredient—the one that is most prominent by weight in the product. The rest of the ingredients are listed in descending order of weight.

There can also be much more to the story, and some food labels provide additional information:

- *Type of product.* Some products are "reduced-fat," "light," or "low-sodium" foods.
- *Health claims.* Allowable claims are strictly defined and regulated by the FDA so that consumers can believe what they say.
- *Description.* This portion may tell how the food is prepared (e.g., baked) or give clues about the texture of the food (e.g., crispy, moist). The description may also reveal what is *not* in the food (e.g., trans fat, gluten). When applicable, the label will also tell whether the food is kosher—that is, prepared according to Jewish ritual law.
- *Dates.* "Sell-by" and "use-by" dates are sometimes included, especially on perishable items and other foods with a short shelf life.
- *Facts Up Front.* These icons give an at-a-glance summary of key nutrients contained in one serving of the packaged food. They include calories along with

Trust the Label

The U.S. Food and Drug Administration tightly regulates the terms and claims that are allowed on food labels. Providing a consistent standard helps consumers place confidence in label claims. For more on the meanings of the terms used on labels, students can visit the FDA website at www.fda.gov/Food/GuidanceRegulation/GuidanceDocumentsRegulatoryInformation/LabelingNutrition/ucm385663.htm#formats (U.S. Food and Drug Administration, 2018b).

three nutrients that need to be limited for good health: saturated fat, sodium, and sugar. Manufacturers may add optional icons for elements such as fiber, vitamins, and minerals if one serving of the food supplies 10 percent or more of the daily recommended amount of that nutrient and therefore is considered a good source of it. Find out more at www.FactsUpFront.org.

For more information, students can visit the FDA's website—specifically, the section about ingredients and packaging, which can be found at www.fda.gov/Food/IngredientsPackagingLabeling/default.htm (U.S. Food and Drug Administration, 2018a).

Nutrition Facts

The Nutrition Facts portion of the label offers need-to-know information that can help students make wise food choices. It is also in transition: New regulations were published by the FDA in 2016, and some companies are currently phasing in the new version of the Nutrition Facts panel; all companies must do so no later than January of 2021.

To help students fully understand the Nutrition Facts portion of the label, refer to the sample label for macaroni and cheese shown in figure 4.5. Differences between the new and old versions of the panel are explained in figure 4.6. When evaluating nutrition facts, students should use the following guidelines:

1. *Check out the serving size.* Students need to start with this information. Is the stated serving size the amount they usually eat? Do they eat more? Twice as much? Half as much? If their serving size is different from the one indicated, then they will need to adjust all of the values on the label accordingly—doubled if they eat twice as much as the stated serving size, divided in half if they eat half of the stated size, and so on.

2. *Consider the calories.* It can be useful to compare the number of calories contained in servings of two similar foods if the products' serving sizes are about equal.

3. *Limit overall intake of fat and sugar:*
   - Fat is quantified in number of grams. Saturated fat and trans fat (also called solid fat) are included as part of the fat total but are listed separately beneath the Total Fat heading. These fats are listed separately because both can be problematic if eaten in excess. Healthier oils—the monounsaturated and polyunsaturated fats—are not required to be listed separately on the Nutrition Facts Label, but they may be. In any case, they are included in the stated amount of total fat.
   - Sugar, listed under the Total Carbohydrate heading, is a simple carbohydrate. On the label being phased out, the Sugars heading includes grams of both

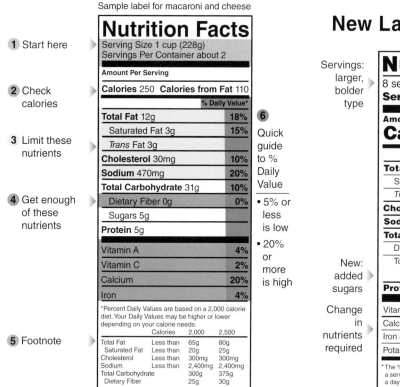

FIGURE 4.5   Components of a Nutrition Facts panel.

Reprinted from U.S. Food and Drug Administration. Available: http://www.fda.gov/Food/IngredientsPackagingLabeling/LabelingNutrition/ucm274593.htm#serving_size

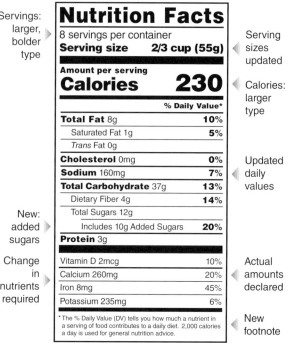

FIGURE 4.6   New Nutrition Facts panel.

Reprinted from U.S. Food and Drug Administration. Available: http://www.fda.gov/Food/IngredientsPackagingLabeling/LabelingNutrition/ucm274593.htm#serving_size

naturally occurring sugars (such as those in fruit and dairy products) and added sugars (such as white sugar or corn syrup), combined into one number. The new version of the label includes an extra line beneath Total Sugars to indicate the amount of added sugar in one serving. It also includes the daily reference value (%DV) for added sugar, based on the 2015-2020 Dietary Guidelines (U.S. Department of Health and Human Services, 2018), which established an upper limit of 10 percent of calories from added sugar. This new labeling makes it easy for consumers to determine how much of the sugar in a given product comes from non-nutritive sources.

4. *Get enough fiber, vitamins, and minerals:*

  ○ Fiber is listed under total carbohydrate. The amount of fiber listed includes both types: soluble and insoluble.

  ○ The old version of the label required listing of two vitamins (A and C) and two minerals (calcium and iron). The new version, in contrast, requires one vitamin (D) and three minerals (calcium, iron, and potassium) because these nutrients are underconsumed by most people. When any vitamins or minerals are added, or when a vitamin or mineral claim is made, those nutrients must be listed on the nutrition label.

5. *Footnote.* This element stays the same on all packages large enough to include it (it can be omitted on small packages). It lists the amounts of nutrients rec-

ommended for a typical person who eats about 2,000 or 2,500 calories per day. The percent daily values (%DVs) are calculated on the basis of a 2,000-calorie intake. The new label eliminates the nutrient recommendations in the footnote and the reference to 2,500 calories. This portion of the label now simply explains the percent daily value: "*The % Daily Value tells you how much a nutrient in a serving of food contributes to a daily diet. 2,000 calories a day is used for general nutrition advice."

6. *Daily value.* Teach students to think of the Daily Value (DV) as the "budget" or "allowance" for a certain nutrient. The Daily Value is the maximum amount recommended. For instance, a label for macaroni and cheese might list three grams of saturated fat, which amounts to 15 percent of the DV for saturated fat. In other words, one serving of the food (1 cup, in this case) uses up 15 percent of one's daily budget or allowance for saturated fat. One serving also provides 20 percent of one's daily calcium needs. In general, if a nutrient provides 5 percent or less of one's Daily Value, then the food is considered low in that nutrient. If a nutrient provides 20 percent DV or more, then it is considered high in that nutrient. Emphasize this 5-20 guideline with your students. Also note, however, that not all foods need to fall within this range. Teach kids that they can balance their food intake throughout the day. For instance, if they eat a food high in fat at lunch, they can balance it by eating foods that are very low in fat for dinner.

Additional changes in the Nutrition Facts panel include the following:

- *Calories and serving sizes are presented more prominently* in order to help address the public health issues of overweight and obesity.

- *Serving sizes are updated* to more accurately reflect amounts that people actually eat. For example, if an item is typically consumed in one sitting, then the label will reflect that reality. A 20-ounce (0.6-liter) bottle of soda, for instance, is typically consumed all at one time, so the FDA's rule on serving sizes will require showing the calories contained in the entire 20 ounces.

- *Larger packages must provide two-column labels* to indicate both per-serving and per-package information about calories and nutrients.

- *Percent of daily value will be displayed more prominently* to help consumers understand how a food fits into their total diet.

- *Total fat, saturated fat, and trans fat must be indicated,* but Calories from Fat will be removed because the type of fat is more important than the total amount.

- *Added sugar is distinguished* from naturally occurring sugar to resolve confusion about how much sugar is added to a food versus how much is naturally found in it. For example, on the old label, a serving of cereal with dried fruit, such as cranberries or raisins, appears to contain the same amount of sugar as a serving of sweetened cereal. The new version of the label clarifies whether the sugar occurs naturally (from the fruit) or is added. Another example involves yogurt. Currently, the naturally occurring sugar in milk and yogurt, called lactose, is listed on the label as sugar, along with any fruit sugar or added sugar. The new label, however, clearly shows consumers the amount of added sugar.

- *Daily Values are updated for sodium, fiber, and vitamin D* to reflect current research and health guidelines. The revisions in Daily Values are based on recommendations published by the Institute of Medicine and other documents such as the Dietary Guidelines. Some daily value amounts (e.g., for saturated fat, cholesterol, and sodium) are meant to convey maximum intake, whereas others (e.g., for iron) help consumers meet a daily required minimum.

- *Potassium and vitamin D are now required on the label* because, along with calcium and iron, they are nutrients of concern. Vitamin D and potassium are added because they play important roles in bone health and blood pressure, respectively, but are often not consumed in adequate amounts. The new label also lists milligram or microgram amounts, as well as %DV, for vitamins and minerals. Vitamins A and C are no longer be required to be listed, because most people regularly consume adequate amounts of these nutrients (U.S. Food and Drug Administration, 2018b).

Equipped with an understanding of food labels, students can inform their families and make choices that benefit their health. For more information, as well as worksheets and take-home materials for kids of age 9 through 13, see www.fda.gov/nutritioneducation (U.S. Food and Drug Administration, 2018c). This site also offers educational materials on other nutrition-related topics.

Vitamins and Minerals (Micronutrients)

Vitamins and minerals are called **micronutrients**, and many of them are essential for normal growth, development, and maintenance of the human body. This section takes a look at some of the major vitamins and minerals, as well as the foods that are rich in them.

The richest sources of the vitamins and minerals we need are fruits and vegetables. With this reality in mind, encourage youth to think of fruits and vegetables as the stars of the nutrition world. They provide a number of nutrients that people tend not to get enough of, including potassium, folate, magnesium, certain vitamins (A, C, and K), and dietary fiber. This nutritional value, along with the fact that they are naturally low in calories, makes them a "green light" or anytime food. In addition, eating them is associated with reduced risk of cardiovascular disease, including heart attack and stroke, and may help prevent certain types of cancer. The many nutrients provided in these foods also help keep parts of the body—the parts that students see—vibrant and glowing. For instance, skin glows, eyes sparkle, and hair shines when kids eat plenty of fruits and vegetables.

It may also be helpful to teach students in some detail about certain key nutrients that are contained in fruits and vegetables and play a large role in human health—namely, vitamins A and C, the mineral potassium, phytonutrients, and fiber.

What Are Phytonutrients?

Phytonutrients, also called *phytochemicals*, are naturally occurring compounds that serve various functions in plants. Many phytonutrients are pigments that provide beautiful colors, as in fruits and vegetables; others may provide a smell, such as that of garlic or cabbage. Phytonutrients are not essential, but they do promote optimal health by playing antioxidant and anti-inflammatory roles. Experts estimate that there are more than 25,000 phytonutrients, but only a handful have been discovered, and even fewer have been researched.

Free Radicals and Antioxidants

Free radicals are molecules that lack an electron; they damage cells, which, in turn, may contribute to cancer, heart disease, cataracts, and possibly aging. Free radicals are formed when the body is exposed to elements such as air pollution, cigarette smoke, X-rays, UV rays from the sun, rancid foods, and over-heated oil, such as that found in many deep-fat fryers in restaurants.

Antioxidants, on the other hand, are substances that neutralize free radicals and stop them from damaging cells. The body makes some antioxidants but also depends on getting more from foods in order to protect cells as much as possible. Antioxidants include the nutrients beta-carotene, certain vitamins (A, C, and E), and the mineral selenium, as well as many phytonutrients (e.g., lycopene).

Vitamin A

Vitamin A helps eyes to see clearly during both the day and the night; it also helps keep them sparkling and healthy. (Note: It does not affect nearsightedness or farsightedness.) Vitamin A is found in plant-based foods and in foods sourced from animals (e.g., fortified milk, liver). The type of vitamin A found in plants is beta-carotene, which can be turned into vitamin A in the body; it also acts as a powerful antioxidant.

Beta-carotene is abundant in orange-colored vegetables (e.g., carrots, yams, sweet potatoes, squash, pumpkin) and in dark green vegetables (e.g., broccoli, romaine lettuce, spinach, kale). The chlorophyll contained in the dark green plants covers up their yellow, orange, and red colors, similar to the case with deciduous tree leaves. The leaves are green all summer, and when the chlorophyll dries up in the fall, the beautiful oranges, reds, and yellows are revealed—but they were always there. The same is true for dark green vegetables rich in beta-carotene.

Vitamin C

Vitamin C helps skin be supple, stretchy, moist, and healthy; it also helps form collagen, which is the foundational structure of our bones, ligaments, skin, hair, and internal organs. Like beta-carotene, vitamin C is also an antioxidant, and research indicates that it may decrease a cold's severity and duration. This vitamin is found in abundance in all citrus fruits, as well as strawberries, cantaloupes, broccoli, bell peppers, potatoes, and many other fruits and vegetables.

Potassium

This mineral keeps the heart healthy, normalizes the heartbeat, and helps keep blood pressure in check. It also helps blunt the adverse effects of sodium on blood pressure, reduces the risk of developing kidney stones, and decreases bone loss. Potassium is abundant in fruits and vegetables. Bananas have a reputation for being high in potassium, but comparable amounts or even more are found in various other foods, such as acorn squash, potatoes, prunes, cantaloupes, oranges, tomatoes, dark leafy greens, and dried beans (e.g., black beans, kidney beans).

Fiber

Fiber is found in plant-derived foods—fruits, vegetables, legumes (dried beans and peas), whole grains, nuts, and seeds. There are two types of fiber. One type is not

Eat a Rainbow

Emphasize to students that it can be both fun and healthy to eat a rainbow of colors provided by the many different fruits and veggies. You might encourage students to appreciate the wide variety of colors in the produce section the next time they visit a grocery store. As shown in table 4.4, the Dietary Guidelines categorize fruits and vegetables into five subgroups based on their nutrient content. People are often concerned about the price of fruits and vegetables, thinking that they are expensive. But when viewed in terms of the vitamins and minerals you get for the money, they provide a nutritional bargain.

TABLE 4.4   Vegetable Examples and Recommended Intakes in Each Subgroup

Vegetable subgroup	Examples	Recommended weekly intake (cup-eq*) based on daily diet of 2,000 total calories
Dark green vegetables	Broccoli, spinach, leafy salad greens (including romaine lettuce), collards, bok choy, kale, turnip greens, mustard greens, green herbs (e.g., parsley, cilantro)	1-1/2 cup-eq
Red and orange vegetables	Tomatoes, carrots, tomato juice, sweet potatoes, red peppers (hot and sweet), winter squash, pumpkin	5-1/2 cup-eq
Legumes (beans and peas)	Pinto, white, kidney, and black beans; lentils; chickpeas; limas (mature, dried); split peas; edamame (green soybeans)	1-1/2 cup-eq
Starchy vegetables	Potatoes, corn, green peas, limas (green, immature), plantains, cassava	5 cup-eq
Other vegetables	Lettuce (iceberg), onions, green beans, cucumbers, celery, green peppers, cabbage, mushrooms, avocados, summer squash (including zucchini), cauliflower, eggplant, garlic, bean sprouts, olives, asparagus, pea pods (snow peas), beets	4 cup-eq
Total fruit and vegetable intake	N/A	17.5 cup-eq per week (2-1/2 cup-eq per day)

*A cup-equivalent (cup-eq) is the amount of a food or beverage product considered equal to one cup from the vegetable, fruit, or dairy food group. A cup-eq for some foods or beverages may differ from a measured cup in volume because the food has been concentrated (e.g., raisins, tomato paste), the food is airy in its raw form and does not compress well into a cup (e.g., salad greens), or the food is measured in a different form (e.g., cheese).

Reprinted from U.S. Food and Drug Administration. Available: http://www.fda.gov/Food/IngredientsPackagingLabeling/LabelingNutrition/ucm274593.htm#serving_size

digestible by the body, so it acts as a broom and thus helps keep the digestive tract free of residual build-up and toxins. It also normalizes bowel function and may help prevent colon cancer. The other kind of fiber helps lower the artery-clogging type of blood cholesterol and stabilize blood sugar levels, thus reducing the risk of cardiovascular disease, obesity, and type 2 diabetes. Fiber also provides a feeling of fullness, which helps prevent overeating.

Calcium

Calcium is one of the most abundant minerals in the body, and 99 percent of it is found in the teeth and bones. Students need to understand that they achieve peak bone mass during adolescence, which makes it vitally important for them to build enough bone during their teen years to last a lifetime. The remaining 1 percent of calcium is used for functions such as muscle contraction, muscle relaxation, blood clotting, and normal heart rhythm. If insufficient calcium is consumed every day to enable these functions, then the body must rob the bones to fill the gap. Doing so over time sets the stage for weakened bones in the present and osteoporosis later in life. In contrast, when young people get enough calcium, vitamin D, and physical activity during their childhood and teen years, they can start out their adult lives with the strongest bones possible.

Thus the bones are like a savings account. We make calcium deposits in our "bone bank" to build up as much calcium as possible. These deposits can be made only while a person is young, and children and teens have the greatest bone-building ability. In fact, about 90 percent of maximum bone size and strength, or **peak bone mass**, is achieved in girls by about age 18 and in boys by about age 20 (National Institutes of Health, 2015). To form a good level of peak bone mass, kids need to get plenty of calcium and weight-bearing physical activity on a daily basis. The remaining 10 percent of bone size and strength is established by age 30, after which bone mass declines, especially if insufficient calcium is consumed during adulthood. It is then that bones are robbed to meet the body's other calcium needs.

Because the bones formed in childhood and adolescence must last a lifetime, we must help students understand the importance of getting sufficient calcium every day. To do so, dairy products and their alternatives are recommended for daily consumption because of their high calcium content. Thus students need to know basic information about dairy products—what they are, how to identify them, and how much to consume—in order to achieve a good level of peak bone mass.

Vitamin D

Vitamin D regulates how the body uses calcium, helping to put it into or take it out of bones as needed. Thus adequate amounts of vitamin D help reduce the risk of bone fractures. Most people do not get enough vitamin D from the foods they eat, but the body makes this nutrient when the skin is exposed to sunlight; as a result, most people have adequate amounts in their bloodstream. Most vitamin D in the United States comes from fortified foods, such as dairy products, breakfast cereals, orange juice, and alternative "milk" beverages. Naturally occurring vitamin D is found in egg yolks and in some fish, such as salmon, tuna, herring, and mackerel. For helpful information about how vitamin D and calcium work together to make strong bones, visit www.niams.nih.gov/Health_Info/Bone/Bone_Health/Nutrition/.

Dairy Foods as a Source of Calcium

Dairy foods contain many nutrients, including calcium, vitamin D, potassium, and protein; as a result, these foods are linked to enhanced bone health. However, they can also be loaded with saturated fat. Therefore, it's important to encourage students to shift from whole or 2 percent milk to low-fat (1 percent) or fat-free milk and milk-based products in order to cut out a significant amount of saturated fat from their

Lactose Intolerance Versus Milk Allergy

Lactose intolerance occurs when a person lacks the digestive enzyme needed to break down lactose, which is a carbohydrate found in milk. People with this condition need to choose either nondairy sources of calcium or dairy products that contain lactase—a natural enzyme that breaks down the lactose in milk. Some people with lactose intolerance are able to eat cheese and yogurt because they contain less lactose. Symptoms of lactose intolerance include cramping, gas, bloating, and diarrhea shortly after consuming dairy products.

Lactose intolerance differs from milk allergy, in which the body mounts an immune system reaction to one or more of the proteins in milk. People who are allergic to milk are *not* helped by using products that contain lactase.

Children with either of these conditions should see their health care provider for guidance in meeting their calcium requirements. School breakfast and lunch programs sometimes offer a lactase-containing milk as a substitute. Alternatively, if a student's physician provides a statement of medical need or allergy and indicates an appropriate alternate source, schools that participate in the National School Lunch program typically provide the product prescribed by the doctor.

daily eating pattern. (Note: Infants should not consume cow's milk or soy milk until after one year of age. In addition, children of age one to two years require full-fat milk for proper brain and nerve development. After age two, children can transition to lower-fat milks.) The Dietary Guidelines recommend three cups of milk per day for everyone who consumes 1,600 or more total calories per day. This recommendation applies to most school-age children.

Some students may choose not to consume milk, or they may be prevented from doing so by a health issue (e.g., lactose intolerance). Such students need to consume other foods that have a similar nutrient profile. Alternatives to milk include *fortified* soy, rice, almond, and coconut beverages. They should choose ones that are fortified with calcium and vitamin D in amounts similar to those found in milk.

An 8-ounce (235 ml) cup of milk contains approximately 300 milligrams of calcium; therefore, consuming three cups of milk (or the equivalent) each day, along with calcium in other foods, will satisfy the body's needs. The Institute of Medicine (2010) recommends the following amounts of calcium per day:

- Girls and boys from 4 to 8 years: 1,000 milligrams
- Girls and boys from 9 to 18 years: 1,300 milligrams

Students need to get enough calcium but not overdo it. If they fill up on milk and milk-based products, then they may skip other foods and nutrients. Milk should be considered a food, not a thirst quencher. Students should use water to quench thirst and milk as a meal or snack component.

The best sources of calcium are dairy and fortified alternate products, but the mineral is also found in dark green leafy vegetables (e.g., broccoli, kale, cabbage, collard and mustard greens) and in tofu made with calcium sulfate. Good amounts of calcium are also found in certain nuts, seeds, and dry beans. Some other foods are fortified with calcium, such as certain fruit juices that are 100 percent fruit juice, cereals, and some milks (e.g., soy, almond, rice). Table 4.5 shows the amount of calcium contained in one cup of milk and how it compares with other calcium-containing foods. Would it be easy or difficult to consume the recommended amount of calcium if one did not eat dairy or fortified foods?

TABLE 4.5   Amount of Calcium in Selected Foods

Amount	Food or beverage	Amount of calcium (mg)
8 oz (about 240 ml)	Cow milk, all types	285-305
8 oz (240 ml)	Calcium-fortified orange juice	300 or more
8 oz (240 ml)	Regular orange juice	3
8 oz (240 ml)	Calcium-fortified soy milk	300 or more
8 oz (240 ml)	Nonfortified soy milk	8
2 oz (60 ml)	American cheese	323
1.5 oz (45 ml)	Cheddar cheese	307
4 oz (120 ml)	Tofu made with calcium	253
6 oz (180 ml)	Fruit yogurt (low fat)	258
3 oz (90 ml)	Pink salmon (canned, with bones)	181
1/2 cup	Collard greens (cooked from frozen)	178
4 oz (114 g)	Ice cream (soft serve)	120
1/2 cup	White beans	96
1 ounce (28 g)	Almonds	80
1/2 cup	Bok choy	80
1/2 cup	Rhubarb (cooked)	75
4 oz (114 g)	Cottage cheese	70
1/2 cup	Red beans	40
1/2 cup	Broccoli (cooked)	35

Recommended calcium intake for children is 1,000 milligrams per day for ages 4 through 8 and 1,300 milligrams per day for ages 9 through 18.

Data from USDA National Nutrient Data Base for Standard Reference. Available: http://ndb.nal.usda.gov/

Water for Health and Performance

Do your students know that people can live for months without food but only a few days without water? In fact, water accounts for 60 percent to 70 percent of the human body. With this reality in mind, teach kids that drinking plenty of water optimizes health and prevents fatigue so that they can play and learn well. In addition, water contains no calories yet helps provide a feeling of fullness. It also offers a number of other benefits:

- It carries oxygen and nutrients to cells via the bloodstream.
- It helps the brain avoid confusion and think clearly.
- Inside of cells, water dissolves nutrients so that cells can use them; indeed, it is used as a solvent in many of the body's chemical reactions.
- It regulates body temperature through sweating.
- It acts as a lubricant and helps cushion joints such as knees and vertebrae.
- It helps prevent fatigue, headaches, and muscle cramps.
- It flushes out wastes and toxins.
- It moves fiber and other food components through the digestive system, thus helping to prevent constipation. The more fiber, protein, or sodium a person eats, the more water the person needs to process what has been consumed.

Bone Bank Relay

Here's a relay game that helps students learn about the amount of calcium contained in various foods. The goal is for each team to get as much calcium as possible into their bone bank as quickly as possible. The bone banks are represented by two clear, plastic gallon-sized (3.8-liter) jars that are labeled as such. The calcium to be deposited into the bone bank is represented by two one-gallon bags of white cornmeal (or flour or powdered milk), each of which contains a half-cup measuring cup. Find pictures of foods with varying amounts of calcium (low, medium, high) and pictures of activities that are either weight-bearing or non-weight-bearing. On the back of each picture, write a 1, 2, or 3. The numbers represent how well the food or activity builds strong bones. For example, a food that is low in calcium gets a 1, as does the activity of swimming; a food that has a moderate level of calcium gets a 2, as does the activity of bicycling; and a food high in calcium (e.g., milk) gets a 3, as do weight-bearing activities.

To begin the activity, explain that students are going to do a bone-building, calcium-bank relay. Show them the bone banks and examples of food models and activities with the numbers on the back. Explain that each picture of a food or activity has a value from 1 to 3 that represents how well the food or activity builds strong bones. Foods are categorized as having a low, medium, or high level of calcium (1, 2, or 3, respectively), whereas activities are categorized according to how well they promote bone formation (i.e., the higher the number, the more weight bearing the activity is and thus better for building bones).

Divide the class into two teams and ask each student to select a food or activity picture. Ensure that students understand the significance of the numbers on the backs of the cards. Make sure they understand that the activity will involve a relay race between the two teams. Students should hop (which is a bone-building activity) to the bone banks and tell the educator at their bank what their food or activity is and what the number is on the back. The educator puts that number of scoops of the calcium product into the bone bank, whereupon the student returns to the team and touches the next person to go. (You will need one adult or student helper at each bone bank.) The team that has the most calcium in their bone bank at the end of the relay has the greatest peak bone mass!

How Much Water Is Needed?

Students need to know that by the time they feel thirsty, mild dehydration has already begun. Sometimes the thirst signal cannot keep up with the body's need for water—for example, on a hot summer day or when performing vigorous physical activity. Even mild dehydration causes a decrease in blood volume and may play a role in headaches. Dehydration affects muscles, can cause fatigue or even cramping, and, if severe enough, can cause confusion and disorientation.

Experts recommend drinking enough water to satisfy thirst. This means that people should drink fluids, preferably water, whenever they begin to feel even slightly thirsty. A person needs extra water in hot climates or when doing a lot of physical activity. Consuming eight cups of water per day is no longer the official recommendation, though it remains a helpful general guideline for adults; there is no such specific guideline for children. Remind students generally to drink water frequently. If they use a water bottle, teach them to use it often—and to clean it with soap and hot water every day.

Children often mistake the feeling of thirst for that of hunger. Therefore, when kids say they are hungry but it's not snack or meal time, it may be helpful to have them drink water and then wait for 15 to 20 minutes. The sensation of supposed hunger often subsides because the body was actually signaling thirst.

Sources of Water

The body obtains water from food, various beverages, and of course water itself. Even foods that seem dry contain some water; for instance, bread is typically about

35 percent water. The main food contributors of water are fruits and vegetables, because most of them are about 90 percent water. (Percentages of water in foods can be obtained from the USDA Food Composition Databases at http://ndb.nal.usda.gov/ndb.) Therefore, by eating the recommended amounts of fruits and vegetables, students also help satisfy their body's need for water.

In most parts of the United States, it is easy to get drinkable water just by turning on the tap because the country has one of the safest and cleanest water supplies in the world. In most communities, there is no need to buy bottled water—tap water is safe to drink unless the water supply has been compromised, in which case government officials issue warnings. Some people prefer bottled water, but from a safety standpoint it is usually unnecessary. Some areas of the country have "hard" water, which is high in calcium and magnesium—minerals that positively affect health. Other areas have "soft" water, either naturally or because the water has been processed by a water softener. Soft water is high in sodium, which can aggravate health issues such as high blood pressure and heart disease; excessive sodium consumption can even leach calcium from the bones. Therefore, it is best to avoid using soft water for drinking. Soft water also tends to dissolve certain metals in pipes, and these metals can be harmful if consumed in large enough quantities. Especially in older buildings with metal pipes, it's a good idea to run tap water for a minute or so before drinking it if the tap hasn't been turned on for six hours or longer. Doing so flushes out unwanted mineral contaminants from the pipes.

Water is also contributed to the body by milk, juices, and the many other types of beverages found in a typical grocery store. Choose ones that are low in added sugar.

Juice as a Source of Water

Juice can contribute to the body's water needs, but students need to know to drink it only in moderation. Juice that consists of 100 percent juice contains only the natural sugar from fruit—no added sugar. Fruit sugar is accompanied by water, vitamins, minerals, and fiber. However, the amount of calories in natural sugar is the same as in added sugar, making juice high in calories, especially since it is concentrated. (Consider how many oranges are squeezed to make one cup of orange juice—usually two or three.) Diluting juice to a half-and-half mixture with water gives children fewer calories yet plenty of flavor and nutrients.

The Dietary Guidelines recommend eating whole fruit rather than juice because a piece of fruit has more fiber and fewer calories than does juice. The guidelines state that no more than half of one's daily fruit intake should be consumed as juice. In 2017, the American Academy of Pediatrics (2017) revised its policy to state that children of ages 4 through 6 years should limit juice intake to 4 to 6 ounces (120 to 180 ml) per day; the Academy further recommended that children of ages 7 through 18 years should limit juice intake to 8 ounces (1 cup) per day. As with milk, juice should be thought of as a food—not a thirst quencher.

Among juices, orange juice contains the most vitamins and minerals; it is especially rich in vitamin C and potassium. Grapefruit and vegetable juices are also good sources of nutrients, but apple and grape juices contain few vitamins and minerals.

Teach kids to limit beverages that consist mostly of added sugar with just a little actual fruit or vegetable juice. Check for wording above the Nutrition Facts portion of the label describing the amount of juice contained in a beverage (e.g., "Contains 100% juice"). Ignore claims on the front of the label that say something like, "100% natural"—sugar is natural (it comes from sugar beets or sugar cane or corn), but it is so highly refined that it contains only calories and no nutrients. Choose beverages that contain 100 percent juice. If kids don't consume the recommended amount of dairy or other calcium-rich foods per day, then they need to choose juices that are calcium fortified to help meet their calcium needs.

Beware of Added Sugar and Sodium

Foods that are high in added sugar and sodium are typically processed, prepared, or fast foods. Tell students that these foods often contain many calories because of the added sugar and may not be particularly abundant in vitamins and minerals. Limiting sugar and sodium helps people maintain a healthy weight, enhances heart health, and may help prevent heart disease, especially when combined with physical activity.

Eating too much added sugar sets the stage for health problems. Foods with significant amounts of added sugar contribute extra calories but provide little nutritional value. Such foods are referred to as "sometimes foods" or "slow" or "whoa" foods because they should be eaten only *some* of the time and in *small* amounts. The Dietary Guidelines recommend choosing foods low in added sugar most of the time.

Some of the more common forms of sugar that may be listed in the ingredients portion of a label include white sugar, brown sugar, turbinado sugar, raw sugar, molasses, honey, corn syrup, high fructose corn syrup, corn syrup solids, fructose, maple syrup, pancake syrup, molasses, evaporated cane juice, concentrated fruit sugar, glucose, maltose, malt syrup, invert sugar, dextrose, anhydrous dextrose, crystal dextrose, and dextrin.

White table sugar is derived from either refined sugar cane or sugar beets. Each of these plants contains a high percentage of natural sugar. When they are processed into white sugar, they retain their calories but lose all of their fiber, vitamins, and minerals, which leaves them with only "empty calories." For instance, high fructose corn syrup is a common sugar substitute in food manufacturing that is derived from the naturally occurring plant sugar in corn. When processed, however, corn loses all of its fiber, vitamins, and minerals.

Excessive intake of added sugar can lead to significant health consequences:

- *Future heart disease.* A CDC report about children's intake of added sugar (Ervin, Kit, Carroll, & Ogden, 2012) stated that high sugar consumption has been associated with measures of cardiovascular disease risk among adolescents, including adverse cholesterol concentrations. This finding is especially disturbing because youthful eating habits tend to carry over into adulthood. A study published in 2014 revealed that eating too much added sugar increases adults' risk of cardiovascular disease (Yang et al., 2014).

- *Increased triglycerides.* Triglycerides are a type of fat in the bloodstream. Eating an excessive amount of added sugar can increase triglyceride levels, which may in turn increase one's risk of heart disease (Mayo Clinic Staff, 2016).

- *Dental caries.* Sugar foods leave a carbohydrate residue on the teeth, and this residue provides food for bacteria in the mouth. As bacteria eat the carbohydrate, an acid forms, which erodes tooth enamel and causes decay. Therefore, brushing (or at least swishing water on) the teeth after eating and drinking sugar foods is critical to preventing cavities.

- *Possible weight gain.* Sweet foods usually taste good and are therefore readily consumed. However, overconsumption may result in more calories being eaten than are used in physical activity. As sugar intake has increased over the past several decades, so have the rates of overweight and obesity.

- *Poor nutritional status.* Filling up on sweets diminishes one's appetite and subsequent intake of foods that provide beneficial nutrients.

- *Weak bones.* Sugar-sweetened beverages often take the place of milk (Gortmaker, Long, & Wang, 2009). When they do, calcium and vitamin D intake decline, and the bones do not have optimum strength, which leaves them at greater risk of fracture, especially among girls.

The 2015-2020 Dietary Guidelines suggest limiting intake of refined sugar to no more than 10 percent of total calories each day. For the average person consuming 2,000 calories per day, that's about 50 grams (12.5 teaspoons). Unfortunately, surveys show that children's and adolescents' total caloric intake from added sugar is significantly higher than is recommended. Children and adolescents typically get 15 percent to 17 percent of their calories from sugar. Nearly half of this sugar comes from sweetened beverages—a typical 12-ounce (0.35 liter) can of soda contains 36 to 40 grams of sugar (9 to 10 teaspoons). An attention-grabbing way to show this reality to kids is to measure out 10 teaspoons' worth of sugar and set it next to a can of pop. For other foods, you can calculate the number of teaspoons of sugar by dividing grams of sugar by four to get the number of teaspoons.

Risky Beverage Choices

All too often, kids and families reach for sugary drinks to satisfy thirst. Making the switch to water is better for everyone's health—and for the family budget. In fact, drinking water instead of sweetened beverages can save money twice. First the grocery bill goes down, and then the reduction in sugary drinks may well result in fewer dental cavities and better weight management, thus helping avoid medical problems that require doctor visits and cost money.

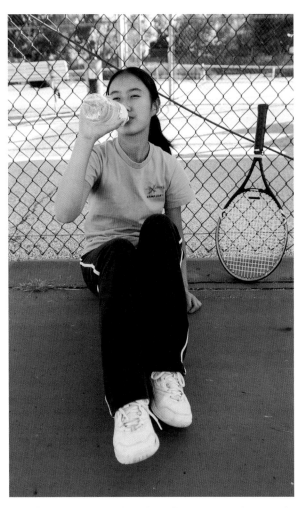

One study showed that as sugar-sweetened beverage consumption increased, so did a child's body mass index and risk of becoming overweight (Ludwig, Peterson, & Gortmaker, 2001). The problem has been compounded over the years by increases in large portion sizes and in the frequency of drinking sweetened beverages (Gortmaker et al., 2009).

Sugary beverages often crowd out more nutritious drinks, such as milk and orange juice, which deliver calcium, potassium, and vitamin C that are lacking in sugary drinks. Even supposedly enhanced beverages contain only tiny amounts of selected vitamins and minerals (often along with sugar or nonnutritive sweeteners). These drinks are not necessary; eating healthy foods provides more vitamins and minerals with fewer calories.

Families can improve health and save money by switching from sugary drinks to water.

Sport Drinks

Sport drinks contain sugar in a special form that can be quickly absorbed. They also contain electrolytes, which are minerals that conduct electricity necessary for cell function; the main ones are sodium, chloride, and potassium. Electrolytes help regulate fluid balance and thereby play a role in maintaining healthy blood pressure; they are also needed for muscle contraction and nerve conduction. Electrolyte consumption may be necessary to replace ones lost through perspiration during exercise or sport participation. However, according to a report on the use of sport drinks and energy drinks among children and adolescents (Schneider & Benjamin, 2011), kids do not need sport drinks in most circumstances, because they get all the electrolytes they need from typical foods. More specifically, kids do not typically need sport drinks unless they are vigorously active for more than an hour or are exercising in an extremely hot climate. Moreover, such beverages contribute extra calories that are unnecessary.

With these understandings in mind, teach students that sport drinks are intended for use only with vigorous activities that last more than an hour or occur in hot conditions. To put it another way, they are necessary only when the body needs to be quickly replenished with glucose and electrolytes. Therefore, they are *unnecessary* during most physical activity and certainly should not be used as a beverage during meals. Instead, water is the best beverage for use before, during, and after most physical activities and sports (Schneider & Benjamin, 2011).

Energy Drinks

Help kids understand that energy drinks differ greatly from sport drinks; specifically, they contain stimulants and additives not found in sport drinks—for example, caffeine, guarana, and taurine. A report by the American Academy of Pediatrics (2011) indicates that caffeine has been linked to a number of harmful health effects in children, including effects on the developing neurologic and cardiovascular systems. It goes on to say that energy drinks are never appropriate for children or adolescents. More generally, research suggests that caffeine in sodas can cause children to get insufficient sleep (Gortmaker et al., 2009), which in turn is linked to weight gain. The 2011 AAP report notes that some energy drinks contain more caffeine than 10 cans of caffeinated soda.

Are Sugar-Free Drinks Better?

Most drinks touted as "sugar free" use artificial sweeteners, which contain no calories. The main ones are aspartame (used in NutraSweet), sucralose (used in Splenda), and saccharin (used in Sweet'n Low). The U.S. Food and Drug Administration considers these sweeteners to be safe for children when used in moderation.

Research, however, has yet to determine conclusively whether artificial sweeteners help with weight loss. Numerous studies indicate that sugar-free beverages do not result in weight loss, but research continues on the issue (Feijo et al., 2013). One reason for this is that when the body tastes something sweet, it expects calories, but since none are provided in sugar-free drinks, the body gets confused and demands calories from another source. This sequence may lead to increased food intake and therefore to increased calorie consumption. On the other hand, some evidence indicates that when nonnutritive sweeteners are used in moderation, they can help reduce consumption of added sugar, thereby reducing caloric intake (Gardner et al., 2012).

Sugar alcohols, which are actually nonalcoholic, are derived from the carbohydrates contained in fruits and vegetables. They contain some calories but fewer than sugar does, and they do not promote tooth decay. They are typically used in chewing gum and sometimes in other foods, such as sugarless candy, fruit spreads, and chocolate. The names of sugar alcohols typically end in "ol"—for example, *xylitol* and *sorbitol.*

Natural sweeteners may or may not contain calories or offer nutritional value. For example, honey and molasses contain calories but few nutrients, though a bit more than are found in white table sugar. Another example, stevia, is a highly processed sweetener derived from a plant; it contains no calories and very few nutrients.

Go Slow With Sodium

Sodium is an essential nutrient and an electrolyte used by the body for fluid balance, which means that it helps the body maintain the appropriate amount of water, both inside and outside of cells. Sodium also plays a role in nerve conduction and muscle contraction. Let students know that in order for their bodies to perform these functions, they need sodium—in small quantities.

Table salt consists of 40 percent sodium and 60 percent chloride; therefore, it is referred to as *sodium chloride*. Only the sodium portion is included in the amount shown on labels and in dietary recommendations. Sodium is not only a flavor enhancer; it also plays numerous other roles in food processing—for instance, in pickling various foods, curing meats, retaining moisture in a product, and stopping yeast from overgrowing in breads.

A report by the Centers for Disease Control and Prevention (2017) found that more than 75 percent of sodium intake in the United States comes from processed, packaged, and restaurant foods. Only about 5 percent of dietary sodium is contributed by home cooking, and only about 6 percent is added at the table. The remaining 12 percent occurs naturally in foods.

Sodium attracts water; therefore, in the body, excess sodium causes fluid retention. It also makes the heart work harder and stresses the blood vessels, thus increasing blood pressure. High blood pressure is known as a "silent killer" because it may have no symptoms but causes severe problems. High blood pressure raises the risk of injury to the heart and arteries and contributes to heart disease, congestive heart failure, stroke, and possibly kidney failure (American Heart Association, 2016).

Sodium is listed on Nutrition Facts labels, which show a %DV based on a limit of 2,300 milligrams for a person consuming 2,000 calories of food per day. As with other nutrients, 5 percent DV is considered low and 20 percent DV is considered high.

Common sources of sodium in the U.S. food supply include the following:

- Packaged foods
- Canned foods
- Pickled foods
- Vegetable juices containing salt
- Cheese
- Ham, bacon, corned beef, luncheon meats, sausages, and hot dogs
- Commercially made main dishes and frozen dinners
- Seasoned salt, meat tenderizers, MSG (monosodium glutamate), spice mixes, and gravy and sauce mixes
- Condiments such as ketchup, mayonnaise, sauces, and salad dressings

The 2015-2020 Dietary Guidelines recommend a sodium intake of 2,300 milligrams per day for people 14 years or older. For younger children, the recommended amounts range from 1,900 milligrams to 2,200 milligrams. To put these numbers into perspective, one teaspoon of table salt contains 2,300 milligrams of sodium.

Sodium's influence on blood pressure can be counteracted in part by increasing one's intake of potassium. This mineral is abundant in fruits and vegetables, especially in potatoes, sweet potatoes, tomatoes, spinach, apricots, bananas, and legumes (dried beans, split peas, and lentils). Other good sources of potassium include fat-free and low-fat (1 percent) dairy products.

Creating a Culture of Health

When teachers invest in youth to help them develop a healthy lifestyle, the rewards are enormous. Habits formed in childhood typically persist into adulthood. As you pursue this endeavor, check out the resources available at the Team Nutrition website, which offers ideas, tips, tools, curricula, handouts, activities, and booklets: https://www.fns.usda.gov/tn/team-nutrition. For instance, if you need ideas for enjoyable, student-tested ways to promote nutrition and physical activity at your school, check out the Team Nutrition Popular Events Idea booklet at https://www.fns.usda.gov/team-nutrition-popular-events-idea-booklet. Or if you want to start a school garden and need ready-made lessons for gardening, download the resources available at https://www.fns.usda.gov/tn/team-nutrition-garden-resources. The Team Nutrition site also offers dozens of other resources to help you build a culture of health in your school.

Many of the ideas provided at Team Nutrition involve little or no cost. However, if you need some funding, consider applying for a $4,000 grant from the Fuel Up to Play 60 program. The application is not difficult to complete, and the funds can be used for events related to nutrition and physical activity at your school. For more information, visit the website at https://www.fueluptoplay60.com/.

Resources are also offered by the Alliance for a Healthier Generation (https://www.healthiergeneration.org/) to help you improve your students' nutritional and physical activity status. And of course, the Physical Best activities in the web resource also demonstrate fun and active ways to teach nutrition concepts to elementary, middle, and high school students.

Summary

The healthy habits that teachers instill in kids will benefit the health of this generation and future generations; as a result, it will benefit the strength of our nation. Physical education teachers are uniquely situated to guide students toward healthy habits in their choices about diet and physical activity. You can create learning opportunities where all students develop the knowledge and skills to live a healthy lifestyle, both now and in their futures. The next chapter introduces the first of the health-related fitness concepts: cardiorespiratory endurance.

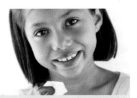

Discussion Questions

1. What are the links between nutrition, physical activity, and academic performance?
2. Design a middle school lesson to introduce the Dietary Guidelines.
3. Describe an activity you might do to help students learn about MyPlate.
4. Carbohydrate is necessary for good health, mental clarity, and physical performance. Create an activity that introduces this concept to elementary students, allows them to identify healthy carbohydrate-rich foods, and requires them to be active.
5. A student challenges you by stating that they eat whatever they want, whenever they want, but have no health problems and still perform well in sports. How would you respond to this student?
6. What is the best age for achieving peak bone mass? Why is this important for students to understand?
7. Which colorful foods are particularly rich in vitamins and minerals? How can physical education teachers encourage students to consume more fruits and vegetables?
8. List three things you think are particularly important to teach students about each of the following:
    1. Calories
    2. Water
    3. Calcium
9. What are three chronic diseases related to poor nutrition? Discuss how you might teach students about this reality by using a Physical Best activity from the web resource.
10. Why is it important to teach students about nutrition labels? Identify key parts to refer to when analyzing a food by its label.
11. Explain what %DV means on a food label. Explain the 5-20 rule.
12. The main risk of eating too much sodium is hypertension, which may seem irrelevant to students who tend to focus on the here and now. How can a physical educator help students develop an appreciation of the risks associated with hypertension?
13. Some students have special dietary needs or conditions (e.g., gluten sensitivity, food allergy, obesity). How can physical educators teach the basics of nutrition while still reaching those with special dietary needs?

Components of Health-Related Fitness

Part II covers basic concepts and applications of the components of health-related fitness for K-12 physical education programming. Each chapter defines a component of health-related fitness and provides teaching guidelines and training methods related to that component. Chapter 5 focuses on cardiorespiratory endurance and provides updated information and research. Chapter 6 focuses on body composition education and measurement; it also addresses the health benefits associated with a healthy ratio of body fat to lean mass while understanding that health can come in all shapes and sizes. Chapter 7 explores flexibility training for youth, as well as best practices for helping students improve their flexibility. Chapter 8 focuses on muscular strength, muscular endurance, and power. Muscular fitness is often taught in the form of separate components with adults, but these components are combined in the Physical Best program because it is developmentally appropriate to do so with children in a physical education setting. These chapters help you prepare to integrate health-related fitness into your physical education program.

CHAPTER 5

Cardiorespiratory Endurance

Jan Galen Bishop and Bette Jean Santos

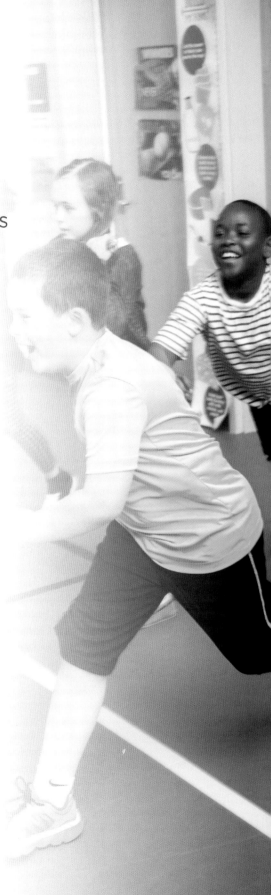

CHAPTER CONTENTS

This chapter focuses on principles of cardiorespiratory endurance and on developmentally appropriate practices and teaching strategies for implementing activities in a physical education program. The chapter will help you share health-related fitness knowledge and concepts with students while providing them with opportunities to participate in a variety of fun and engaging activities that benefit cardiorespiratory endurance. You can help students find cardiorespiratory endurance activities that they enjoy and help them value the benefits of these activities so that they choose to participate in them beyond the school day and beyond their school years.

Cardiorespiratory Endurance and Related Terms

Before examining how to develop, teach, and benefit from cardiorespiratory endurance, we need to discuss its many names and decide which to use, both in this chapter and when teaching K-12 classes. This component of health-related fitness is often referred to by means of a number of terms. Two of these describe it in terms of the circulatory system (*cardiovascular endurance* and *cardiovascular fitness*), two others describe it in terms of both the cardiovascular and respiratory systems (*cardiorespiratory endurance* and *cardiorespiratory fitness*), and four more describe it in terms of metabolic function (*aerobic fitness, aerobic power, aerobic capacity*, and *aerobic endurance*). SHAPE America chooses to use the term **cardiorespiratory endurance** following the lead of the Institute of Medicine (2012, pp. 1-2), which recommends defining cardiorespiratory endurance for field tests (based on a definition by Saltin [1973]) as "the ability to perform large-muscle, whole body exercise at a moderate to high intensity for extended periods of time." Because the term *cardiorespiratory endurance* reflects the ability to "perform functional fitness activities of daily life associated with the three principal systems supporting performance (cardiovascular, respiratory, muscular)" (Corbin et al., 2014, p. 28), it is used in this text and is appropriate to use in physical education with students.

When working with elementary students, however, it may be appropriate sometimes to use the term *aerobic fitness*, which may be more easily understood. *Aerobic fitness* is easier for young children to articulate and remember, along with terms such as *cardio* and *heart-healthy activities*. In contrast, older students who are studying anatomy and physiology can benefit from hearing both versions. They can link the word *aerobic* to the concept of producing energy using oxygen, and they can link the phrase *cardiorespiratory endurance* to the biological systems involved in supplying the muscles with oxygen. When working with students, be sure to educate them about the appropriate terms and definitions to help them become informed consumers who can advocate for and improve their own health-related fitness. Students themselves, however, will be more likely to recognize and use slang terms such as *cardio* and *aerobics*. It is fine for students to use these terms as long as they also understand the scientific terms and definitions.

A more technical term is **aerobic capacity**, which refers specifically to the maximum amount of oxygen that the body is able to use to produce work. Aerobic capacity is usually expressed in terms of maximal oxygen uptake ($\dot{V}O_2$max), which is considered the best way to measure aerobic capacity (Corbin et al., 2014). This term is discussed in more detail later in the chapter, and more in-depth treatments of aerobic capacity can be found in the *FitnessGram Administration Manual* (Cooper Institute, 2017) and the *FitnessGram Reference Guide* (Plowman & Meredith, 2013), which are available at www.cooperinstitute.org/fitnessgram.

We must also distinguish between the terms *physical activity*, *aerobic activity*, and *anaerobic activity*. **Physical activity**, the broadest term, refers to "any bodily movement produced by skeletal muscles that increases energy expenditure" (Caspersen, Powell, & Christenson, 1985, p. 126). Therefore, physical activity includes everything from washing dishes to running a marathon. Two subgroups, or types, of physical activity are aerobic activity and anaerobic activity. *Aerobic* means "with oxygen"; therefore, **aerobic activity** requires the use of oxygen to produce energy for movement. Engaging in aerobic activity improves cardiorespiratory endurance. People who have good cardiorespiratory endurance can sustain this kind of movement better than those who do not. Examples of aerobic activity include jogging, swimming, and snow-shoeing—all of which involve large muscles in repeating a motion rhythmically. For a more complete list of aerobic activities, see table 5.1.

TABLE 5.1　Examples of Moderate and Vigorous Aerobic Activities and Muscle- and Bone-Strengthening Activities for Children and Adolescents

Type of physical activity	AGE GROUP	
	Children	Adolescents
Moderate-intensity aerobic	• Active recreation (e.g., hiking, skate-boarding, in-line skating) • Bicycle riding • Brisk walking	• Active recreation (e.g., canoeing, hiking, skateboarding, in-line skating) • Bicycle riding (stationary or road) • Brisk walking • Housework and yardwork (e.g., sweeping, pushing a lawnmower) • Games that require catching and throwing (e.g., baseball, softball)
Vigorous-intensity aerobic	• Running and chasing games (e.g., tag) • Bicycle riding • Rope jumping • Martial arts (e.g., karate) • Running • Sports (e.g., soccer, ice or field hockey, basketball, swimming, tennis) • Cross-country skiing	• Running and chasing games (e.g., flag football) • Bicycle riding • Rope jumping • Martial arts (e.g., karate) • Running • Sports (e.g., soccer, ice or field hockey, basketball, swimming, tennis) • Vigorous dancing • Cross-country skiing
Muscle strengthening	• Games (e.g., tug-of-war) • Modified push-ups (knees on floor) • Resistance exercises using body weight or resistance bands • Rope or tree climbing • Curl-ups or crunches • Swinging on playground equipment or bars	• Games (e.g., tug-of-war) • Push-ups and pull-ups • Resistance exercises with exercise bands, weight machines, hand-held weights • Wall climbing • Curl-ups or crunches
Bone strengthening	• Games (e.g., hopscotch) • Hopping, skipping, jumping • Rope jumping • Running • Sports (e.g., gymnastics, basketball, volley-ball, tennis)	• Hopping, skipping, jumping • Rope jumping • Running • Sports (e.g., gymnastics, basketball, volleyball, tennis)

Note: Some activities, such as bicycling, can be either moderate or vigorous, depending on the level of effort.

Based on U.S. Department of Health and Human Services, 2008, *Physical Activity Guidelines for Americans*. Washington, DC. https://health.gov/paguidelines/guidelines.

Anaerobic means "without oxygen" or "in the absence of oxygen." Accordingly, **anaerobic activity** consists of movements fueled by energy stored in the body. Because this supply is limited, these activities involve short bursts of moderate- to high-intensity activity, such as sprinting or performing a short series of push-ups. The anaerobic systems—phosphagen and anaerobic glycolysis (lactic acid)—provide most of the fuel for activities lasting from a few seconds to about 90 seconds. Both anaerobic and aerobic activity train cardiorespiratory function, though in different ways, and they provide some overlapping health benefits. This topic is discussed further when interval training is described later in the chapter.

Importance and Benefits
of Cardiorespiratory Endurance

The National Physical Activity Plan Alliance (2018, p. 28) reports that cardiorespiratory endurance levels are decreasing in U.S. youth of ages 12 to 15; specifically, the percentage of those with adequate cardiorespiratory endurance fell from 52 percent in 1999 to 42 percent in 2012. SHAPE America's *SHAPE of the Nation 2016* report (2016) found that 32 percent of children and adolescents between the ages of 2 and 16 are overweight or obese, are sedentary, do not meet physical activity recommendations, and do not receive adequate physical education. The increase in obesity parallels the decrease in cardiorespiratory endurance. Without intervention, the increased risks associated with a sedentary lifestyle will exert an extremely negative effect on health and quality of life.

Cardiorespiratory endurance is one of the most important indicators of good health and physical condition and has a well-established association with health outcomes in adults (see figure 5.1). But since children and adolescents are not adults, we must consider the research specific to this age group before assigning benefits. In a literature review, the Committee on Fitness Measures and Health Outcomes in Youth (Pillsbury, Oria, & Pate, 2012, p. 145) acknowledges that "the measurement of cardiorespiratory endurance and its relationship to health outcomes in youth is relatively new to the literature." It also reports, however, that "sufficient relationships have been established between cardiorespiratory endurance and several health risk factors in youth, including adiposity and cardiometabolic risk factors (blood pressure, blood lipids and glucose, and insulin sensitivity). A few studies have established a relationship with other, less-studied pediatric health risk factors, such as pulmonary function, depression and positive self-concept, and bone health" (p. 145).

In addition, an increasing body of research supports a connection between physical activity (especially aerobic activity) and cognition. For instance, a systematic review of the research on children (ages 5 to 13 years) found that "PA has a positive influence on cognitive function as well as brain structure and function" (Donnelly et al., 2016, p. 1197). However, that same research review also indicated that some studies of physical activity, fitness, physical education, and academics have provided mixed results. Thus, more research needs to be done in this area, but there are encouraging studies. As figure 5.2 illustrates, physical activity increases brain activity. It seems to wake up the brain and prime it for learning. Neurosurgeon John Medina, author of *Brain Rules*, captures the significance of this growing body of research with his catchy phrase, "Physical activity is cognitive candy" (2014, p. 31), playing off the idea that the brain loves physical activity as much as most of us love candy. He points out that physically active students are healthier and can better transport oxygen and nutrients

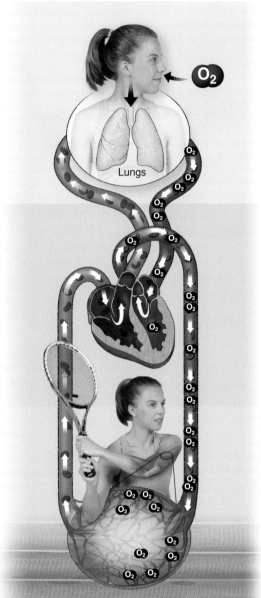

- Lungs work more efficiently
- Deliver more oxygen to blood
- Healthy lungs allow deeper and less frequent breathing

- Healthy elastic arteries allow more blood flow
- Less risk of atherosclerosis
- Lower blood pressure
- Less risk of a blood clot leading to heart attack
- Development of extra blood vessels
- Healthy veins with healthy valves

- Use oxygen efficiently
- Get rid of more wastes
- Use blood sugars and insulin more effectively to produce energy

- Heart muscle gets stronger
- Pumps more blood with each beat (stroke volume)
- Beats slower
- Gets more rest
- Works more efficiently
- Helps the nerves slow your heart rate at rest
- Builds muscles and helps them work more efficiently

- Less bad cholesterol (LDL) and other fats in the blood
- More good cholesterol (HDL) in the blood
- Reduces inflammatory markers in the blood
- Fewer substances in the blood that cause clots

FIGURE 5.1   Research has proved many health benefits of physical activity for the cardiorespiratory system in adults.

to all parts of the body, including the brain. Moreover, according to the *Shape of the Nation 2016* report (SHAPE America, 2016, p. 3), "Studies show that active and fit children consistently outperform less active, unfit students academically in both the short and the long term. They also demonstrate better classroom behavior, greater ability to focus, and lower rates of absenteeism."

According to Gomez-Pinilla and Charles Hillman (2013), research over the past decade has shown that physical activity can improve cognitive health throughout a person's life. People who are aerobically fit have protection from age-related loss of brain tissue. They also show enhanced functionality in some higher-order areas of the brain that deal with cognition; increased attention and faster information processing occur when people are more active with high fitness levels. There is also a

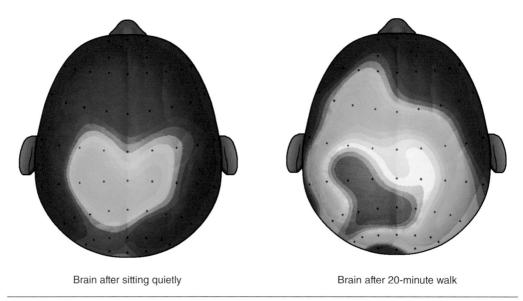

Brain after sitting quietly   Brain after 20-minute walk

FIGURE 5.2 After 20 minutes of physical activity, brain activity has increased.

Reprinted by permission from C.H. Hillman et al., "The Effect of Acute Treadmill Walking on Cognitive Control and Academic Achievement in Preadolescent Children," *Neuroscience* 159, (2009): 1044-1054.

growing body of evidence that physical activity interventions can reduce the severity of ADHD symptoms in children and adults (Pontifex, Saliba, Raine, Picchietti, & Hillman, 2013; Smith et al., 2013).

Physical activity, and particularly aerobic activity, can also play a role in ameliorating depression, enhancing self-esteem, and lifting spirits. *Healthy People 2020* reports that between 2008 and 2016, the proportion of adolescents (aged 12 to 17 years) who had experienced a major depressive episode in the past 12 months increased by more than half, from 8 percent to 13 percent (U.S. Department of Health and Human Services, 2010). Psychiatrist John Ratey, author of *Spark: The Revolutionary New Science of Exercise and the Brain*, shares evidence that "exercise is as effective as certain medications for treating anxiety and depression" (Ratey & Hagerman, 2008). Our young people need the positivity and energy that can be derived from games and activities that enhance cardiorespiratory endurance, and schools can provide such opportunities through physical education, before- and after-school programs (e.g., running clubs, dance teams), and chances for students to connect with community programs. School and community programs are particularly important for students who live with the stress of unsafe neighborhoods, poverty, or homelessness.

Developing good physical activity habits early in life can also help our young people achieve and maintain a healthy body composition and set the pattern for an active adult life. Cardiorespiratory endurance training has a positive effect on obesity because it burns calories from stored fat to fuel aerobic metabolism. This effect is critical given that in recent years the national obesity rate for children (ages 2 to 19 years) has remained all too high. Results from the 2015-2016 National Health and Nutrition Examination Survey (Fryar, Carroll, & Ogden, 2018), using measured heights and weights, indicate that an estimated 18.5 percent of U.S. children and adolescents aged 2 to 19 years have obesity, including 5.6 percent with severe obesity, and another 16.6 percent are overweight. A closer look shows that the prevalence in obesity in 2- to 5-year-olds, which had declined in 2011-2012 to 8.4 percent, rose to 13.9 percent in 2015-2016. The rates among 6- to 11-year-olds and 12- to 19-year-olds are relatively stable but they are holding around 18 percent and 20 percent, respectively, which is alarmingly high.

Lack of physical activity during adolescence may carry long-term health implications for adulthood. Indeed, there is a known increase in morbidity and mortality in adults attributable to chronic disease and sedentary lifestyles (U.S. Department of Health and Human Services, 2000). Research shows an association between overweight in adolescence and an increased risk of being overweight as an adult (Guo et al., 1994); it also shows that maintenance of health-related fitness through puberty provides health benefits in later years (Janz et al., 2002). Data from the National Health and Nutrition Survey, Phase 1, 1988-91 (McDowell et al., 1994) indicate that increased caloric intake is not solely responsible for the increased prevalence of overweight among youth and that lack of physical activity may also be a contributing factor. Behaviors that influence excess weight gain include consuming high-calorie, low-nutrient foods and beverages; not getting enough physical activity; engaging in sedentary activities, such as watching television or using other screen devices; using certain medications; and having poor sleep routines. In contrast, consuming a healthy diet and being physically active can help children grow well; avoid excess weight gain by balancing calories consumed with calories burned during activity; and avoid chronic diseases, including cancer, heart disease, and type 2 diabetes, the latter of which is increasing in prevalence among youth (Centers for Disease Control and Prevention, n.d.).

Many organizations, including SHAPE America, the Centers for Disease Control and Prevention (n.d.), the American Academy of Pediatrics (2000), and the U.S. Department of Health and Human Services (2018), advocate increasing childhood physical activity that will carry into adulthood, thereby reducing health problems associated with inactivity. *Healthy People 2020* (Office of Disease Prevention and Health Promotion, 2016) lists physical activity as one of the nation's 12 leading health indicators, and two of the plan's objectives specifically target increased physical activity for children and adolescents. Objective PA-3 specifically calls for increasing the proportion of adolescents who meet current federal guidelines for aerobic physical activity and muscle-strengthening activity from 29 percent to 32 percent, and objective PA-6 calls for increasing the requirement for regularly scheduled recess sessions in U.S. elementary schools from 7 states to 17 states.

50 Million Strong by 2029

SHAPE America's 50 Million Strong by 2029 initiative makes a commitment to increasing health and physical literacy through effective health and physical education programs. In part, this initiative is based on research and evidence of a clear need to make substantial changes to impact the current and future health of our students. As of 2017, the current generation of young people may have a lower life expectancy than their parents (SHAPE America, 2016). Physical education and health in schools is an ideal way to reach every student in the United States. The national physical education standards are set to guide physical educators in helping students become physically literate. Two of the five national physical education standards reflect the importance of cardiorespiratory endurance.

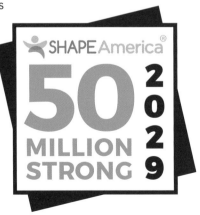

We cannot overemphasize the importance of increasing physical activity and enhancing health-related fitness among youth. This need is the reason that Physical Best sets its mission as providing students with the knowledge, skills, values, and confidence they need in order to engage in physical activity—both now and in the future—through fun and enjoyable activities.

Physical Activity and Cardiorespiratory Endurance Guidelines

Over the years, a number of guidelines have been offered for how much physical activity one needs in order to be healthy and fit. Many physical education teachers were raised on the American College of Sports Medicine (ACSM) gold standard of 20 to 60 minutes of vigorous aerobic activity on three to five days per week. This standard, however, was for healthy adults, not children and adolescents. As a result, the U.S. Department of Health and Human Services (HHS) formed an advisory committee to rethink the guidelines and broaden them to include recommendations for ages six years and older. As of 2018, the guidelines extend down to children ages three years and older. This advisory committee examined the relationship between health benefits and aerobic activity measured in both absolute and relative terms. The goal was to translate scientific evidence about intensity into user-friendly guidelines. The committee concluded that guidelines expressed in accrued minutes of moderate- and vigorous-intensity activity would be easy to follow and would result in substantial health benefits for people who followed them.

The resulting guidelines, the *2018 Physical Activity Guidelines for Americans* (U.S. Department of Health and Human Services, 2018) are endorsed by a number of professional organizations, including ACSM, the Centers for Disease Control and Prevention (CDC), and SHAPE America. This chapter examines the guidelines with a specific focus on how they relate to the health-related component of cardiorespiratory endurance. As you read the relevant sections of the guidelines, note the role played by aerobic activity.

Children and adolescents should perform 60 minutes or more of physical activity per day. Most of those minutes should involve either moderate- or vigorous-intensity aerobic activity, and vigorous-intensity physical activity should be included on at least three days per week.

- Adolescent students should aim for at least 20 continuous minutes of exercise in the target heart rate zone (THRZ) three or more times per week. Following these recommendations, exercise in the THRZ is cumulative and can yield improvements in cardiorespiratory endurance.

- Elementary students need moderate- to vigorous-intensity activity in bouts of approximately 15 minutes that add up to at least 60 minutes.

In the portions of the *2018 Physical Activity Guidelines for Americans* that address recommendations for children and adolescents, aerobic activities are described as "those in which young people rhythmically move their large muscles. Running, hopping, skipping, jumping rope, swimming, dancing, and bicycling are all examples of aerobic activities" (U.S. Department of Health and Human Services, 2018, p. 49). However, children's normal movement activity is not prolonged; to the contrary, children like to engage in intermittent activity with short rests. In recognition of this tendency, the guidelines for aerobic activity among children and adolescents expand the definition to include "activities in short bursts, which may not technically be aerobic" (U.S. Department of Health and Human Services, 2018, p. 49). In other words, let kids be kids, and do not try to tie them to prolonged activity at one pace. In fact, children commonly combine aerobic movement with muscle- and bone-building movement. For example, a child may dash across the playground, swing across the monkey bars, jump to the ground, and then chase a friend. In this context, cardiorespiratory endurance can be thought of as the ability to exercise or play for an extended period without getting tired (U.S. Department of Health and Human Services, 2018).

The 2018 Guidelines for Physical Activity Reports cite strong evidence of the health benefits of 60 minutes daily of moderate to vigorous physical activity. They also support the idea that three of those days should include muscle-strengthening, bone-strengthening, vigorous physical activity and that children who are three to five years old benefit from physical activity involving jumping, leaping, and gymnastics. The health benefits of increased moderate to vigorous physical activity include improved bone density and health, increased cardiovascular and muscular fitness, and a healthier weight status (U.S. Department of Health and Human Services, 2018).

Also note that *any* amount of physical activity is beneficial (Medina, 2014). If a student can go from refusing to participate (that is, being sedentary) to even five minutes of movement, the health benefits kick in. You can help students by focusing on improvement, consistency, and persistence rather than using a narrow focus of passing or failing the guidelines. One way to do so—and to shift control from teacher to students—is to have students keep a log of activity both in and out of class and reflect on how they are doing.

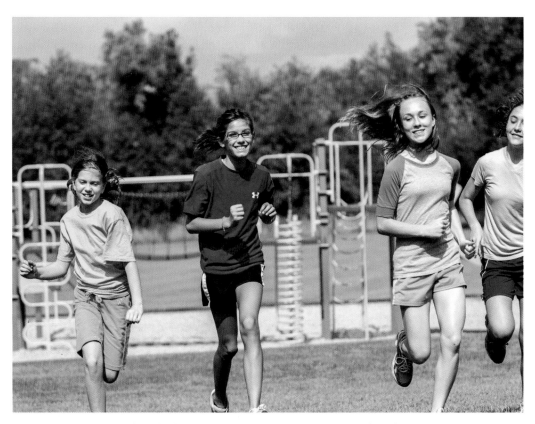

The stop-and-go play that children love gives them the health benefits of aerobic activity.

Given that class time in physical education is limited (sometimes as little as 30 minutes per week), many physical educators cannot provide enough aerobic activity for students. In that case, we must go beyond doing aerobic activities with students. We must also educate them about how to recognize and select aerobic activity and how to apply the principles of health-related fitness to optimize their participation and enjoyment outside of school.

Teaching Cardiorespiratory Endurance

Before beginning any lesson with new students, work with the school nurse to determine which students have medical conditions that you should be aware of, such as orthopedic issues, asthma, epilepsy, diabetes, or disabilities. This knowledge will help you reduce students' risk of injury or medical complications. Proper screening of your students will also help you develop a well-rounded program that addresses the needs of all students, including those who should use extra caution when engaging in aerobic activities.

The concept of cardiorespiratory endurance can be taught to students of all ages, but the practice of cardiorespiratory endurance training must take into consideration developmental differences. As suggested earlier, children and adolescents are not little adults; therefore, strategies of continuous exercise, use of the FITT guidelines, and interpretation of test results are not the same for them. Developmental differences are major determinants of how to teach the concept of cardiorespiratory endurance in physical education class.

The score that a young student attains on a cardiorespiratory endurance test does not correlate well with the amount of aerobic activity that a child gets. Aerobic capacity is affected by age, heredity, and maturation. Therefore, be careful *not to assume* that children with strong PACER or mile-run scores are more active than others, or that students with weaker scores are less active. Indeed, a child with favorable individual genetics may be minimally active and still have a good score (Pangrazi & Corbin, 2008). In an example from outside of physical education, a person who has inherited an aptitude for spelling does not have to practice much in order to spell words correctly, whereas another individual may practice a great deal and still not do well. In physical activity, however, the sheer act of doing it provides benefits, and students who regularly accumulate appropriate amounts of moderate and vigorous activity (regardless of test scores) will benefit from being active.

As students go through puberty, their bodies become more capable of responding to training. In the meantime, trying to force increases in $\dot{V}O_2$max by increasing training regimens among prepubescent children can result in injury and burnout. Therefore, performance scores should be deemphasized, especially for elementary students; instead, highlight participation and improvements in technique. Focus less on training and scores and more on providing students with opportunities for moderate and vigorous activities that match the go-and-stop nature of child's play—that is, periods of vigorous activity followed by recovery time, as in station work or circuit training.

When teaching prepubescent children, reinforce the health benefits of physical activity (increased bone density, improved lipid profile, and healthy body composition); help students understand that increased respiration and heartbeat are desirable; and create opportunities for them to experience joy in movement. Movement that produces sweat, faster breathing, and a pounding heart needs to be fun in order to appeal to children. You can include activities that develop motor skills both for the application of cardiorespiratory endurance and for an enjoyable experience. For instance, low-skill, low-organization invasion games build the skills of throwing and catching while getting students' heart rates into the THRZ; examples include variations of ultimate and team handball. You can alternate sport skill stations with cardiorespiratory endurance stations to provide recovery time for deconditioned students. These students need safe bouts of exercise to build endurance—not extended periods of activity that compromise their chance of success (Alleyne, 1998).

As students enter middle school, growth and maturation go into high speed. Rapid growth comes with physiological changes that affect test scores for aerobic capacity and cardiorespiratory endurance. The heart gets bigger and stronger and can pump more blood; that is, it can produce more cardiac output. Height and weight increase, which means longer limbs as well. Longer legs with more muscle translate to longer stride lengths and stronger propulsion, which can help students run faster or farther with less fatigue. Thus growth and maturation result in improved aerobic capacity as measured in terms of $\dot{V}O_2max$ (ml $\cdot$ kg^{-1} $\cdot$ min^{-1}).

As a result, during rapid-growth years, it is more difficult to determine how much improvement in cardiorespiratory endurance is due to growth and physiological maturation and how much is due to training. The existing research (which is not abundant) suggests that aerobic training can bring modest improvements in aerobic capacity in adolescents. Until about age 10, the genders are pretty similar, but as maturation occurs, boys tend to gain more lean body mass while girls add a greater percentage of adipose tissue. This divergence tends to give boys an advantage and is one reason that gender differences are seen in raw test scores in secondary school. FitnessGram adjusts the raw scores to account for gender difference. Therefore, gender and age must be entered in the software in order to determine the estimated $\dot{V}O_2max$ and the associated category of health-related fitness for the three assessments of cardiorespiratory endurance.

To promote optimal physical activity among students, encourage participation in a wide variety of enjoyable and available activities (see figure 5.3). To make the best use of your class time with older students, help them connect the lesson to their real lives, enjoy what they are doing, and understand the importance of cardiorespiratory endurance for their personal health. Emphasize helping students discover physical activities that benefit cardiorespiratory endurance and are personally enjoyable so that they will want to continue being active into adulthood. Lessons can include segments in which you help students explore real-world applications for tracking and training cardiorespiratory endurance, such as logging free-time aerobic activities in a journal, tracking and looking for trends in heart rate, and organizing health-related fitness night at school for families and friends.

In general, SHAPE America recommends sport sampling over sport specialization early in life (National Association for Sport and Physical Education, 2004). Early specialization can be beneficial to athletes who epitomize the body structure requirements in certain sports, as long as proper dietary habits and recovery time are incorporated into the training. Some evidence suggests that early sport specialization is the preferred approach in sports where elite performance is achieved before puberty (e.g., figure skating, gymnastics), but this research is sparse, and caution should be used in drawing any conclusions (Carson, Landers, & Blankenship, 2010).

Moreover, most physical education students do not aspire to perform at the elite level, and a focus on sport sampling can help them find activities that they enjoy and will continue for a lifetime. As students move through middle school and high school, the opportunity to choose activities and develop their own health-related fitness plan is central to maintaining motivation. They can use FitnessGram and ActivityGram

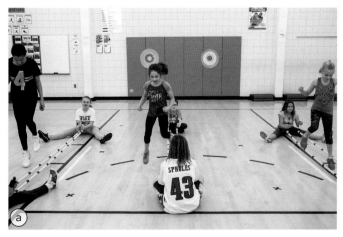

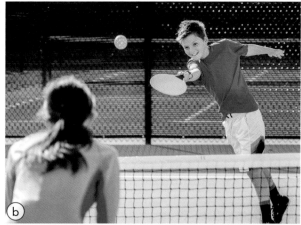

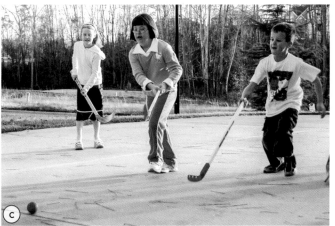

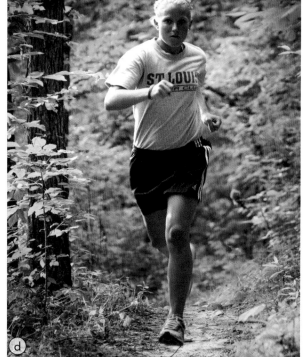

FIGURE 5.3   Sample activities that can help students improve cardiorespiratory endurance.

Photo b © Rich Legg/Getty Images; photo c © Bold Stock/age footstock; photo d © Chris Mautz/fotolia.com

to log and track their activity. High school activities should be taught in more depth and with a lifetime orientation. For students who participate in sport programs (at school or in the community), care should be taken not to overtrain them by requiring similar training in physical education and sport practice.

For all ages, the Physical Best philosophy emphasizes teaching health-related fitness concepts through physical activity and designing lessons that minimize the number of inactive students at any given time (for example, waiting for a turn), especially if the class meets only once or twice per week. In addition, when all students are engaged simultaneously, they are less likely to feel that they are being watched and may be ridiculed. Focus on a single concept each day rather than trying to force-feed multiple concepts. Use the Physical Best activities from the web resource to teach key concepts through activity. For example, the concept of venous return can be taught while performing an aerobic cool-down, and the circulatory system can be simulated by using a jogging course in which students act as blood traveling through the heart, arteries, or veins.

Another powerful motivator for exercise is music. It can provide a distraction from fatigue, elevate mood, increase endurance, and reduce perceived effort. Choice of music is a personal matter, but a tempo between 120 and 140 beats per minute seems to optimize the positive effects of music for exercise. Including a variety of musical genres at the recommended tempo may meet the needs of most students.

When we teach health-related fitness, we must also consider the social and emotional dimensions of our students. As students try to navigate a socially challenging world, as well as the physiological changes that come with maturation, we need to present aerobic activity to them in a way that is both emotionally and physically safe. The sidebar titled Keeping Students Emotionally Safe provides some tips for preventing embarrassment and promoting a classroom climate in which everyone feels safe. Using health-related fitness activities (such as running laps) as punishment sends the wrong message, whereas getting to run an extra "birthday" lap (in elementary school) or developing health-related fitness for a hiking field trip (secondary school) puts health-related fitness in a positive light.

When you teach students about cardiorespiratory endurance, remember that differences in performance on assessments are affected not only by activity levels but also by various other influences, including genetics, developmental factors, body composition, and psychological factors such as motivation. The goal of the Physical Best program is to promote noncompetitive, self-enhancing, and enjoyable activities that encourage students to be physically active. Even if the relationship is not strong between increased physical activity and cardiorespiratory endurance in children

Keeping Students Emotionally Safe

- When students make fun of other students who are less fit, make a point of teaching about individual differences and relative intensity. Help students think about their different strengths (e.g., math, writing, flexibility), their weaknesses, and the fact that the world needs people with all kinds of talents working together.

- Cultivate an atmosphere of acceptance by using cooperative games and health-related fitness challenges that require the help of the whole team. Model empathy and teach students to encourage each other.

- Have students pair up and become advocates for one another. Ask them to share their goals and develop helping relationships. Reward both students when one succeeds.

- Don't publicly announce or post fitness test results; instead, have students privately record their results in their health-related fitness logs and use them to set effective goals.

- When students do the mile run or warm-up jog, use staggered starts or have students run for a set amount of time (e.g., 10 minutes) rather than a set distance (e.g., three laps). Use the PACER test, because lower-scoring students will finish first, not last, and can continue to walk the course, rest, and then rejoin the activity. They can also cheer on classmates who are still testing.

- Instead of expecting all students to complete a set number of pedometer steps, ask students to find out how many steps they typically take and then set a goal to improve by 10 percent.

- Use fitness tracking data to set goals and design and implement an improvement or maintenance plan—not to grade.

- Provide variety through stations or self-selected options for the day. Be aware that heavier (overfat) individuals may experience joint pain and impact stress when running or doing extended rope jumping. Allow for low-impact activities such as brisk walking, cycling, elliptical stepping, swimming, and outdoor winter choice activities such as skating and cross-country skiing.

(Rowland, 2016; Pangrazi & Corbin, 2008), the program aspires to promote active children to become active adults for whom cardiorespiratory endurance training (following the FITT guidelines) yields improvements in cardiorespiratory endurance and enhanced health benefits.

Principles of Exercise and Cardiorespiratory Endurance

The principles of exercise introduced in chapter 3 will now be specifically applied to cardiorespiratory endurance. Table 5.2 provides information about how to apply the FITT guidelines for younger children (5 to 12 years old) and adolescents (11 years and older), as well as older youth who participate in athletics. Because the table includes some overlap in age, it allows for changes in the guidelines based on individual developmental age rather than chronological age. As noted by Welk and Blair (2008), the fact that "children *can* adapt to physical training does not mean they should be encouraged or required to do so." Rather than emphasize the adult exercise prescription model, the aim with children should be to foster and maintain a physically active lifestyle.

As the FITT principles are applied, remember that students who are new to aerobic activity need to start slowly. The recommended approach is to gradually increase a single variable (frequency, intensity, time, or type) rather than increasing multiple variables. For less-fit individuals, it is better to increase time (duration) or frequency first, instead of intensity, because students are less likely to become discouraged and more likely to stick with an activity or exercise program if it does not cause extreme fatigue or soreness. Long periods of continuous vigorous activity are not recommended for children of ages 6 through 12 unless they are freely chosen by the child (NASPE, 2004).

Exercise intensity should follow a bell curve. Training bouts for cardiorespiratory endurance begin with a warm-up period to prepare the body for exercise. Range-of-motion movements should mimic the exercise mode while increasing heart rate, respiration, and core body temperature. After the main activity, the cool-down period of low-intensity work allows the heart rate and breathing to return to a slightly elevated, preexercise state.

The basis of a training program for cardiorespiratory endurance is formed by the training principles of specificity, progression, overload, regularity, individuality, and FITT guidelines.

- **Specificity principle.** Students need to be able to recognize and select aerobic activities if they wish to improve their cardiorespiratory endurance. Teach students that doing 10 push-ups will not improve their ability to sustain a run without breathing hard. Nonaerobic exercises may, however, help support an aerobic activity such as running. For example, strengthening the legs can help with stride propulsion, and sprint work can improve a mile run. Type of exercise should be specific to the goals of cardiorespiratory endurance training; in other words, the exercise should increase oxygen consumption by increasing heart rate and respiration. Cardiorespiratory endurance comes from meeting the energy demands of a working muscle.

- **Progression and overload principles.** These two principles work together. Progression should be purposefully provided by manipulating frequency, intensity, and time. To overload is to do a little more than normal in order to

TABLE 5.2 FITT Guidelines Applied to Cardiorespiratory Endurance

	Children (5-12 years)[a]	Adolescents (≥11 years)[b]	Middle school and high school youth who participate in athletics[c]
Frequency	• Developmentally appropriate physical activity on all or most days of the week • Several bouts of physical activity lasting 15 min or more daily	• Activity daily or nearly every day • Three or more sessions per week	• Five or six days per week
Intensity	• Mixture of moderate and vigorous intermittent activity • Moderate: low-intensity games (hopscotch, four-square), low-activity positions (goalie, outfielder), some chores, yardwork • Vigorous: games involving running or chasing; playing sports (level 2 of Physical Activity Pyramid)	• Moderate to vigorous activity (not expected to maintain target heart rate at this level) • Rating of perceived exertion: 7-10 (Borg)[d], 1-3 (OMNI)[e]	• 60%-90% max heart rate (MHR) or 50%-85% heart rate reserve (HRR) • Rating of perceived exertion: 12-16 (Borg), 5-7 (OMNI)
Time	• Accumulated activity of at least 60 min and up to several hr • Up to 50% accumulated in bouts of 15 min or more	• 30-60 min of daily activity • 20 min or more in a single session	• 20-60 min
Type	• Variety of activities selected from first three levels of Physical Activity Pyramid (continuous activity not expected for most children)	• Play, games, sports, work, transportation, recreation, physical education, or planned exercise (in the context of family, school, or community activities) • Brisk walking, jogging, stair climbing, basketball, racket sports, soccer, dancing, lap swimming, skating, lawn mowing, cycling	• Activities that use large muscles rhythmically (e.g., brisk walking, jogging, stair climbing, basketball, racket sports, soccer, dancing, lap swimming, skating, cycling)

[a]National Association for Sport and Physical Education. (2004). *Physical activity for children: A statement of guidelines for children ages 5–12*, 2nd ed. Reston, VA: Author.

[b]Corbin, C.B., and Pangrazi, R.P. (2002). Physical activity for children: how much is enough? In G.J. Welk, R.J. Morrow, & H.B. Falls (Eds.), *FitnessGram Reference Guide* (p. 7 Internet Resource). Dallas, TX: The Cooper Institute.

[c]American College of Sports Medicine. (2000). *ACSM's guidelines for exercise testing and prescription*, 6th ed. Philadelphia: Lippincott, Williams, and Wilkins.

[d]Borg, G. (1998). *Borg's perceived exertion and pain scales.* Champaign, IL: Human Kinetics, 47.

[e]Robertson, R.J. (2004). *Perceived exertion for practitioners: Rating effort with the OMNI pictures system.* Champaign, IL: Human Kinetics, 141-150.

From National Association for Sport and Physical Education 2004; Corbin and Pangrazi 2002; American College of Sports Medicine 2000; Borg 1998.

encourage adaptation (improvement), and progression involves doing so in gradual increments over time. Students who are sedentary or have low fitness need to start off easy and build up stamina. For example, a progressive overload might work first on walking longer without having to stop and then on picking up the pace of the walking. The next step would be to alternate walking with some jogging. The following list offers some ways to increase cardiorespiratory endurance activities in order to provide an overload. In each case, the overload should follow a gradual progression.

○ Increase the distance covered.

○ Increase the duration of the activity (e.g., game with a cardiorespiratory endurance component, cardiorespiratory endurance activity such as Zumba).

○ Increase the frequency—that is, do it more often (increasing from two times per week to three times).

○ Pick up the pace.

○ Increase the incline (on mixed terrain or on a cardio machine).

When planning for progression, take care not to undercut enjoyment by increasing a variable too quickly. In the initial stages of an exercise program, increase duration first. Then, after the individual has been exercising regularly for a month or more, you can gradually increase frequency, intensity, or time (American College of Sports Medicine, 2014). How to adjust the variable depends on the student, who should be involved in setting goals and planning the exercise.

• **Regularity principle.** Cardiorespiratory endurance is not something you can do a lot of all at once and then "put it in the bank and save it." Children and adolescents need to engage in moderate to vigorous aerobic activity for at least 60 minutes every day. High school students who are 18 years or older need to meet the adult guidelines of 150 minutes per week (75 if vigorous).

• **Individuality principle.** Genetics, growth, and maturation all play sizable roles in how young people respond to cardiorespiratory endurance training. Therefore, it is much more important to focus on participation, fun, and confidence building than it is to measure health-related fitness changes. As students approach adulthood, we must also remember that the guidelines are established for an average healthy individual and should be adjusted to accommodate individuals with health conditions or disabilities. We must also recognize that aerobic response follows a normal curve and that there are actually a few people who are nonresponders insofar as their $\dot{V}O_2$max does not improve with training. Even so, they receive health benefits from being active.

• **FITT guidelines** (U.S. Department of Health and Human Services, 2018):

○ For children and adolescents: F = most days of the week, I = moderate to vigorous intensity, T (time) = 60 minutes or more per day, and T (type) = a wide variety of aerobic activities.

○ For adults: F = three days or more per week, I = moderate to vigorous intensity, T (time) = 150 minutes per week at moderate intensity or 75 minutes at vigorous intensity, and T (type) = a wide variety of aerobic activities.

○ Intensity can be estimated and monitored in a number of ways (e.g., heart rate monitoring, rating of perceived exertion), which are discussed in a later section.

FITT-VP Principle

For years, the acronym has been FITT, or occasionally FITTE (*E* for *enjoyment*), but now you may also see it written as FITT-VP. The last two letters stand for *volume* and *progression*. Progression and overall volume (how much) of exercise one performs both play important roles in training. This text stays with the simpler acronym but not without the appropriate nod to the VP criteria, which become increasingly specific as one trains for competition. For example, a competitive swimmer will increase the volume of a workout during the off-season, then shorten it as competition days draw near in order to be rested and in peak condition. Progressions can move more quickly some of the time and require more rest and smaller increments at other times. Personal trainers and coaches work hard to find the right balance for their clients and athletes. For health purposes, gradual progression is generally employed; volume is increased when health-related fitness gains are desired and held steady when maintenance is the objective. Varying the way in which the desired volume is attained can be a good way to prevent boredom and optimize training results.

Although the lifetime physical activity model emphasized in Physical Best provides guidelines for cardiorespiratory endurance training that are sufficient for good health, teachers will encounter students who want to achieve higher levels of health-related fitness. We must provide these students with accurate information that helps them reach their goals for cardiorespiratory endurance in a safe manner. We should always take care not to train children and youth as if they were "little adults." Too many young people experience burnout from overtraining, whereas healthful lifetime patterns are encouraged when physical activity is enjoyable.

Monitoring Intensity

The concept of intensity is one of the most important to teach. You can use several methods to teach about and monitor the intensity of cardiorespiratory endurance activity. This section discusses monitoring with heart rate, the talk test, and ratings of perceived exertion. As with all Physical Best concepts, the way in which intensity is presented must grow with the students. It is exciting to watch young children recognize the beating of their heart and realize that it is more than a Valentine shape; it is just as fun to watch teenagers stare with curiosity at a heart rate monitor as it picks up their heartbeat.

Intensity can be assessed in either absolute or relative terms (U.S. Department of Health and Human Services, 2018). An absolute measure involves, for example, walking at 3 to 4 miles (4.8 to 6.4 kilometers) per hour or running a 12-minute mile (7.5-minute kilometer). In contrast, a relative measure determines intensity as a percentage of **maximal heart rate (MHR), heart rate reserve (HRR),** or aerobic capacity reserve. In the first case, everyone works at a specified speed—for instance, a brisk walk. In the latter, the intensity is adjusted to the individual's level of cardiorespiratory endurance; that is, it uses an individualized training heart rate zone. To motivate students to do their best and to account for individual differences among students, relative measures should be used. Relative measures using heart rate and ratings of perceived exertion are explained in the next two sections. Monitoring intensity is important because health benefits are associated with reaching moderate and vigorous levels of physical activity.

Heart Rate

Heart rate can be a useful indicator of exercise intensity, and it should be taught, measured, and used differently with children, adolescents, and adults. Monitoring heart rate can be as simple as counting beats for young children, whereas older students can learn how to calculate a target heart rate zone.

Measuring Heart Rate in Children

Young children can be taught to find their heart rate by placing their right hand on the left-center of their chest and feeling for the "bump, bump" or "flub dub." If they start by playing an active game (e.g., tag) or doing a warm-up jog, the beating of the heart will be more pronounced and easier for them to find. Once they are good at feeling their heartbeat with the one hand, they can use the other hand to open and close a fist to the tempo of the heartbeat. If they raise their tempo hand overhead, then you can easily monitor their responses. This approach provides a great visual. Students can note the general speed of the heartbeat using terms such as *slow*, *medium*, and *fast* or *turtle* and *race car*. Once they can do this, you can teach a lesson that progresses in intensity from a gentle warm-up to vigorous activity and have students make the connection between an increasing heart rate and increasing exercise intensity. You can use stations at which students check their heart rate and decide whether the station is a low-, medium-, or high-intensity aerobic activity.

In addition to heart rate, students can learn to recognize heavier breathing as a sign of intensity. Sweat, on the other hand, is a tricky characteristic. Children may connect it with exercising hard, but it is not a reliable indicator of cardiorespiratory intensity. Indeed, it is common for people to sweat in different amounts—some a lot, others hardly at all—even when exercising at the same relative intensity in the same environment (e.g., hot or cool; humid or dry).

You can introduce older children to the ideas of aerobic and anaerobic exercise. They can start to distinguish between short high-intensity (anaerobic) activities that leave them out of breath and aerobic activities during which they can breathe evenly and keep going for a while. You can ask them to think about the games they play, and whether they are moving for short or long periods of time before resting, and relate these patterns to either aerobic or anaerobic activity. Students can also begin to feel for their pulse and learn more about the anatomy of the circulatory system.

In addition, you can ask children of all ages to report back on heart-healthy activities they do at home. The goal is for them to understand the concept of intensity, learn about which activities are good for their heart, and then be moderately to vigorously active for at least an hour per day.

It is *not* age-appropriate for younger students to sustain a specific target heart rate zone for a designated amount of time. As mentioned earlier, interval-style activity is natural for younger children. When they play tag, they often run hard and fast for a bit and then look for the safety of a "base" or a location far from the tagger so that they can rest. Once rested, they are off again at top speed.

Measuring Heart Rate in Adolescents

The 2018 Physical Activity Guidelines (U.S. Department of Health and Human Services, 2018) call for 60 minutes of moderate to vigorous activity per day. They do *not* call for continuous minutes in a designated heart rate zone. The important thing for adolescents is to continue teaching the concept of intensity by having students compare levels of intensity between activities and helping them understand what moderate to vigorous intensity feels like. Teaching this concept can be facilitated by monitoring heart rate and using ratings of perceived exertion. At the same time, it is appropriate to allow adolescents to train for longer continuous periods of time if they choose to do so of their own accord. In addition, as students move toward adulthood, the relationship between heart rate and oxygen consumption becomes more valid. It is therefore appropriate to introduce and monitor the cardiorespiratory endurance training zone in high school, particularly in the upper grades. Teach students that an increasing heart rate correlates with an increase in oxygen consumption, which is the measure of aerobic capacity.

Taking the Pulse

To use heart rate as an estimate of aerobic intensity, students first need to learn how to take their pulse accurately. (If using heart rate monitors, teach students that the monitor is counting the pulse for them.) Two common sites used to count heart rate are the carotid artery (in the neck) and the radial artery (in the wrist, on the thumb side). To begin, teach students to locate the pulse by placing the first two fingers of the right hand lightly on the right side of the neck, below and to the right of the Adam's apple (figure 5.4a). The Adam's apple is not prominent in children, especially girls. In an alternate method, the student looks straight ahead and places two fingers on the

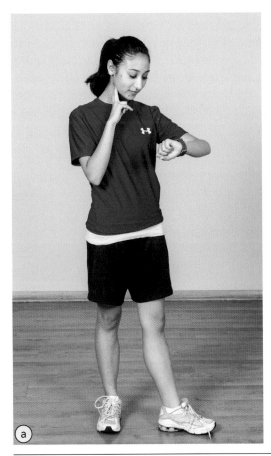
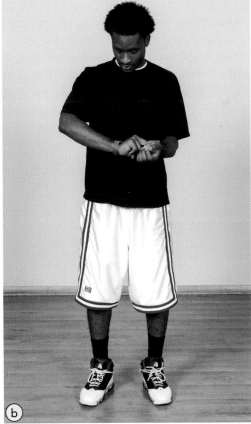

FIGURE 5.4 Two methods of taking a pulse: *(a)* at the carotid artery (neck) and *(b)* at the radial artery (wrist).

bone behind the earlobe (the mastoid process). They then gently press and slowly slide the fingers down and forward until they feel the heartbeat. The fingers will naturally follow the angle of the jaw and end up to the right of the Adam's apple. Be sure that each student is capable of feeling his or her heartbeat. Make sure that students do not press too hard or massage the neck, because doing so will slow the heart rate. In addition, they should never palpate both carotid arteries at the same time, because reduced blood flow to the brain may cause them to become dizzy or faint.

Teach older students to use the radial artery at the wrist by placing the first two fingers of either hand on the opposite wrist (with the palm facing up), just below the base of the thumb (figure 5.4b). Students should move their fingers around until they locate the pulse. Students should not use the thumb to palpate the pulse because the thumb has a pulse in itself, which means that a double count could occur. When students are first learning to palpate the pulse, it is helpful to have them be active for a couple minutes first so that the heartbeat is more pronounced. If younger students cannot find their carotid pulse, they can try finding their radial pulse instead.

The pulse is often counted for one minute when measuring resting heart rate; shorter intervals are used to measure the heart rate during exercise. If the first heartbeat is counted while simultaneously starting the stopwatch, the first beat should be counted as zero. If the stopwatch is already running, the first beat should be counted as one (Heyward, 2010). Students may either count their pulse for 6 seconds and multiply by 10 (simply add a zero to the number they counted), count for 10 seconds and multiply by 6, or count for 15 seconds and multiply by 4. Fitness professionals generally prefer the 10-second count because it tends to be the most accurate. To avoid having to multiply the 10-second count by 6, which can be difficult to do in your head, students can either refer to a chart (see table 5.3) or divide their training target heart rate zone (see next section) by 6 and use a range for beats per 10 seconds. For example, a training range from 153 to 165 beats per minute translates to about 25 to 27 beats per 10 seconds.

Target Heart Rate Zone

The **target heart rate zone (THRZ)** indicates the optimal range of exercise intensities for improving cardiorespiratory endurance when using continuous aerobic

TABLE 5.3   Heart Rate Based on 10-Second Count

Beats per 10 seconds	Heart rate (beats per minute)	Beats per 10 seconds	Heart rate (beats per minute)
10	60	22	132
11	66	23	138
12	72	24	144
13	78	25	150
14	84	26	156
15	90	27	162
16	96	28	168
17	102	29	174
18	108	30	180
19	114	31	186
20	120	32	192
21	126	33	198

Maximal Heart Rate Method

To use the maximal heart rate method, first calculate the maximal heart rate (MHR) using the following formula: 207 − (0.7 × age). Then select a range of intensity between 55 percent and 90 percent of MHR by referring to table 5.4. For example, a student who is 18 years old at a marginal level of health-related fitness would select 65 percent to 75 percent of MHR and find the THRZ by first finding MHR and then finding the proper percentages of MHR:

$$MHR = 207 - (0.7 \times 18) = 194.4 \text{ or simply } 194$$

Next, calculate the THRZ by changing the selected percentages to decimals and multiplying them by the MHR:

$$0.65 \times 194 = 126.1 \text{ or } 126$$
$$0.75 \times 194 = 145.5 \text{ or } 146$$

Thus, rounded to the nearest whole number, this student's THRZ ranges from 126 to 146 heartbeats per minute.

TABLE 5.4 Progression of Frequency, Intensity, and Time Based on Health-Related Fitness Level

	Low health-related fitness	Marginal health-related fitness	Good health-related fitness
Frequency	3 days per week	3 to 5 days per week	3 to 6 days per week
Intensity			
Heart rate reserve (HRR)	40%-50%	50%-60%	60%-85%
Maximal heart rate (max HR)	55%-65%	65%-75%	75%-90%
Rating of perceived exertion (RPE)	12-13 (Borg)[a], 5 (OMNI)[b]	13-14 (Borg), 5-6 (OMNI)	14-16 (Borg), 6-7 (OMNI)
Time	10-30 min	20-40 min	30-60 min

[a]Borg, G. (1998). *Borg's perceived exertion and pain scales* (Champaign, IL: Human Kinetics), 47.

[b]Robertson, R.J. (2004). *Perceived exertion for practitioners: Rating effort with the OMNI pictures system* (Champaign, IL: Human Kinetics).

From Corbin et al. (2004).

Karvonen (Heart Rate Reserve) Method

The Karvonen or heart rate reserve (HRR) method of calculating target heart rate zone takes into account an individual's health-related fitness and resting heart rate. For high school students, this method can be taught and used to demonstrate how intensity can be modified as health-related fitness improves and resting heart rate decreases. Students calculate maximum heart rate by subtracting age from 220. This is the theoretical maximum heart rate.

$$220 - age = MHR$$

To find a target heart rate zone, subtract the RHR from the MHR and multiply it by a minimal percentage (50%) and add the RHR to get the low end of the zone. To get the high end of the zone, subtract the RHR from the MHR and multiply by the maximal percentage (85%).

$$[(MHR - RHR) \times 0.50] + RHR = \text{Low end of THRZ}$$
$$[(MHR - RHR) \times 0.85] + RHR = \text{High end of THRZ}$$

A 15-year-old student with a resting heart rate of 70 beats per minute would have a target heart rate zone of 138 to 185.

$$220 - 15 = 205 \text{ (MHR)}$$
$$[(205 - 70) \times 0.50] + 70 = 138 \text{ (137.5; low end of THRZ)}$$
$$[(205 - 70) \times 0.85] + 70 = 185 \text{ (184.75; high end of THRZ)}$$

endurance training. The low end of the zone is the threshold of aerobic training, and the upper end (often referred to as the *top* or *ceiling*) is the anaerobic threshold. Maintaining a heart rate within the zone will result in aerobic conditioning. High school students can begin to use the THRZ to guide them in monitoring intensity of activity.

The THRZ is based on a percentage of maximal heart rate (MHR), which can be determined by means of several formulas based on age, resting heart rate, and numeric value differences between males and females. These formulas often assume different theoretical maximal heart rates.

The most frequently used method for calculating THRZ is the maximal heart rate method, which uses an age-predicted theoretical MHR as a starting point. Despite its popularity, however, this method is limited in that it does not accommodate for different resting heart rates that reflect varying levels of cardiorespiratory endurance. Another method sometimes used to calculate THRZ is the Karvonen or heart rate reserve (HRR) formula. This approach accounts for the individual's level of health-related fitness in determining the target heart rate zone by factoring in resting heart rate (RHR). Both of these methods are described in the sidebar titled Calculating Target Heart Rate Zones. For younger students, it is appropriate to simply count and compare the difference between resting heart rate and exercise heart rate.

Talk Test and Rating of Perceived Exertion

In addition to heart rate, there are two other ways to monitor intensity. The talk test simply stipulates that your intensity is appropriate if you can talk but not sing. If you are too out of breath to talk, then the intensity is too high; if you can sing, then the intensity is too low. This method is particularly useful when students have difficulty finding their heartbeat.

The second alternative, rating of perceived exertion (RPE), estimates how hard or easy a person feels that she or he is working. Table 5.5 depicts the OMNI scales for rating of perceived exertion for children (ages 8 through 15) and adults (ages 16 and older). These scales were developed using pictures of exertion, as well as words and numbers. The pictures, provided in reproducible form in the web resource, are especially helpful with elementary and middle school children (see figure 5.5). Specifically, they can rate their level of perceived exertion more accurately by pointing to a picture than by selecting a number or word phrase. Note that the children's word phrases are different from the adult's phrases. The OMNI scales can be used to determine an RPE for the whole body, for the limbs, or for the chest. Therefore, they are useful for teaching about intensity in both cardiorespiratory endurance and resistance exercise. RPE is a valid measure of intensity, and a rating of four to six correlates with the target heart rate zone.

TABLE 5.5   Verbal Cues for OMNI RPE Scales

Adults	Children
Extremely easy = 0	Not tired at all = 0
Easy = 2	A little tired = 2
Somewhat easy = 4	Getting more tired = 4
Somewhat hard = 6	Tired = 6
Hard = 8	Really tired = 8
Extremely hard = 10	Very, very tired = 10

Reprinted by permission from V.H. Heyward, *Advanced Fitness Assessment and Exercise Prescription*, 7th ed. (Champaign, IL: Human Kinetics, 2014), 84.

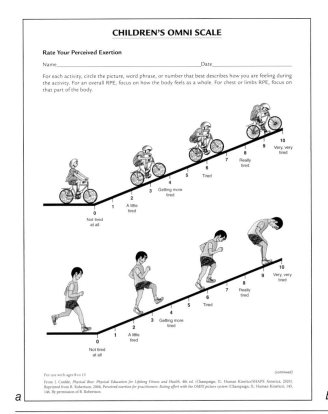

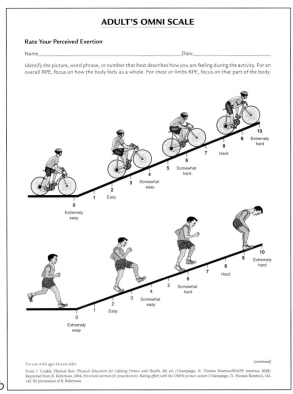

a   b

FIGURE 5.5   The *(a)* children's and *(b)* adult's OMNI RPE scales allow students to use the scale pictorially. Reproducible versions of these scales are available in the web resource.

Reprinted from R. Robertson, 2004, *Perceived exertion for practitioners: Rating effort with the OMNI pictures system* (Champaign, IL: Human Kinetics), 141, 142, 145, 146. By permission of R. Robertson.

Training Methods for Cardiorespiratory Endurance

The cardiorespiratory system can be trained in a number of ways. The main method for improving cardiorespiratory endurance is steady state training, or continuous training. In this approach, the heart rate follows a bell curve of increasing intensity to a leveling peak, followed by decreasing intensity to the cool-down period. Other methods explored in this section are interval training and circuit training.

The standard exercise prescription is to perform 15 to 20 minutes of cardiorespiratory endurance exercise in the target heart rate zone on three or four days per week. Adjust the application of training methods depending on the age, ability, and health-related fitness of each student. Building personal choice into each type of training can provide students with a way to individualize it to meet their needs. For example, your students might choose between a run for time and a run for distance during continuous training, take a shorter or longer rest option during interval training, and select a lower or higher step bench at a station during circuit training. You can also give students the opportunity to create their own workouts.

Continuous Training

Continuous training, or steady state training, involves performing the same activity or exercise over an extended period. This style of activity is most associated with aerobic exercise and is not common among children. **Continuous activity** is defined as "movement that lasts at least several minutes without rest periods" (NASPE, 2004,

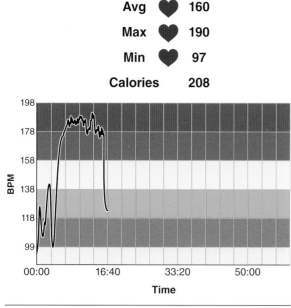

Avg	♥	160
Max	♥	190
Min	♥	97
Calories		208

FIGURE 5.6 Heart rate graph for a cardio workout for a 16-year-old female.

p. 6). As stated previously, vigorous continuous activity is not recommended for children 6 to 12 years old, but some continuous moderate activity is appropriate (NASPE, 2004). If you use continuous activity at the elementary level, incorporate plenty of rest periods. Continuous activity of 3 to 5 minutes at moderate intensity may be the limit for primary-grade or low-fit students, whereas 10 minutes may be a good limit for older elementary students (grades 3 through 5). Students in middle school and high school might perform 20 minutes or more of continuous activity, depending on their health-related fitness and goals.

For students at the high school level, it is important to calculate and monitor exercise heart rate. See figure 5.6 for an example of continuous training and associated heart rates for a high school female during physical education. Specifically, this graph shows a cardio workout for a 16-year-old female that lasts 16 minutes 40 seconds. She started class with her cardio work and implemented a gradual upward curve of intensity. At the end of the workout, she removed the monitor to complete her weightlifting workout.

At the middle school level, students can calculate heart rate but should not be required to maintain a set range. Because activity at high intensity can become discouraging for some students, it is best to limit the required time spent performing high-intensity activity, which is often more appropriate for training and conditioning athletes (unless students choose it). Middle school and high school students can either use the adult model and calculate target heart rates or simply perform the activity at a pace at which they can comfortably converse.

One way to provide continuous physical activity is through active, low-organization games. Teach games and activities that students will want to play in their free time. For middle school and high school students, mixing aerobic activities that sustain a moderate to vigorous level of intensity for a designated period may be more enjoyable and therefore more beneficial to their overall health-related fitness.

Fartlek training is a modification of continuous training in which periods of increased intensity are interspersed with continuous activity over varying and natural terrain. The word *fartlek* comes from the Swedish word for "speed play," and the bursts of higher-intensity exercise are spontaneous, not systematically controlled as in interval training. Fartlek training can help students develop aerobic power and focus on pacing, effort, and development of mental toughness (Greene & Pate, 2014). By adding variety, fartlek training can also increase motivation (Virgilio, 2011, p. 40). Although high-end fartlek training can be very demanding, this approach can also be used at a lower level to provide variety and fun in the workout. One simple option is to have students jog in lines of about six students (in a follow-the-leader style) and then, on a signal (or by student choice), have the person at the end of the line sprint to the front and become the leader. Figure 5.7 shows a sample fartlek training course appropriate for older, active elementary students. A similar modified activity can be designed for older students, especially if choice of intensity is built into the activity.

Interval Training

Interval training involves alternating moderate- to high-intensity effort with recovery periods. It includes high-intensity interval training, Tabata training, and anaerobic

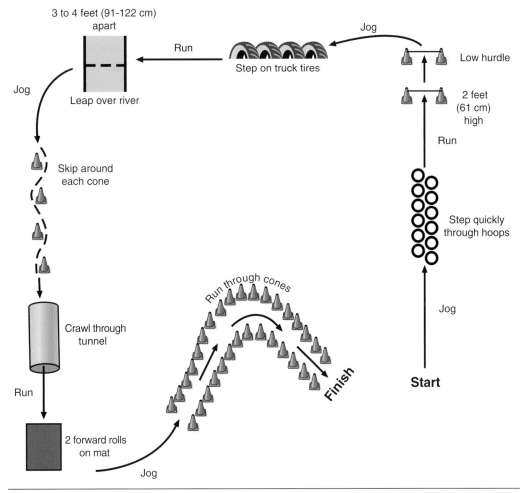

FIGURE 5.7 Sample fartlek training course. In order to use such a course, students should be of older elementary age and accustomed to being active at this level.

Adapted by permission from S. Virgilio, *Fitness Education for Children* (Champaign, IL: Human Kinetics, 1997), 149.

threshold training. By cycling through the target heart rate zone, students work for a short burst at their highest intensity with a recovery period at the low end of the zone. The ratio of work to rest is often 1:1, meaning the same length of time for activity as for rest, but it may be 1:2, 2:1, or another variation. An example of a 1:1 ratio would be to sprint for one minute and then rest or recover for one minute. In contrast, a two-minute hard run followed by one minute of rest would be an example of a 2:1 interval.

An alternative method is to have students determine their preexercise heart rate, do a designated amount of hard exercise, and then rest until they return to the preexercise heart rate. Once recovered, they can start the next interval. If using this approach, set up the exercise space so that students can restart without waiting in line behind someone or waiting for equipment at a station.

Intervals can be varied in length depending on the desired training effect. In physical education, the keys are to make the activity fun and to make high intensity a choice rather than a requirement. Leave wind sprints to the track coach! Instead, have your students (for example) play games that encourage fast breaks. For instance, they might pass a soccer ball between partners while running downfield as fast as they can. Students can also be given a choice between continuous and interval activity; remember, choice helps motivate students.

Aerobic interval training involves alternating the intensity of an activity between the low and high ends of the aerobic zone without using rest interval intensities outside the zone. For example, this approach might involve alternating medium and fast rope jumping as long as the intensity remains at a level where students can keep going rather than getting winded and having to stop for rest. Interval programs are often available on exercise equipment such as treadmills and stationary bikes.

High-intensity interval training (HIIT) has become a popular form of exercise in the adult fitness world. Workouts consist of very hard bouts of exercise followed by a rest or active-recovery interval. One form of HIIT is known as *Tabata*, after the Japanese researcher who partnered with coach Irisawa Koichi to develop HIIT for elite speed skaters. This method uses a four-minute workout consisting of eight rounds of 20 seconds of maximal effort and a 10-second rest. Tabata et al. (1996) rocked the fitness world with their research finding that four minutes of HIIT was as good as an hour of traditional endurance aerobic training!

A meta-analysis of HIIT research concluded that endurance training and HIIT both elicit large improvements in the $\dot{V}O_2$max of healthy individuals ranging from young adults to middle age; in fact, the gains in $\dot{V}O_2$max were greater with HIIT when with endurance training (Milanović, Sporiš, & Weston, 2015). In addition to providing aerobic conditioning, HIIT participants also improve their anaerobic conditioning. This wonderful news is tempered by the fact that the intervals of near-maximum to maximum effort are very strenuous, can result in considerable muscle soreness, and are not enjoyable for everyone. Fortunately, additional research has provided evidence that a lower level of exertion with a longer rest interval provides sedentary adults with similar aerobic benefits (Hood et al., 2011). In response to this research, a variety of exercise protocols have emerged. Depending on the goal, the high-intensity interval can be very short or up to about eight minutes.

HIIT was developed for and researched among adults, and caution must be employed when considering this type of training for youth. Interval training that is safe for all participants in a physical education class is individually flexible. For instance, a modification for high school students might allow students to maintain a self-selected high intensity for as long as possible (say, 15 to 30 seconds) with adjustments based on the individual student's condition. When the student can no longer maintain the exercise, intensity is reduced to allow the heart rate to return to the low end of the target heart rate zone. This type of interval training can be used, for example, with rope jumping that starts with a slow jump and progresses to a hard-as-you-can jump for a set (e.g., 25 reps) and then returns to slow jumping until the individual is ready for another intense bout. If you watch children play tag, their activity mimics HIIT with its all-out bursts followed by rest to catch their breath.

To prevent injuries and prepare for HIIT, it is recommended that an individual be at least moderately fit. With this mind, remember that one in six school children and adolescents are obese (Office of Disease Prevention and Health Promotion, 2016) and that many are not moderately fit, thus making HIIT an inappropriate workout for them. Note also that HIIT is not as lifetime oriented as are many other cardiorespiratory activities. Nonetheless, for students who are motivated to train this way, you can help them build their fitness by using continuous training and then ease them into an appropriate version of HIIT. Using a mix of interval and continuous training keeps workouts fresh. In all cases, it is important to warm up and cool down.

Circuit Training

Circuit training alternates cardiorespiratory endurance training with noncardio activity. Stations for noncardio work may include exercises for muscular endurance or strength, stretches for flexibility, sport skill work, or a short cognitive assignment. This approach offers a natural fit for developing children, because intermittent activity mixed with short rest periods is necessary for normal growth and development (Bailey et al., 1995). Students can do the exercise at one station and get a brief rest as they move to the next one. Stations can be designed to work well for every age, and they offer a great way to add variety and keep the workouts fresh. They can be set up with various challenge levels, and students can explore and self-select activities to promote success.

This type of activity removes the element of competition and the resulting necessity to determine winners and losers. Many Physical Best activities use stations and are designed so that all students can be active at the same time. In addition, once students have learned the basic routine (e.g., how and when to rotate, how to make choices at stations), the stations offer an efficient way to use class time in order to maximize physical activity with minimal need to explain the activity. To keep the circuit aerobic, however, the stations must involve variations of aerobic activity. Older elementary students and middle school and high school students can help design the stations as a practical application of the health-related fitness knowledge that they are learning. Figure 5.8 shows an example of a circuit appropriate for elementary-age children, and figure 5.9 shows one for secondary students; note that aspects of each circuit can work for all ages, as long as the equipment is sized properly.

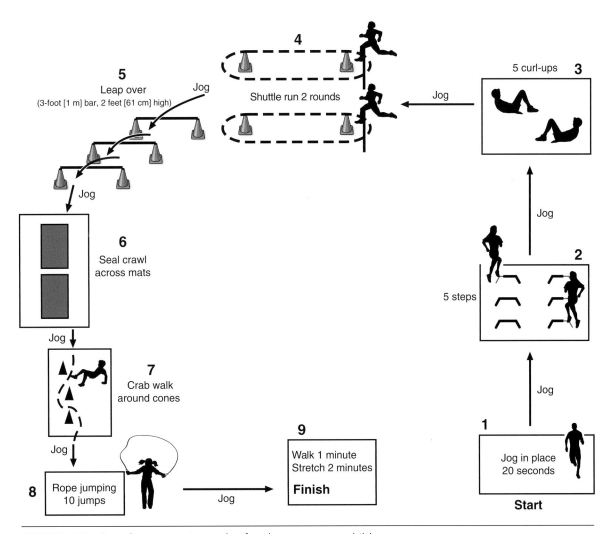

FIGURE 5.8 Sample circuit training plan for elementary-age children.

Adapted by permission from S. Virgilio, *Fitness Education for Children* (Champaign, IL: Human Kinetics, 1997), 158.

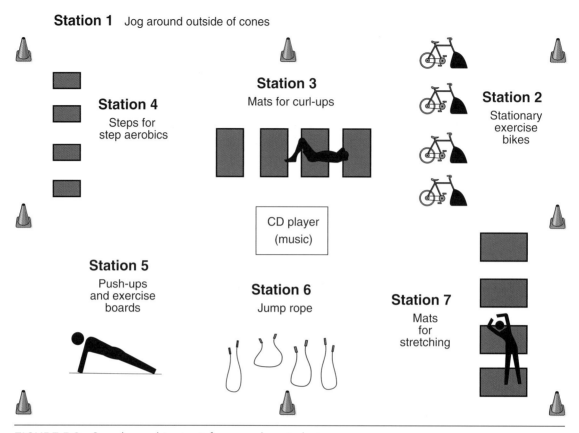

Station 1 Jog around outside of cones

Station 4
Steps for
step aerobics

Station 3
Mats for curl-ups

Station 2
Stationary
exercise
bikes

CD player
(music)

Station 5
Push-ups
and exercise
boards

Station 6
Jump rope

Station 7
Mats
for
stretching

FIGURE 5.9 Sample aerobic circuit for secondary students.

From Mosston and Ashworth (2002); Grineski (1996).

A circuit can be completed in a continuous fashion by spacing the students well enough that they do not have to stop. They can either move through it continuously (obstacle-course style) or complete timed stations with brief rests as they move from one station to the next. Instead of walking between stations, students can also be asked to jog a lap around the gym as they transition to the next station. Well-designed obstacle courses can provide both cardiorespiratory endurance and muscular fitness as long as students can maintain a moderate to vigorous pace. For example, you can intersperse aerobic activities such as agility runs and low hurdles with activities such as crawling through a tunnel and swinging across a space using a hanging rope. Stations arranged on a circuit also provide a good way to stretch the equipment that you have a little further. For example, if you have only four stationary bikes, you can place them in one station on a circuit and divide the class into groups of four.

Each student's level of health-related fitness should dictate the intensity and duration of the circuit. You can enable this individualization by providing options at the stations or by allowing students to move between stations at their own pace. To keep the activity organized and moving quickly, consider using task cards and arrow signs to help facilitate students' movement through the activities.

Safety Guidelines

Safety concerns for children differ from those for adults. For children, they focus mostly on joint safety and maintenance of appropriate body temperature. Younger children should experience lifetime activities and avoid highly structured, high-intensity training. Exercising in heat is a concern for children, especially in the spring and early summer, when temperatures rise before children's bodies have acclimated to the heat. Special attention must be paid to children who are obese or who have asthma, diabetes, cardiac issues, or orthopedic concerns. School nurses and district policies may provide guidance and protocols. To paraphrase the Hippocratic oath: Above all, do no harm. Help students become lifelong learners and active, healthy adults.

Many safety issues must be considered when helping children increase their cardiorespiratory endurance. Keep in mind the following information about physiological differences between adults and children when manipulating the principles of training (Bar-Or, 1984; Rowland, 1996):

- Children produce more heat than adults do relative to body size, both at rest and during exercise (i.e., with equal absolute workloads).

- Children sweat less than adults do and therefore have difficulty using evaporation as a method of heat dissipation.

- Prepubertal children cannot sustain exercise in hot environments as well as adults can.

- Children also fatigue sooner than adults do when exercising in the heat.

- Children are less economical in their activity and use more oxygen than adults do at any given submaximal exercise intensity.

- Children's heart rates are generally higher than those of adults, both at rest and across all levels of exercise.

- Children's maximal heart rates generally vary from 195 to 205, and large variability is present between individual subjects.

- Children have less efficient **ventilation** (volume of air moved) than do adults.

- Children have higher breathing frequencies and lower **tidal volume** (volume of air either inhaled or exhaled in a normal resting breath) than do adults.

- Children have higher pulmonary ventilation (breathing frequency × tidal volume) per liter of oxygen consumed than adults do during submaximal and maximal exercise.

- Children hyperventilate during exercise more than adults do.

Thus we must recognize the physiological differences between adults and children in order to support children and help them safely improve their cardiorespiratory endurance. Children have smaller organs in proportion to body size than do adults; they also have less efficient metabolism. As a result, they may experience less of a training effect in terms of ventilatory oxygen uptake. In addition, because their ratio of body surface area to body mass is higher than that of adults, children are at risk for heat gain when exercising

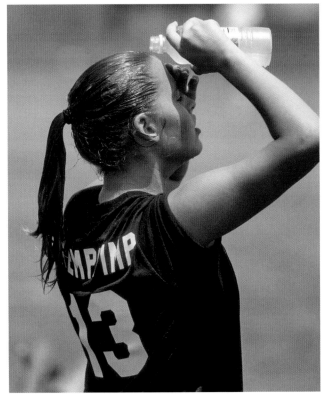

Adjust exercise intensity and take hydration breaks when children are participating in cardiorespiratory endurance activities in warm temperatures.

in temperatures above body temperature. The capacity to cool themselves is also inhibited by their lower rate of sweat production (Rowland, 2008).

Because of these physiological factors, we must build in frequent rest periods, especially for younger students, and provide water before, during, and after physical activity. In hot and humid weather, avoid conducting sessions with elementary children and consider slowing down or canceling activity with middle schoolers and high schoolers. Although most students in your classes will handle cardiorespiratory endurance activities safely, you will encounter a few who will need special guidance and modified activities. Be sure that you know which students have medical conditions and special needs so that you can modify health-related fitness activities to be as inclusive as possible. Not all of these conditions will be obvious, so review school records, consult with the school nurse, talk with parents and classroom teachers, and carefully follow school or district policies to ensure that you are fully informed. Ask for input about what each student in question can handle and seek advice about how to safely apply the overload and progression principles and the FITT guidelines. If in doubt, obtain written parental permission to talk with the student's health care provider.

Technology

Many wearable devices, as well as smart phone apps, can be used to monitor intensity and track distance, speed, steps, and calories. Some are good only for rough estimates, whereas others provide data that are precise, accurate, and reliable. The way in which a device monitors and calculates physical activity makes a difference in how reliable and valid the measures will be. For example, less accurate data will be obtained from a heart rate monitor that depends on picking up the pulse in a finger placed on a button on a wrist-only monitor or from an app on a device that reads heart rate by placing the finger over a light. In contrast, more accurate data will be obtained from a heart rate monitor with a sensor on a band worn around the chest. The accuracy level needed may be dictated by a lesson's purpose. For instance, in a lesson on the change in heart rate during various activities, the technology needs only to be accurate enough to rank-order the activities. On the other hand, a lesson using THRZ requires more accuracy. Therefore, when selecting which technology to use, one must consider not only cost but also purpose.

Technology should also be matched to the developmental level of the students. For example, young children who cannot count above 20 are not able to compare pedometer steps in the hundreds and thousands, and students who don't yet understand percentages are not able to calculate or fully understand the concept of a heart rate zone of 60 percent to 80 percent of HR max. Finally, given the wide array of apps available, we should also teach students to be good consumers. It can be very instructional to walk them through apps that prescribe cardiorespiratory endurance programs and ask them if the activities are being presented correctly. You might also ask them how the activities might be modified for different levels of health-related fitness or to make physical accommodations for individuals with disabilities.

Technology can also facilitate gamification, which is another fun way to integrate cardiorespiratory endurance. Students can play computer-generated games, download motivational apps, or get out for a walk or hike while using geocaching, letterboxing, or a version of Pokémon Go.

Heart Rate Monitors

Heart rate monitors (HRMs) are useful because they quantify intensity, provide students with immediate feedback, and help students more accurately rate perceived exertion and understand what their target zone feels like. These monitors provide accurate information, whereas some students may have difficulty manually palpating the pulse, especially children below the fourth grade. If you are using heart rate monitors at the elementary level, make sure to use them for fun and for teaching cardiorespiratory endurance concepts—not for attaining a specified target heart rate zone. You might try activities such as asking students, "Who can get their heart rate to 140 beats per minute? How about 150 beats per minute?" Follow the activity with a rest period, then repeat the sequence using different heart rate goals. This routine provides short bursts of activity, is considered vigorous activity when higher heart rates are used, and provides a goal for elementary students to attain for brief periods. At the middle school and high school levels, using monitors to check calculated target heart rate or exercise intensity can help teach students about individualizing their cardiorespiratory endurance workout.

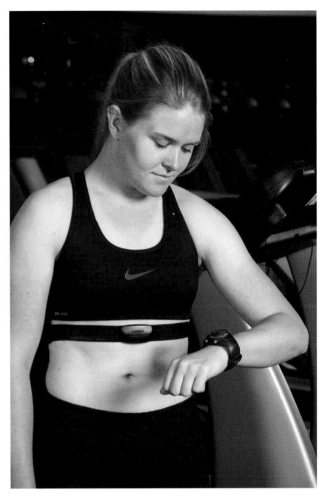

Heart rate monitors can help older students check their target heart rate or exercise intensity, and they are a fun way for younger students to learn cardiorespiratory endurance concepts.

Heart rate monitors are also useful for teaching students of all ages about pacing. Students can run, try to guess their heart rate, and then check their estimates against the monitor. They can also learn pacing by trying to traverse a certain distance in a designated time; for example, jogging one-eighth of a mile (one-fifth of a kilometer) in one minute is equivalent to the pace of an eight-minute mile (five-minute kilometer). Students can set the stopwatch on the HRM, jog, and then see whether they are close to a 1-minute time. Using this self-testing, older students can try various pacing levels and see what pace keeps them in their target heart rate zone. For more information about heart rate monitors, see chapter 13.

Step Count Devices

The many wearable step count devices, including wristbands and pedometers, offer a fun and motivating way to challenge students to be more active. Both practitioners and researchers endorse the usefulness of pedometers for measuring and promoting physical activity (Beighle, Pangrazi, & Vincent, 2001; Cuddihy, Pangrazi, & Tomson, 2005; Tudor-Locke et al., 2004). These devices can record steps taken, miles traveled, calories used, and time spent exercising. Some also use an accelerometer to measure the amount of time spent in moderate to vigorous activity, which is an indication of cardiorespiratory endurance exercise.

Pedometers are so useful because they are inexpensive and easy to obtain and provide an objective measure of physical activity. Using pedometers is especially helpful when working with children, who often have difficulty discerning how much moderate to vigorous activity they perform. Although not all pedometers perform equally well, the research generally finds electronic pedometers to be reliable and valid indicators of physical activity (Beets, Patton, & Edwards, 2005; Crouter, Schneider, Karabulut, & Bassett, 2003; Schneider, Crouter, & Bassett, 2004; Schneider, Crouter, Lukajic, & Bassett, 2003). More specifically, they tend to be accurate in assessing number of steps, less accurate in assessing distance, and even less accurate in assessing kilocalories used (Crouter et al., 2003).

Wristbands range in capability from simple step counters to sophisticated devices that can track steps, heart rate, and sleeping stages and provide GPS data and information about health-related fitness. The cost of these devices varies greatly. They can serve as excellent tools for teaching students how to monitor activity time and intensity and track personal data, but the cost may prevent many physical education programs from purchasing a class set. Fortunately, these devices are not necessary in order to provide students with the tools they need for developing physical literacy. At the same time, introducing students to them can help students prepare for self-monitoring and self-motivating in the future. Many fitness apps are available to educate and motivate exercisers and to quantify the amount and intensity of exercise; see the list provided in the web resource.

Students will often ask how many steps they should take in a day. In the same vein, a number of studies including both adults and children have been conducted in an attempt to link daily step counts to health benefits and recommended levels of physical activity. Because children are naturally more active than adults are, the adult standard of 10,000 steps (Hatano, 1993; Welk et al., 2000) may be low for them. Tudor-Locke and colleagues (2004) examined the relationship between steps per day and body mass index (BMI). They found that girls and boys aged 6 through 12 who accumulated 12,000 and 15,000 steps, respectively, tended to be under the international BMI standard for being overweight or obese. Additional research is needed to address questions such as whether healthier children simply take more steps or whether taking a certain number of steps results in healthier children. Note that pedometers and some wristbands do not log physical activity done during activities such as biking and swimming; however, some of the more sophisticated wearable devices are waterproof and can be used during a variety of activities.

To address individual differences, Pangrazi, Beighle, and Sidman (2003) suggest the following baseline and goal-setting approach. A baseline count is determined by wearing the step counter for four days (for children) or eight days (for adolescents and adults) and determining the average number of steps per day. A 10 percent increase in steps is then calculated and added to the step goal every two weeks. The overall goal is to achieve about 4,000 to 6,000 steps above baseline. For example, a student whose baseline is 6,000 steps will increase that amount by 600 steps every two weeks to work up to 10,000 to 12,000 steps per day.

Assessing Cardiorespiratory Endurance

As students learn about health-related fitness and move toward becoming physically literate people, the teaching and learning process involves assessment of cardiorespiratory endurance. As you may recall, cardiorespiratory endurance is the ability to perform large-muscle, dynamic movement at a moderate to vigorous level of intensity for a prolonged period. The oxygen needs of working muscles are supported by the cardiovascular and respiratory systems through the process of oxygen uptake. Measured in terms of $\dot{V}O_2$, oxygen uptake increases proportionately with an increase in intensity of exercise. When $\dot{V}O_2$ cannot increase, it has reached its maximum level, which is known as $\dot{V}O_2$max, or aerobic capacity, and serves as a quantification of cardiorespiratory endurance. $\dot{V}O_2$max can be improved with training, but it also is influenced by genetics (Centers for Disease and Control and Prevention, n.d.).

$\dot{V}O_2$max is usually determined in a laboratory setting by measuring the oxygen and carbon dioxide levels of inspired and expired air. In physical education settings, it can be estimated as a proxy for cardiorespiratory endurance, or aerobic capacity, through field tests, such as FitnessGram's PACER (progressive aerobic cardiovascular endurance run; developed by the Cooper Institute), and the mile-run and mile-walk tests. Choosing the appropriate test is important to the outcome. You (or the students) should choose the test that is appropriate for both the age group and the current levels of activity and cardiorespiratory endurance of the participants. The PACER test (15- or 20-meter) is recommended at all levels and is especially suited to the go-and-stop activity preferences of young children. The PACER test is recommended for all ages, and it is the preferred test for participants in grades K through 3, with whom it should be administered with an emphasis on having fun. There are no health-related fitness standards for this age group; participation should be a pleasant experience. When practicing the PACER (at any age), you can add age-appropriate music and allow students to have more than one miss and to reenter after a rest. These approaches encourage students to build endurance, not to view the test as a pass-or-fail endeavor. The PACER also serves as an excellent tool for teaching the concept of pacing for the mile run.

For older, orthopedically compromised, or obese students, other test options may be more appropriate or additionally useful. The mile-walk test, which levels the field to the mode of walking, is individualized because it incorporates the participant's weight and heart rate into the calculation of $\dot{V}O_2$max. In addition, it does not favor those with a tendency toward fast-twitch muscle fibers. The mile run, in contrast, may not be a safe choice for deconditioned or obese students. It is possible to test the mile walk and mile run concurrently by giving students a choice of exercise mode. Regardless of the test used, make sure that students understand the field-test scores in terms of $\dot{V}O_2$max.

The Cooper Institute provides a free web-based version of the *FitnessGram/ActivityGram Reference Guide* at www.cooperinstitute.org/fitnessgram/components. FitnessGram also provides the capability to compare results ($\dot{V}O_2$max estimates) among the three cardiorespiratory endurance tests. Note that it uses the term *aerobic capacity* instead of *cardiorespiratory endurance* because *aerobic capacity* refers more specifically to the volume of oxygen consumed, whereas *cardiorespiratory endurance* refers to the amount of exercise that can be sustained using that oxygen.

Physical Best also supports the use of the Brockport Physical Fitness Test (BPFT) for youngsters with disabilities. The BPFT is a health-related fitness assessment that can be easily customized through selection of any of its 27 items, which are organized in three domains: aerobic function, body composition, and musculoskeletal function. To test cardiorespiratory endurance, use the PACER, the target aerobic movement test, or the one-mile run or walk. The test protocols and standards are available at https://www.pyfp.org/doc/brockport/brockport-ch5.pdf. The BPFT can be used to identify current level of performance, identify unique needs, and establish annual goals, including short-term objectives (Winnick & Short, 2014). Therefore, it can serve as a valuable tool not only for health-related fitness testing but also for the development of an individualized education plan for students with disabilities. For more information, refer to the *Brockport Physical Fitness Test Manual: A Health-Related Assessment for Youngsters with Disabilities* (Winnick & Short, 2014).

Cardiorespiratory Endurance and the Curriculum

Cardiorespiratory endurance can be infused into the curriculum in several ways. One way is to design a separate health-related fitness segment for every lesson. This segment might be an extension of the warm-up, where students perform an extended run or a series of stations that include items such as step boxes, agility ladders, jump ropes, and low hurdles. Warm-ups can also include moving (e.g., jogging, shuffling) between specified lines on a court or field. Another option is to make aerobic exercise an integral part of a sport activity by having students jog while, for instance, dribbling or passing a ball back and forth, playing running games (e.g., capture the flag), or playing in small-sided games (e.g., 3v3) in relatively large spaces so that they have to move a lot. A third way to incorporate cardiorespiratory endurance is to center a unit on it. This approach might involve outdoor activities such as treasure hunts, geocaching, hiking, and track and field, or it might take place in a fitness facility with cardio equipment. It might also take the form of group fitness activities, such as Zumba or cardio kickboxing.

Cardiorespiratory endurance can be taught effectively in many ways. Regardless of your approach, one key element is vertical curriculum. You should introduce concepts at the elementary level and build on them all the way through high school graduation. The following two unit examples incorporate best practices; each step can be used for one or several lessons.

Teaching Motor Skills and Cardiorespiratory Endurance

The importance of skill development should not be underestimated, especially at the elementary level. Happily, many of the Physical Best activities provide opportunities to simultaneously develop motor skills and cardiorespiratory endurance. For example, Around the Block is an elementary activity available in the web resource that requires students to walk, jog, and leap to practice pacing and focusing on time while simultaneously developing cardiorespiratory endurance.

Sample Ideas for the Elementary Level

- *Step 1.* Introduce terms that will be used to learn about cardiorespiratory endurance. Introduce the idea of cardiorespiratory endurance and the concept of intensity from the FITT principle. Focus on deeper and faster breathing and on speeding up the heart rate. Have students perform some activities that grow in intensity, such as starting with a turtle walk, moving to a bear walk, and eventually galloping like a horse and soaring like an eagle. Between the animal movements, ask students to place a hand on their chest and check to see if their heartbeat is going slower, the same, or faster. Reverse the order for a cool-down.

- *Step 2.* Set up stations with a variety of activities. Ask students to identify which activities will improve cardiorespiratory endurance; to help them decide, ask them about increased breathing and heart rate. Add the guideline of being physically active every day and ask students to do cardiorespiratory endurance activities at home and draw pictures of them for the bulletin board.

- *Step 3.* Reinforce the idea of being active, including cardiorespiratory endurance activity every day per the frequency element of the FITT principle. Then add the *T* for time by adding the 60 minutes a day. The station activity for the day should consist completely of cardiorespiratory endurance activities in order to show students the many ways in which they can be active. Stations might include, for instance, a variety of rope-jumping stations, step aerobics boxes, agility ladders, and scooter traverses. Periodically ask students to stop and check how fast their hearts are beating and whether they are breathing faster. Then have them cool down and check breathing and heart rate again.

- *Step 4.* Reinforce the FITT elements of frequency, intensity, and time. Then add type. Students have experienced many types of cardiorespiratory endurance activity in the circuit. Now, introduce the use of game play to work on cardiorespiratory endurance. A variety of activities can be used here, including traditional team sports (e.g., soccer), tag games, and dance routines. Periodically ask students to check for faster breathing and heart rate. Then have them cool down and check breathing and heart rate again.

A cardiorespiratory endurance unit can also be tied in with a Kids Heart Challenge Event or a healthy-heart unit keyed to Valentine's Day. Here are some additional approaches:

- Rather than do a straight cardiorespiratory endurance unit, consider developing a unit that teaches all four of the health-related components of fitness and the characteristics and benefits of activities that fall into each category.

- Instead of (or in addition to) a stand-alone unit on health-related fitness, build cardiorespiratory endurance activities into every lesson plan through instant activities, health-related fitness stations, and use of aerobic movement in skill-based activities.

Sample Ideas for the Middle School and High School Levels

Here again, cardiorespiratory endurance can be taught in multiple ways, and the optimal choice depends on a number of factors, which may include facility, teaching staff, equipment, weather, and class length. Some schools have state-of-the-art fitness centers replete with a variety of cardio machines, whereas others have dance or fitness spaces that work well for group fitness, and some have appropriate weather for activities such as snowshoeing or outdoor cycling. Class length, for instance, may vary from 40 to 90 minutes. Shorter lesson times work well with group fitness and station work, whereas longer lesson times allow for extended activities such as orienteering. Regardless of the activity used, teach the exercise principles and the FITT guidelines. Here are four options:

- *Cardiorespiratory endurance unit.* In this option, the entire unit is focused on cardiorespiratory endurance. Students can learn or review the definition of it, as well as the FITT guidelines and how to apply the principles of exercise. You can then establish a baseline to inform students' goals either by assessing them now or, if FitnessGram tests are conducted on a regular basis, by using their last PACER or mile-run score. To reach their goals, students can be guided in how to set up a plan using the FITT guidelines. To increase motivation, allow students to select one or more activities to work toward their goals. Options might include following (or creating) a group fitness routine (e.g., cardio kickboxing, Zumba), using a cardio machine (e.g., treadmill, spin bike, elliptical machine, rower), completing an interval routine, or playing a game with a sufficient level of activity (e.g., 3v3 soccer or basketball). The choices may be determined in part by the facilities available. For example, if the class space is a fitness room, then the choices must all be doable in that space. If team teaching is available, more options in a second space can be offered while still maintaining supervision and feedback opportunities. Students can monitor their use of the FITT guidelines by logging their accomplishments, either in a paper journal or in a digital program or app. Journal entries can include items such as minutes of moderate to vigorous activity, distance (e.g., laps), number of pedometer steps, heart rate information, and talk-test levels or ratings of perceived exertion.

- *Elected activities.* This option offers students several activity choices, all of which enhance cardiorespiratory endurance. This model differs from the individualized approach presented in option 1 in that, in this option, all students who make the same choice will engage in the chosen activity as a group. Units of this type might range from swimming to spinning to hiking to Zumba and might encompass both indoor and outdoor possibilities, depending on weather and climate.

- *Embedded cardiorespiratory endurance.* This option requires you to plan skill practices and games in a way that embeds cardiorespiratory endurance into the activity. For example, tennis students might try to achieve a certain number of pedometer steps by keeping their feet "alive" while waiting for return shots, running or walking briskly to pick up balls, and rushing the net whenever possible. You might also engage students in a scavenger hunt tied to health-related fitness by trying to find the items as quickly as possible or establishing specific rules for other games that keep players moving. For instance, the goalie rule in Sabakiball requires the goalie to start play with a new ball within three seconds after the game ball goes out of bounds. Sports such as Ultimate Frisbee and soccer can also be made even more aerobic by using small groups (e.g., 3v3).

- *Lesson segment on health-related fitness.* In this option, a portion of class time is allocated to working on cardiorespiratory endurance. This segment might involve students in doing a series of cardiorespiratory endurance stations, either before or after a skill- or game-based lesson or by participating in one of the Physical Best activities that teaches a concept (e.g., continuous rope jumping). An individualized approach can be used by allowing students to select a cardiorespiratory endurance activity from a list and complete a number of minutes or a number of pedometer steps before moving on to the rest of the lesson. For example, students might perform 3,000 steps by jumping rope, following a group fitness video, or running on a treadmill before moving on to a weight training activity.

Summary

Cardiorespiratory endurance activities can and should be enjoyable at every age. Young children who thrive on intermittent, playful activities can learn which activities are heart healthy and what it feels like to exercise at moderate and vigorous intensities. Middle school students can start to improve pacing and learn how to determine intensity by using ratings of perceived exertion and heart rate, but they still should not be held to target heart rate zone criteria. High school students can learn how intensity relates to oxygen consumption, heart rate, and perceptions of exertion and how to create individualized workouts to improve or maintain cardiorespiratory endurance. The joy of cardiorespiratory endurance movement can be created or sustained by teaching a wide variety of activities and allowing students to work at their own level. Simply getting moving can start an upward spiral of positive health behaviors.

Cardiorespiratory endurance can be combined with skill development and built into many activities already offered in the curriculum. Students can also learn about technologies that can support their attainment of healthy levels of cardiorespiratory endurance. In addition, they can learn to assess their cardiorespiratory endurance using the PACER test, mile walk, or mile run. The ultimate goal is for students to find activities that they enjoy, develop a healthy activity pattern, and understand how to apply the FITT guidelines and other training principles to reach their physical best!

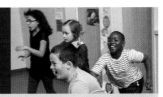

Discussion Questions

1. List the benefits of developing cardiorespiratory endurance and explain how to describe these benefits in terms that students can understand.

2. Since most programs do not provide enough time to meet physical activity guidelines in physical education class, how can you encourage your students to meet them outside of class?

3. What are some factors that influence $\dot{V}O_2$max in students (especially young children) and make it difficult to determine how much improvement results from participation and training?

4. How can teachers design cardiorespiratory endurance activities and assessments in a way that protects the emotional safety of all students and are fun for all?

5. Why is it important to include relative measures (e.g., THRZ, percent increase in pedometer steps) rather than depending on absolute measures (e.g., 10,000 steps, time of a completed mile run) when building up a student's cardiorespiratory endurance?

6. Pedometers can be great motivators, but students are often told to reach a one-size-fits-all number of steps. How can you use goal setting and individualize step counts?

7. Choose a sport skill activity that is not aerobic and modify it into an activity that supports the improvement or maintenance of cardiorespiratory endurance.

8. What kinds of things interfere with getting an accurate heart rate count? When heart rate is not a good indicator during exercise, what are some alternative methods that one can use to estimate exercise intensity?

9. Children are physiologically different from adults. How will these differences influence your teaching and assessment of cardiorespiratory endurance?

10. Create a circuit training workout that includes cardiorespiratory endurance training, sport-specific skills, and a short cognitive assignment for elementary, middle school, and high school students (one for each level).

CHAPTER 6

Body Composition

Scott Going and Melanie Hingle

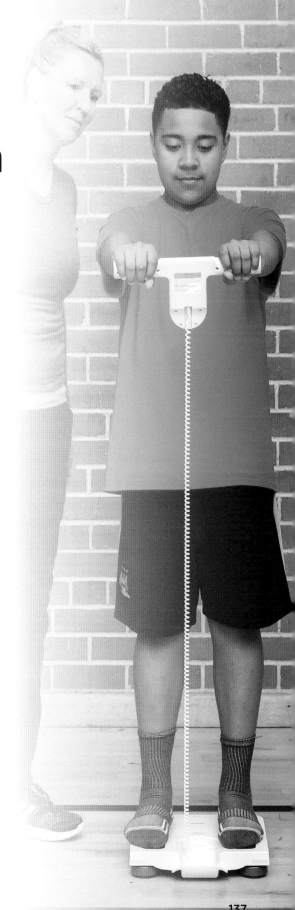

Few physical educators would deny that teaching about body composition is one of the most sensitive areas of health-related fitness education. The topic is complicated by factors related to cultural, social, and personal beliefs and attitudes, and the temptation to avoid the subject may be strong. Nonetheless, understanding body composition—including what affects it and what benefits are provided by a healthy body composition—is critical to overall health-related fitness. The importance of this topic is underscored by the current obesity epidemic among children and adolescents, with its attendant health issues, especially in adolescents. Although it is not important to calculate exact indicators of body composition for very young children, these children still need to explore the related concepts and understand how body composition is affected by an active lifestyle. Older children also need this information, as well as tools to monitor and affect body composition positively throughout life. This information is critical for preventing chronic disease.

Teaching Guidelines for Body Composition

The term **body composition** refers to the amounts and proportions of body constituents—that is, the atoms, molecules, and tissues that make up the body mass (Going, Hingle, & Farr, 2013). In practice, in a health setting, body composition is typically assessed in terms of the amount of body fat and the amount of lean body mass, which includes all tissues other than fat (e.g., bone, muscle, organs, and body fluids). It is usually expressed in terms of percent body weight. Excess fat and high fat-to-lean ratio represent health risks. Several methods are available for gauging whether body composition is healthy, and value ranges have been identified that represent healthy percent body fat. Recommended ranges for boys and girls are presented in tables 6.1 and 6.2, respectively (Plowman & Meredith, 2013).

TABLE 6.1   FitnessGram Body Composition Standards for Boys

	PERCENT BODY FAT				BODY MASS INDEX			
Age	Very lean	HFZ	NI (some risk)	NI (high risk)	Very lean	HFZ	NI (some risk)	NI (high risk)
5	≤8.8	8.9-18.8	≥18.9	≥27.0	≤13.8	13.9-16.8	≥16.9	≥18.1
6	≤8.4	8.5-18.8	≥18.9	≥27.0	≤13.7	13.8-17.1	≥17.2	≥18.8
7	≤8.2	8.3-18.8	≥18.9	≥27.0	≤13.7	13.8-17.6	≥17.7	≥19.6
8	≤8.3	8.4-18.8	≥18.9	≥27.0	≤13.9	14.0-18.2	≥18.3	≥20.6
9	≤8.6	8.7-20.6	≥20.7	≥30.1	≤14.1	14.2-18.9	≥19.0	≥21.6
10	≤8.8	8.9-22.4	≥22.5	≥33.2	≤14.4	14.5-19.7	≥19.8	≥22.7
11	≤8.7	8.8-23.6	≥23.7	≥35.4	≤14.8	14.9-20.5	≥20.6	≥23.7
12	≤8.3	8.4-23.6	≥23.7	≥35.9	≤15.2	15.3-21.3	≥21.4	≥24.7
13	≤7.7	7.8-22.8	≥22.9	≥35.0	≤15.7	15.8-22.2	≥22.3	≥25.6
14	≤7.0	7.1-21.3	≥21.4	≥33.2	≤16.3	16.4-23.0	≥23.1	≥26.5
15	≤6.5	6.6-20.1	≥20.2	≥31.5	≤16.8	16.9-23.7	≥23.8	≥27.2
16	≤6.4	6.5-20.1	≥20.2	≥31.6	≤17.4	17.5-24.5	≥24.6	≥27.9
17	≤6.6	6.7-20.9	≥21.0	≥33.0	≤18.0	18.1-24.9	≥25.0	≥28.6
>17	≤6.9	7.0-22.2	≥22.3	≥35.1	≤18.5	18.6-24.9	≥25.0	≥29.3

HFZ = healthy fitness zone
NI = needs improvement

Reprinted by permission from Cooper Institute, *Fitnessgram/Activitygram Test Administration Manual*, 5th ed. (Dallas, TX: Cooper Institute), 86.

TABLE 6.2   FitnessGram Body Composition Standards for Girls

Age	PERCENT BODY FAT				BODY MASS INDEX			
	Very lean	HFZ	NI (some risk)	NI (high risk)	Very lean	HFZ	NI (some risk)	NI (high risk)
5	≤9.7	9.8-20.8	≥20.9	≥28.4	≤13.5	13.6-16.8	≥16.9	≥18.5
6	≤9.8	9.9-20.8	≥20.9	≥28.4	≤13.4	13.5-17.2	≥17.3	≥19.2
7	≤10.0	10.1-20.8	≥20.9	≥28.4	≤13.5	13.6-17.9	≥18.0	≥20.2
8	≤10.4	10.5-20.8	≥20.9	≥28.4	≤13.6	13.7-18.6	≥18.7	≥21.2
9	≤10.9	11.0-22.6	≥22.7	≥30.8	≤13.9	14.0-19.4	≥19.5	≥22.4
10	≤11.5	11.6-24.3	≥24.4	≥33.0	≤14.2	14.3-20.3	≥20.4	≥23.6
11	≤12.1	12.2-25.7	≥25.8	≥34.5	≤14.6	14.7-21.2	≥21.3	≥24.7
12	≤12.6	12.7-26.7	≥26.8	≥35.5	≤15.1	15.2-22.1	≥22.2	≥25.8
13	≤13.3	13.4-27.7	≥27.8	≥36.3	≤15.6	15.7-22.9	≥23.0	≥26.8
14	≤13.9	14.0-28.5	≥28.6	≥36.8	≤16.1	16.2-23.6	≥23.7	≥27.7
15	≤14.5	14.6-29.1	≥29.2	≥37.1	≤16.6	16.7-24.3	≥24.4	≥28.5
16	≤15.2	15.3-29.7	≥29.8	≥37.4	≤17.0	17.1-24.8	≥24.9	≥29.3
17	≤15.8	15.9-30.4	≥30.5	≥37.9	≤17.4	17.5-24.9	≥25.0	≥30.0
>17	≤16.4	16.5-31.3	≥31.4	≥38.6	≤17.7	17.8-24.9	≥25.0	≥30.0

HFZ = healthy fitness zone

NI = needs improvement

Reprinted by permission from Cooper Institute, *Fitnessgram/Activitygram Test Administration Manual*, 5th ed. (Dallas, TX: Cooper Institute), 87.

To teach students about body composition in a sensitive and professional manner, you should be mindful of four main considerations:

- Project an attitude of acceptance toward individual differences and demand that students follow your lead with their peers.
- Respect each person's privacy (e.g., collect and discuss individual measures in private).
- Relate body composition to the other components of health-related fitness in meaningful ways.
- Acknowledge whether or not you can help a student who is over or under an appropriate body fat and refer the student and parents to professional help if body composition suggests high risk for health concerns.

Accepting Individual Differences

You should avoid asserting that there are absolute indicators of good and poor health related to body composition. Remember, all methods (laboratory and field) have some degree of error, and the healthy range is wide. In addition, explain to students that genetics plays a role in body composition (this topic is discussed in detail later in the chapter). Never use a student as a positive or negative model of body composition. Instead, encourage students to find personal satisfaction with their overall health, wellness, nutrition, and physical activity habits rather than struggling to measure up to a rigid standard or to cultural expectations. Remind students that "normal" comes in all shapes and sizes. With adolescents, it may be helpful to discuss unrealistic images of ideal body types portrayed in the media, as well as the resulting emphasis on appearance rather than health.

Respecting Privacy

Never publicize a student's measurements or percent body fat; to the contrary, secure the information where other students cannot access it. Some students may be reluctant to be measured in front of their peers. With this potential for sensitivity in mind, conduct weighing, skinfold caliper assessment, and any other measurement in private and as a voluntary activity. Explain to students that body composition is a personal matter and that they should focus only on their own information. Remember that individual student data are protected by the Family Educational Rights and Privacy Act (FERPA; U.S. Department of Education, 2011). In addition, check with a school administrator about any other guidelines that may be in place. For example, parental permission may be needed (or parental notification completed) before conducting for body mass index or skinfold assessment. It may also be prudent to have another adult present during assessment to prevent any potential harassment issues.

Relating Body Composition to Other Health-Related Fitness Components

As with any component of health-related fitness, a person's body composition does not exist in isolation from the other components. Show students the connections between all of the components so that they can see clearly how their personal choices in various areas affect this particular area. Although genetics plays a significant role, body composition can be modified with regular participation in activities designed to improve other health-related fitness components (e.g., cardiorespiratory endurance, muscle strengthening). Here are some specific connections:

- *Cardiorespiratory endurance.* Aerobic activities burn calories and help maintain a healthy weight.
- *Muscular strength and endurance.* Lean tissue with its high muscle fraction burns (metabolizes) more calories at rest than does adipose (fat) tissue. Moreover, the most significant source of calorie burning is resting metabolism. Thus physical activity that follows the principles of training (chapter 3) and is designed to promote muscle strength and endurance burns calories and helps maintain an appropriate body composition. In contrast, a low level of muscle, like excess body fat, is associated with higher levels of risk factors for chronic disease (Kim & Valdez, 2015).
- *Flexibility.* A flexible body can better tolerate activities that support cardiorespiratory endurance and muscular strength and endurance and thus contribute

Selecting Apps to Help Improve Physical Activity and Dietary Behaviors

Look for an app that has the following functionality:

- Self-monitoring (tracking, feedback, visualization)
- Goal setting (with customization)
- Connecting with others (social support)
- Credibility (trustworthy source?)
- Evidence-based information aligned with national recommendations

Finally, try out the app before recommending it to others.

to a desirable body composition. Flexibility enables a student to participate in activities more easily, thus increasing the likelihood of participation in the first place.

Strive to point out connections between physical activity, diet, and body composition related to daily life, recreational pursuits, and physical education activities. Emphasize, too, that a student who is overfat because of genetics can still greatly reduce health risks by being physically active even in the absence of significant changes in body weight and composition (Bell et al., 2007; Shaibi et al., 2006). Even without calorie restriction, physical activity helps reduce a person's risk for chronic disease, regardless of the person's level of obesity (Ross, Freeman, & Janssen, 2000; U.S. Department of Health and Human Services, 2001). Several studies have now shown that overfat people who exercise regularly are at no greater health risk than thin people who don't exercise (Allen et al., 2007; Boreham et al., 2001; Haskell et al., 2007).

Body composition concepts can be integrated into classes designed to teach other concepts and skills. In elementary school, it is appropriate to emphasize that one's body is made of different types of tissues (e.g., muscle, bone, organs, adipose tissue) that are all important and that can be kept in the right proportions by being physically active and eating healthy foods. In middle school and high school, it is reasonable to discuss healthy ratios of lean mass and fat mass, their relationship to disease risk (e.g., diabetes, heart disease), and their contribution to and effect on various skills, locomotor activities, and health-related fitness activities. At this level, it is appropriate to engage students in projects related to self-assessment, personal goal setting, and personal logging, all of which can be facilitated by a variety of apps and other resources.

On the elementary level, concepts related to body composition can be incorporated into the curriculum through simple games that help younger students understand that their bodies need a balance of different types of tissues. Examples of two games are given in the sidebar titled Activities for Teaching Body Composition Concepts to Younger Students. Both of these activities should be used only after a supportive class climate has been established and students are ready to care for each other. Classes where teasing or remarks about individual students might be made should first spend time building a class culture of respect.

Activities for Teaching Body Composition Concepts to Younger Students

Simple games can be used to help younger students understand concepts of body composition. Activity 1 helps students understand that their bodies need different types of tissues. Activity 2 lets them experience what it might feel like to carry extra weight and how it might affect their engagement in physical activity.

Activity 1

Depending on student and equipment numbers, provide one hoop to each student, pair of students, or group of students. Make piles of colored beanbags around the area, each pile a different color. Blue bags represent bone, red bags represent muscle, green bags represent organs, and yellow bags represent fat. The object of the game is for students to assemble a healthy body in their hoop.

To get a beanbag, students must perform prescribed activities:

- *Blue beanbag.* Perform a jumping activity—for example, jump rope or jump up and down 10 times, hop on one foot 10 times, or jump off of a sturdy box (of age-appropriate height) 5 to 10 times.

(continued)

- *Red beanbag.* Perform a muscle-strengthening activity, such as push-ups, curl-ups, planks, or squats.
- *Green beanbag.* Name an organ in the body.
- *Yellow beanbag.* Pretend to eat (students could view cards of high-calorie or fatty foods) and sit down for a count of 10.

When the game begins, start a timer. Set the number of minutes based on the size of the area and how long it will take students to collect four or more beanbags (at least one of each color). Collecting more than four allows older students the opportunity to consider an appropriate number of each colored bag. Students run to a pile of bags, do the prescribed activity, and return to their hoop with the bag. Then they go after another bag. If students must take turns going for a beanbag, then all group members can still complete the prescribed activity while waiting, in order to attain more physical activity during the class period. The goal is to get at least one bag of each color in the hoop. When time runs out (i.e., when the timer stops), movement stops and students check to see what bags they have in their hoop. Winners are those who managed to collect a healthy body (one bag of each color) in their hoop before the timer went off. The teacher can ask how they did and whether they got a healthy body with a bag of each color.

Discussion might address the following questions:

- What do bones do, and what activities are good for building bones?
- Why is it important to have strong muscles? What activities help make muscles strong?
- Why is body fat needed? What can happen if you have too much? Too little?

One beanbag of each color would mean that body fat accounted for 25 percent of body composition, which for elementary school is reasonably accurate. In middle school, the same activity can be done with more precise levels and with accounting for gender differences. This increase in precision gives these older students an opportunity to visualize the fact that fat is needed, but not too much. It also gives them a chance to discuss what types of activity are good for building healthy bones and muscles and burning calories to maintain a healthy weight and body composition. Asking students to explain what they have in their hoop, and why it would or would not be considered to form a healthy body composition, can help you evaluate students' understanding.

Activity 2

The backpack activity is designed to help students understand some of the problems associated with carrying around extra weight. To enable this activity, set up a series of stations with activities—some skills (e.g., line dancing, dribbling a basketball, throwing a ball against a wall) and some health-related fitness activities (e.g., rope jumping, aerobic steps). Either ask students to bring their backpacks or provide a number of backpacks containing 5 to 10 pounds (about 2.3 to 4.5 kg) of sandbags or other relatively soft objects as well as padding around the objects.

Divide the class into groups and assign each group to a station. At each station, half of the students wear the backpacks on their front sides, where excess weight is often felt, while they do the activity. The other half does the activity without the backpack. The groups then switch roles and repeat the station activity (or switch at the next station). It is extremely important to discuss safety with students during this learning activity. Ensure that students take proper precautions to avoid injury. For example, caution them to avoid using too much weight in the backpack. They should start with a lower amount, such as 3 to 5 pounds (1.4 to 2.3 kg), and then add weight once they have tried the activity and come to understand it. Instruct students to maintain an upright posture; adjust each backpack to fit the child.

After doing the stations, students discuss what it felt like to carry the extra weight; whether their weight was more like extra muscle or extra fat; and how it would feel different if it were extra muscle (e.g., making everything easier instead of more difficult). You can also initiate discussion about what students can do to increase or decrease extra body fat.

Strength Training
and Body Composition Management

Strength training can be a valuable adjunct to a body composition management program (Faigenbaum, 2007). A weight-reduction program that is limited to caloric restriction can cause loss not only of body fat but also of lean tissue, which is primarily muscle. Strength training can prevent significant loss of lean body mass, which in turn prevents a decrease in **resting energy expenditure (REE)**, or the amount of energy used by the body at rest. Resting energy expenditure is the single largest component of daily energy expenditure. Each additional pound (0.5 kg) of muscle tissue can raise REE by about 35 kilocalories per day (Campbell, Crim, Young, &

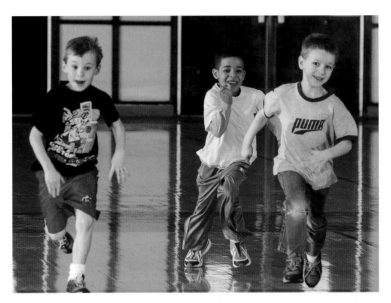

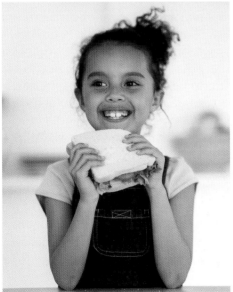 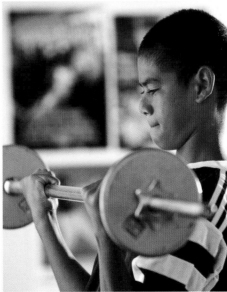

When teaching about health-related fitness, it is important to ensure that students develop a thorough understanding of body composition, the factors that affect it, and the benefits of a healthy body composition.

Bottom left photo © Stockdisc Royalty Free Photos; bottom right photo © Photodisc

Evans, 1994), which over the course of a year makes a significant contribution to total energy expenditure and weight control.

Students need to know that although resistance training burns calories, the effect is relatively small as compared with that of aerobic exercise. The difference in caloric expenditure can be explained by the fact that resistance exercise tends to be more intermittent than aerobic exercise; thus, over the same duration, aerobic exercise requires greater energy expenditure. Students must also understand that it is physiologically impossible for muscle cells to turn into fat, and vice versa—a common misconception. A combination of aerobic exercise and resistance training is the best approach for body composition management and health.

Methods of Measuring Body Composition

Several field methods for estimating body composition can be used in the physical education setting. Field methods are indirect and validated against more direct laboratory methods. They are not as accurate as laboratory methods, but they do give reasonably accurate results and are especially useful for screening at-risk individuals. You will need to learn about the sources of error and understand the limitations of the methods and choose a method that gives the most accurate estimate, considering what can be done in your school environment. Teach elementary students the basic concepts of body composition, as well as the variables that affect it. Teach middle school and high school students specific methods of assessing body composition, as well as the pros and cons of each method.

FitnessGram Body Composition Conversion Chart
This chart is to be used with the two-site skinfold measurements. Measure the triceps and the calf skinfolds. Add the values of triceps and calf skinfolds and find the number in the Total MM column. Look in the % Fat column for the level of fatness associated with that total value.

GIRLS

Total MM	% Fat	Total MM	% Fat	Total MM	% Fat	Total MM	% Fat	Total MM	% Fat
1.0	5.7	16.0	14.9	31.0	24.0	46.0	33.2	61.0	42.3
1.5	6.0	16.5	15.2	31.5	24.3	46.5	33.5	61.5	42.6
2.0	6.3	17.0	15.5	32.0	24.6	47.0	33.8	62.0	42.9
2.5	6.6	17.5	15.8	32.5	24.9	47.5	34.1	62.5	43.2
3.0	6.9	18.0	16.1	33.0	25.2	48.0	34.4	63.0	43.5
3.5	7.2	18.5	16.4	33.5	25.5	48.5	34.7	63.5	43.8
4.0	7.5	19.0	16.7	34.0	25.8	49.0	35.0	64.0	44.1
4.5	7.8	19.5	17.0	34.5	26.1	49.5	35.3	64.5	44.4
5.0	8.2	20.0	17.3	35.0	26.5	50.0	35.6	65.0	44.8
5.5	8.5	20.5	17.6	35.5	26.8	50.5	35.9	65.5	45.1
6.0	8.8	21.0	17.9	36.0	27.1	51.0	36.2	66.0	45.4
6.5	9.1	21.5	18.2	36.5	27.4	51.5	36.5	66.5	45.7
7.0	9.4	22.0	18.5	37.0	27.7	52.0	36.8	67.0	46.0
7.5	9.7	22.5	18.8	37.5	28.0	52.5	37.1	67.5	46.3
8.0	10.0	23.0	19.1	38.0	28.3	53.0	37.4	68.0	46.6
8.5	10.3	23.5	19.4	38.5	28.6	53.5	37.7	68.5	46.9
9.0	10.6	24.0	19.7	39.0	28.9	54.0	38.0	69.0	47.2
9.5	10.9	24.5	20.0	39.5	29.2	54.5	38.3	69.5	47.5
10.0	11.2	25.0	20.4	40.0	29.5	55.0	38.7	70.0	47.8
10.5	11.5	25.5	20.7	40.5	29.8	55.5	39.0	70.5	48.1
11.0	11.8	26.0	21.0	41.0	30.1	56.0	39.3	71.0	48.4
11.5	12.1	26.5	21.3	41.5	30.4	56.5	39.6	71.5	48.7
12.0	12.4	27.0	21.6	42.0	30.7	57.0	39.9	72.0	49.0
12.5	12.7	27.5	21.9	42.5	31.0	57.5	40.2	72.5	49.3
13.0	13.0	28.0	22.2	43.0	31.3	58.0	40.5	73.0	49.6
13.5	13.3	28.5	22.5	43.5	31.6	58.5	40.8	73.5	49.9
14.0	13.6	29.0	22.8	44.0	31.9	59.0	41.1	74.0	50.2
14.5	13.9	29.5	23.1	44.5	32.2	59.5	41.4	74.5	50.5
15.0	14.3	30.0	23.4	45.0	32.6	60.0	41.7	75.0	50.9
15.5	14.6	30.5	23.7	45.5	32.9	60.5	42.0	75.5	51.2

From J. Conkle, *Physical Best: Physical Education for Lifelong Fitness and Health*, 4th ed. (Champaign, IL: Human Kinetics/SHAPE America, 2020). Reprinted from The Cooper Institute, *FitnessGram Administration Manual: The Journey to MyHealthyZone*, 5th ed. (Champaign, IL: Human Kinetics, 2017).

FIGURE 6.1 Guidelines for measuring skinfolds are available in the web resource.

Skinfold Caliper Assessment

Skinfold caliper assessment is a commonly used method for determining body composition in the field. It involves using a **skinfold caliper** to take **skinfold** measurements at specific sites on the body. This method is one of the more accurate ways of measuring body composition that is generally available to physical educators, and it is relatively inexpensive to implement. Still, in order to take accurate and reliable measurements, a tester must be well trained. The time needed to take the measurements is another potential limitation, because obtaining the measurements takes more time and teacher attention than do other methods. In addition, because this method involves touching a student, other sensitivities may arise. If a teacher does not feel comfortable with or qualified to use this method, the teacher can seek further training or arrange for help from more qualified personnel (perhaps someone from the physical education or athletic training department of a local university). Age-specific guidelines for skinfold measurement are published in the latest *Fitness-Gram Administration Manual* (The Cooper Institute, 2017); the current guidelines are also available in the web resource and shown in figure 6.1.

Tips for Conducting Skinfold Assessment

Many teachers feel uncomfortable measuring percent body fat. Reasons for this discomfort may include the following:

- A teacher may be reluctant to touch students in any manner.
- Students may be reluctant to let teachers touch them in any manner.
- A student may feel embarrassed by the assessment results.
- Training and practice are required in order to measure skinfolds accurately.

These concerns can be addressed in several ways.

- Get the training and practice you need in order to take accurate measurements. Alternatively, invite a qualified fitness instructor, university physical education instructor, school nurse, or certified athletic trainer to conduct the assessment.
- Teach older students to use the skinfold calipers. This approach allows them to assume responsibility and self-assess. Measurement of absolute skinfold thickness without conversion to percent body fat is informative and can be used both to track changes over time and to educate students about the importance of physical activity and good nutrition for body composition. Self-assessment can be performed at sites on the trunk (e.g., abdominal site, near the umbilicus, and suprailiac site), as well as the thigh and calf. Self-assessment is recommended for high school students but not for younger students. Measuring sites on the trunk and leg support the opportunity to discuss the differential contribution of truncal (central) versus leg (peripheral) fat deposition for disease risk. For comparison to national distributions, refer to national skinfold data from the NHANES survey (Centers for Disease Control and Prevention, 2012). This activity provides a good opportunity to reinforce with students the fact that people come in different shapes and sizes and that regardless of positive habits, people inherit different body types with different capacities for change.
- Focus on helping students understand the personal choices that all people make that can affect their body composition. This perspective helps students set goals based on the process of living a physically active and healthful lifestyle rather than on the product. In addition, teach students that both too much and too little body fat can be harmful. If students are of the appropriate age, discuss eating disorders.
- If possible, conduct skinfold assessment in a separate room or behind a privacy screen and assess one student at a time. This protocol may relieve some students' discomfort with the process.
- If touching a student may raise concerns, arrange to have a knowledgeable second adult attend the assessment. Remember also that Physical Best provides options for estimating body composition—for example, bioelectrical impedance analysis or body mass index calculations.

Body Mass Index

Although the attention paid by the media to **body mass index (BMI)** has risen recently, this method of determining body composition is not new. In fact, it has been used for decades as a measure of overweight and obesity in population studies. Pediatricians use BMI to assess weight-for-height status, and federal agencies generally use this measure when reporting obesity statistics. By convention, body mass index is expressed in units of kilograms per meter squared (kg/m^2) and calculated from weight in kilograms and height in meters. In adults, the following definitions are used:

- BMI less than 18.5: underweight
- 18.5 to 25: optimal
- 25.1 to 29.9: overweight
- 30 or more: obese
- 40 or more: morbidly obese

In adults, the health risk from excess weight increases with BMIs over 30 and especially over 35. In both youth and adults, as BMI increases above recommended levels, health risk also increases (Li, Ford, Zhao, & Mokdad, 2009).

Although BMI does not directly measure body composition, this ratio of weight to height correlates with body fat in the general population. BMI is a measure best used for postpubescent students and adults. In children and adolescents, BMI standards are age and gender specific. Girls and boys mature at different ages and in different ways. As a result, the Centers for Disease Control and Prevention (CDC) has created age-specific BMI tables that account for gender differences, growth spurts, and the changing relationship between BMI and body composition as boys and girls mature. These charts exist for children of ages 2 through 20 years and are available in the web resource (figure 6.2). The CDC also offers a pediatric BMI calculator at https://www.cdc.gov/healthyweight/bmi/calculator.html. In children and adolescents (up to age 18 years), gender- and age-specific percentiles are used to define desirable ranges of BMI. Ranges defining underweight, overweight, and obesity are as follows:

- Less than 5th percentile: underweight
- Greater than 85th percentile to 94.9th percentile: overweight
- Greater than or equal to 95th percentile: obese

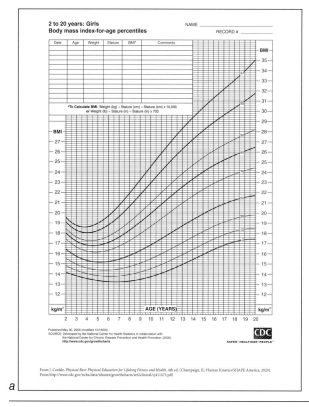
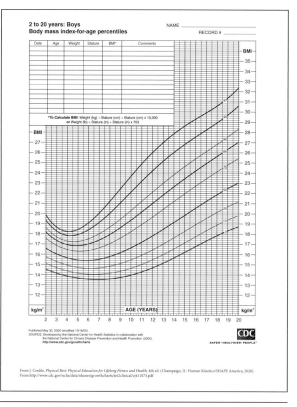

FIGURE 6.2   BMI charts for *(a)* girls and *(b)* boys of ages 2 through 20 are available in the web resource.

The BMIs that correspond to CDC percentiles are based on national distributions of weight-for-height for boys and girls who were measured in the 1960s and 1970s, before the onset of the childhood obesity epidemic. In contrast, FitnessGram standards are based on health-related criteria (e.g., risk factors for cardiovascular disease) linked to desirable ranges of percent body fat. Early FitnessGram standards were derived from data produced by the Bogalusa Heart Study, a long-term study of the natural history of heart disease (Williams et al., 1992). More recently, measures of percent fat have become available from the National Health and Nutrition Examination Survey, the longest ongoing surveillance study with a nationwide sample of the U.S. population. As a result, for the first time, it is possible to derive standards for youth from a nationally representative sample with measures of body composition and disease risk factors (Going et al., 2011; Laurson, Eisenmann, & Welk, 2011a, 2011b; Welk, Going, Morrow, & Meredith, 2011).

The body composition standards shown in tables 6.1 and 6.2 were developed by determining the values of percent fat that best discerned youth at higher risk for chronic disease from those at lower risk (Laurson et al., 2011b). These revised standards have been incorporated into the FitnessGram software. The corresponding BMI standards shown in tables 6.1 and 6.2 were derived by finding the BMI that best identified the various percent fat zones (Laurson et al., 2011c). BMIs that identify very lean boys and very lean girls are equivalent to the CDC-defined 5th percentile of age- and gender-specific BMI, which is the accepted definition for underweight and could indicate future health risks.

In the FitnessGram software, the BMI standards were set to correspond with the established health-related body fat standards. Further analyses determined that the widely used CDC growth chart values had similar clinical utility as the FitnessGram BMI standards for determining metabolic syndrome. Based on these findings, the FitnessGram Scientific Advisory Board decided to modify the FitnessGram standards to coincide with the CDC cut points. The alignment of BMI standards enabled youth to receive consistent information from FitnessGram and the CDC growth charts, which are commonly used by pediatricians. The FitnessGram HFZ standards now coincide with the CDC categorization of "normal weight." The two associated "needs improvement" zones—NI (Needs Improvement) and NI-HR (Needs Improvement Health Risk)—in FitnessGram also match the respective CDC values used to categorize youth as "overweight" or "obese." This correspondence is reflected in the current online version of FitnessGram.

In summary, BMI provides a quick body-composition check that a person can self-administer. It takes little class time and teacher attention and is easy for a student to use outside of a physical education program; it is also commonly used by pediatricians. Its primary disadvantage is that it oversimplifies body composition because it does not distinguish lean mass from body fat. For example, two people with the same BMI and the same level of health-related fitness may have different fat-to-lean mass ratios (based on genetic factors and differences in other body components, such as bone mass) and different percentages of body fat (see the sidebar titled Percent Body Fat Versus Body Mass Index). Moreover, a person can be fit and healthy or be unfit and unhealthy at levels of BMI that define underweight, overweight, or obesity. Even so, BMI gives people one indicator of health and wellness, and it has been used widely in epidemiological studies. When indicated, help students who have a BMI at one of the extremes look for causes and solutions, and encourage them to complete a more accurate assessment of body composition. To help postpubescent students calculate their own body mass index, use the steps provided in the sidebar titled Calculating BMI.

Calculating BMI

To calculate a person's BMI, simply divide weight in pounds by height in inches squared, then multiply the result by 703 to convert the units to metric. Here is the formula:

$$\text{BMI} = (\text{weight in pounds} \div [\text{height in inches} \times \text{height in inches}]) \times 703$$

For example, a boy who weighs 150 pounds and is 5 feet 5 inches tall would calculate his BMI as follows:

$$\text{Step 1: BMI} = (150 \div [65 \times 65]) \times 703$$
$$\text{Step 2: BMI} = (150 \div 4{,}225) \times 703$$
$$\text{Step 3: BMI} = 0.0355 \times 703 = 25$$

If you are using the metric system, simply divide the weight in kilograms by the height in meters squared.

$$\text{BMI} = \text{weight in kilograms} \div (\text{height in meters} \times \text{height in meters})$$

The same boy is 165 centimeters (1.65 meters) tall and weighs 68 kilograms; thus he would calculate his BMI as follows:

$$\text{Step 1: BMI} = 68 \div (1.65 \times 1.65)$$
$$\text{Step 2: BMI} = 68 \div 2.72 = 25$$

Percent Body Fat Versus Body Mass Index

Body mass index (BMI) does not estimate percent fat; it merely gives an indication of the appropriateness of weight relative to height. The following example demonstrates how two students who fall into the healthy fitness zone (HFZ) based on body mass index calculations can have quite different levels of body fat. In this example, Jane's percent body fat is 35 and outside of the HFZ, whereas Jeanette's percent body fat is 19 and within the HFZ.

Jane and Jeanette are both 16 years old, weigh 130 pounds (59 kg), and are 5 feet 6 inches (168 cm) tall. Although both girls have the same body mass index (BMI), body composition assessments show that Jane carries about 45 pounds (20.4 kg) of fat, whereas Jeanette carries about 25 pounds (11.3 kg) of fat.

Jane's percent body fat is calculated as follows:

$$45 \div 130 = 0.35 \ (\text{metric: } 20.4 \div 59 = 0.35)$$
$$0.35 \times 100 = 35 \text{ percent body fat}$$

And here is Jane's BMI calculation:

$$(130 \div 66^2) \times 703$$
$$(130 \div 4{,}356) \times 703$$
$$0.0298 \times 703 = 21$$

Or, using metric units:

$$59 \div 1.68^2$$
$$59 \div 2.82 = 21$$

Meanwhile, Jeanette's percent body fat is calculated as follows:

$$25 \div 130 = 0.19 \ (\text{metric: } 11.3 \div 59 = 0.19)$$
$$0.19 \times 100 = 19 \text{ percent body fat}$$

Jeanette's BMI is calculated as follows:

$$(130 \div 66^2) \times 703$$
$$(130 \div 4{,}356) \times 703$$
$$0.0298 \times 703 = 21$$

Or, using metric units:

$$59 \div 1.68^2$$
$$59 \div 2.82 = 21$$

Thus, although height–weight charts and BMI may provide general indications of health, they do not provide measures of percent fat and therefore do not tell the complete story of body composition.

Weight–Height Chart

Weight–height charts (also known as weight-for-height charts) were created by Louis Dublin, an actuary for the Metropolitan Life Insurance Company. They arose because insurance companies try to predict scientifically which clients have lower or higher risks and when and whom to insure for how much. Similar to BMI, weight–height charts do not measure body composition, and the ratio of body fat to lean tissue can vary substantially at a given weight. Due to the current trend toward more body fat at a higher weight for a given height, weight-for-height charts have been used as a guideline for determining appropriate weight ranges. However, BMI is preferred over simple weight-for-height charts because BMI is more strongly related to body fat. As a result, use of these wall charts is not recommended. Although they may simplify teaching, they do not provide accurate information, and they have often led to public postings that compare students' body compositions—something to be avoided at all costs.

Waist-to-Hip Ratio

Because research has shown that the distribution of body fat relates to its adverse effects, scientists have investigated the correlation between waist-to-hip ratios and health risks. The findings indicate that being pear shaped carries less health-related risk than does being apple shaped; that is, it is better to have excess weight on the hips and thighs than around the waist (Wickelgren, 1998). In fact, research indicates that the excess abdominal fat that creates an apple shape increases a person's risk for heart disease and diabetes later in life (Ziegler & Filer, 2000). Waist-to-hip ratio is a simple way to evaluate whether a person is pear- or apple-shaped. For example, a person with a waist measurement of 28 inches (71.1 cm) and a hip measurement of 38 inches (96.5 cm) would have a waist-to-hip ratio of 0.74 (28 ÷ 38, or 71.1 ÷ 96.5). Ratios above 0.86 in women and 0.95 in men indicate a waist-to-hip ratio considered to be apple shaped and therefore associated with higher levels of heart disease, diabetes, and cancer. These numbers have not been adjusted or validated for children, so the usefulness of this assessment is limited in a health-related physical fitness education program. Moreover, the ratio alone does not indicate whether the numerator (waist circumference) or denominator (hip circumference) is high or low, which limits its utility as an index of disease risk.

Waist Circumference

Although the concept of apple and pear shapes is useful for explaining fat distribution to children and youth, the waist-to-hip ratio can be difficult to interpret. For example, a ratio more than 1 could occur due to a large waist or a small hip circumference. Given this uncertainty, it is becoming more common to use waist circumference alone, which is significantly associated with abdominal fat and adverse health risk and may be more easily obtainable in both adults and children (Katmarzyk et al., 2004). Analyses based on U.S. data support the conclusion that children above the 90th percentile for age and gender are at increased risk for obesity comorbidities (Bassali, Waller, Gower, Allison, & Davis, 2010; Fernandez, Redden, Pietrobelli, & Allison, 2004). Until more definitive standards are developed, a waist circumference above the 90th percentile can be used to refer a child for further screening (McDowell, Fryar, Ogden, & Flegal, 2008; Sharma, Metzger, Daymont, Hadjiyannakis, & Rodd, 2015). Adults and youth with high percent fat (or high BMI) and high waist circumference have the greatest risk for high levels of disease risk factors and chronic disease. See the sidebar titled Measuring Waist Circumference for guidelines on how to properly measure student waist circumferences. Waist percentile charts for boys and girls can be found at https://cpeg-gcep.net/sites/default/files/upload/bookfiles/Pediatr%20 Res%202015;78(6)723-729.pdf. In addition, waist circumference charts for boys and girls are included in the web resource and presented in figure 6.3.

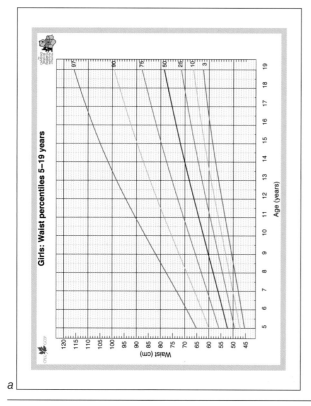

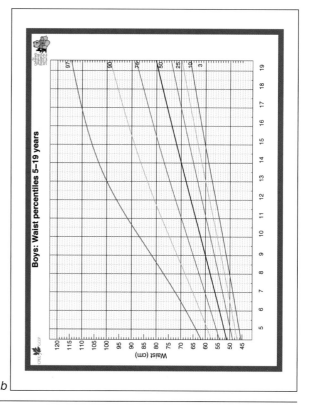

a   b

FIGURE 6.3   Waist circumference charts for *(a)* girls and *(b)* boys.

Based on Sharma et al. (2015).

Measuring Waist (Minimal) Circumference

- Ask the student to stand erect, with the feet together and the abdomen relaxed.
- Ask the student to gather his or her shirt above the waist, cross the arms, and place the hands on the opposite shoulders. It may help to tell the student to give himself or herself a hug. Demonstrate the desired position of the arms.
- Stand behind the student and locate the narrowest part of the torso.
- Then move to the front of the student to take the measurement.
- Ask the student to lift the arms while you place the measuring tape around the narrowest part of the torso. Hold the zero end of the tape in your right hand and the rest of the tape in your left hand.
- Once the tape is around the student's torso, ask the student to relax the arms at the sides.
- Be sure that the tape is in a horizontal plane, evenly placed around the body and not catching on any clothing. If possible, an adult volunteer can check to ensure that the tape is horizontal; alternatively, position the student in front of a mirror so that you can see the tape and ensure that it is horizontal.
- Once the tape position is set, switch the zero end of the tape to your left hand and the rest of the tape to your right hand, or cross your hands to overlap the tape.
- Pull the tape lightly with your left hand until appropriate tension is achieved. Hold the tape in place with your right hand. The tape should lie snugly against without compressing the skin.
- Record the measurement to the nearest 0.1 centimeter.

Figure 6.4 shows proper measurement.

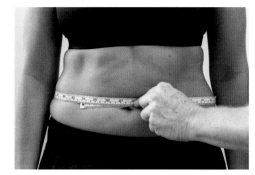

FIGURE 6.4 Waist circumference provides an index of abdominal fat, which is related to adverse health risk.

Bioelectrical Impedance Analysis

Bioelectrical impedance is a noninvasive technique for measuring body composition that requires little skill to administer. Research has shown that impedance can be used to predict fat-free mass and percent body fat in children and adults with errors that are about the same as those accompanying skinfold measurements, provided that population-specific equations are used to estimate composition (Heyward & Wagner, 2004; Silva, Fields, & Sardinha, 2013). A variety of analyzers are available; all are based on introducing a low-level electrical current (800 or 500 microamperes) of different frequencies into the body. Early, single-frequency (e.g., 50-kilohertz) analyzers introduced the current through four electrodes placed on the wrists and ankles while the person being measured lay supine. Today, a number of single-frequency and multiple-frequency devices can measure impedance across multiple axes of the body, including handheld devices, as well as bathroom-type scales that measure weight and impedance in order to estimate composition (see figure 6.5).

Impedance is based on the simple premise that tissues containing a lot of water and electrolytes readily conduct electricity, whereas tissues storing a lot of fat are poor conductors of electricity. Multiple-frequency devices and those that measure impedance across multiple axes (e.g., ipsilateral, contralateral) and segments (e.g., arms, legs, trunk) tend to be more accurate than do simpler devices, but they are also more expensive. The rapid administration and ease of use of simple-impedance devices may be offset by the need to control hydration status and timing of the last preceding meal in order to avoid higher errors. Also, it is generally recommended *not* to use the manufacturer's equations unless the population that you are assessing is a subgroup of the population in which the equation was validated and then cross-validated.

If you decide to use impedance instead of skinfold measurements, follow these recommendations:

- Purchase an impedance instrument that offers multiple equations, including equations for children, that have been shown to provide accurate estimates of percent fat against a more accurate laboratory method.
- Standardize the measurement protocol according to the manufacturer's recommendations.
- Require the student to remove metal jewelry.
- Make sure that the student is well hydrated.
- Avoid assessment soon (less than two hours) after a meal or exercise.
- If multiple equations are not available, or if the accuracy of the equations is uncertain, the alternative is to purchase an instrument that provides the user with the resistance, reactance, and impedance readings, to which you then apply an appropriate equation based on the age, gender, and population group of the student you are assessing.

Heyward and Wagner (2004) have published decision trees to guide the selection of equations for different groups. Even so, bioelectrical impedance is limited by the fact that few cross-validated equations are available for minority children and adolescents; in addition, the manufacturer's equations are usually not provided for review (Silva et al., 2013; Talma et al., 2013).

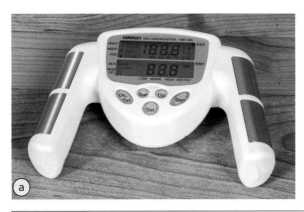
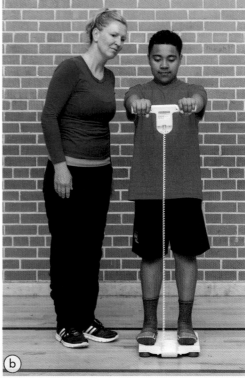

FIGURE 6.5 *(a)* Handheld and *(b)* scale-type bioelectrical impedance analysis instruments.

Helping Students Who Are Overfat or Underfat

Body composition assessment provides an opportunity to discuss how body composition affects health and how it can be affected by behavioral factors such as eating a healthy diet and engaging in regular physical activity. Through formal assessment, you will identify students who appear to be either over or under an appropriate percent body fat. As a physical educator, you should not attempt to treat serious problems, such as eating disorders or extreme obesity, or prescribe a diet. Instead, you should refer such students to their parents with a recommendation for professional help. The following sections discuss the symptoms and causes of obesity and eating disorders to help you identify contributing factors and develop a factual discussion.

Obesity

According to the Centers for Disease Control and Prevention, about 65 percent of all adults in the United States are overweight or obese (Ogden, Carroll, Fryar, & Flegal, 2015). In addition, the percentage of youth who are overweight or obese has more than doubled in the last three decades. Current estimates indicate that 17 percent to 20 percent of U.S. children and youth aged 6 to 19 are obese (Ogden et al., 2016). Given these statistics, physical educators are likely to have overweight children in their classes. **Obesity** is defined as 120 percent or more of ideal body weight or as a BMI greater than 30 in adults. In children and adolescents (those younger than 18 years old), obesity is defined as a BMI equaling or exceeding the 95th percentile for one's age and gender. Obesity is associated with three main contributing factors: genetics, diet, and physical activity. Keep this in mind when preparing lesson plans.

- *Genetics.* Research suggests that genetics contributes about 30 percent to a person's body weight (Ziegler & Filer, 2000). The genetic component is multiple in nature: It determines metabolism, placement of excess fat (e.g., hips, arms, abdomen), effectiveness of the gastrointestinal tract, level of appetite, preferences for certain types of food (e.g., sweets, salty snacks), and response to exercise. Many factors are involved, and research is still exploring the exact genes, their products, and the exact biochemical mechanisms.

- *Diet.* The average American diet contains more calories than it did 30 years ago. Contributing factors include eating more meals away from home (particularly fast food), consuming larger portion sizes of both foods and beverages, consuming more sugar-sweetened beverages, and snacking in less healthy ways (Briefel & Johnson, 2004). Given these trends, it should not be surprising that the diet quality of youth falls far short of recommendations. More than 70 percent of youth do not meet recommendations for dietary fat intake, and less than half eat the recommended servings of vegetables on a daily basis (U.S. Department of Agriculture, 2013). In addition, poor eating habits that are developed during childhood may continue to be reinforced throughout adulthood.

- *Physical activity.* Physical activity increases the body's use of calories, which decreases energy storage and helps maintain a normal weight and body composition and optimize overall health. Unfortunately, the level of physical activity continues to decrease in the United States. Despite the widely documented benefits of exercise, including better long-term health, improved body image, and reduced risk of depression, most American adults do not achieve recommended levels of physical activity (Troiano et al., 2008). Nor is this inactivity limited to adults: Fewer than 50 percent of children and youth participate in the recommended daily amount of physical activity, and screen time has

Teaching Body Composition Concepts

In addition to the many activities provided in the web resource, consider the following ideas for teaching nutritional concepts related to body composition.

Teaching Models

Create class fat models to supplement lectures and stimulate class discussion. Start by obtaining nutrition information from local fast-food chains; to do so, consult the Verywell Fit website at https://www.verywellfit.com/weight-loss-dining-out-advice-4157001. Then label clear plastic cups with various food types and add the appropriate amount of shortening or margarine to demonstrate the food's fat content (one teaspoon is equivalent to five grams of fat). This activity helps students visualize the fat content in their favorite fast-food items.

Journaling

Ask students to complete a dietary journal noting all foods eaten in the previous 24 hours. They should record how they felt (in terms of emotions) when they ate, as well as why they ate each item. The objective is to demonstrate how often people eat for reasons other than hunger and why they choose the foods that they do. Food choices are often more about convenience, taste, and availability than about making healthy choices. Although younger children may not get to choose their food daily, they do get some choice with school lunches and at restaurants.

Finding a Menu

A majority of restaurant menus can be found online. Ask students to provide names of restaurants that they frequent. Then ask them to work in small groups or as a class to select the most-healthy and least-healthy menu items from local restaurants. Ask them also to explain why they labeled certain choices as either healthy or unhealthy. Next, engage them in a discussion of strategies they can use to make healthier choices when eating out. For more information and activity ideas, visit the Choose MyPlate website at www.choosemyplate.gov and look at the tips for eating out at https://www.choosemyplate.gov/ten-tips-eating-foods-away-home.

---

replaced much of the after-school yard play in which many children used to engage. In addition, daily participation rates in physical education classes are woefully low (Institute of Medicine, 2013).

The number of calories ultimately used during physical activity depends on the intensity and duration of the activity. Lower-intensity activity must be done for a longer time than higher-intensity activity in order to achieve the same energy expenditure. Therefore, moderate to vigorous activity is recommended for its health benefits, including significant energy expenditure in a feasible time (e.g., 30 to 60 minutes). Significantly overweight children may find it difficult to engage in higher-intensity activity or to sustain activity for more than a few minutes at a time. Therefore, they may need to engage in lower-intensity activity and increase the intensity progressively as their body composition and health-related fitness improve. Lower-intensity and intermittent activity still provides health benefits; the key is to accumulate 30 to 60 minutes of activity throughout the day.

Eating Disorders

Although obesity is now the most prevalent nutritional problem among youth, psychological and social pressures to look thin have contributed to the development of eating disorders that also pose serious health risks. Three eating disorders are common in the school-age population—anorexia nervosa, bulimia, and binge eating—and physical educators and coaches must be able to recognize the warning signs of each. To help students achieve and maintain good body composition, teach them about the importance of healthy eating and regular physical activity for optimal growth and health. Stress that healthy people come in all shapes and sizes, and discuss the unrealistic images that are often portrayed in the media. If an eating disorder is suspected, discuss your concern with the school nurse and refer the child and parents to an appropriate professional.

Anorexia Nervosa

Anorexia nervosa is a serious and potentially fatal disease characterized by self-induced starvation and extreme weight loss (see the sidebar titled Warning Signs of Anorexia). According to the National Eating Disorders Association (2016), anorexia nervosa has four primary symptoms:

- Inadequate food intake, leading to a weight that is clearly too low (generally, less than 85 percent of ideal body weight)
- Intense fear of weight gain, obsession with weight, and persistent behavior to prevent weight gain
- Self-esteem overtly related to body image
- Inability to appreciate the severity of the situation

These are two types of anorexia nervosa. The first type is characterized by **binge eating** or **purging** behaviors during the past three months. The second type, known as **restrictive anorexia nervosa**, does not involve binge eating or purging.

Warning Signs of Anorexia

- Dramatic weight loss
- Preoccupation with weight, food, calories, fat grams, and dieting
- Refusal to eat certain foods
- Progression to restrictions on whole categories of food (e.g., no carbohydrate)
- Frequent comments about feeling fat or overweight despite weight loss
- Anxiety about gaining weight or being fat
- Denial of hunger
- Development of food rituals (e.g., eating foods in certain orders, excessive chewing, rearranging food on a plate)
- Consistent excuses to avoid mealtimes or situations involving food
- Excessive, rigid exercise regimen despite inclement weather, fatigue, illness, or injury; felt need to "burn off" calories taken in
- Withdrawal from usual friends and activities
- Generally, behaviors and attitudes indicating that weight loss, dieting, and control of food are primary concerns

Reprinted by permission from the National Eating Disorders Foundation, "Warning signs of anorexia nervosa." [Online]. Available: http://www.nationaleatingdisorders.org [April 1, 2010].

About 90 percent to 95 percent of people with anorexia nervosa are female. The disease can carry extremely negative health consequences, including abnormally slow heart rate, reduction in bone mass, hair loss, dry hair, and severe dehydration (which can result in kidney failure). People with anorexia nervosa also experience growth of a downy layer of hair called **lanugo**; its purpose is to help the body to keep warm. Among persons with anorexia nervosa, statistics indicate that 5 percent to 20 percent will die. Experts in eating disorders have found that prompt, intensive treatment significantly improves the chances of recovery; therefore, it is crucial to be aware of the warning signs of anorexia nervosa.

Bulimia

Bulimia (see the sidebar titled Warning Signs of Bulimia) is a serious, potentially fatal eating disorder characterized by a destructive cycle of bingeing and purging. According to the National Eating Disorders Association, bulimia has three primary symptoms:

- Eating large quantities of food in short periods, or bingeing, typically in secret
- After binges, performing a compensatory behavior to account for the caloric intake (e.g., vomiting, laxative abuse, diuretic abuse, fasting, compulsive exercise)
- Extreme concern with body weight and shape

Roughly 1 percent to 5 percent of the U.S. population has bulimia. Estimates vary because bulimia can go undetected for long periods. About 80 percent of people with bulimia are female. Unlike those with anorexia nervosa, most people with bulimia have a normal weight or even slightly above. Health consequences of bulimia can include tooth decay, ulcers, electrolyte disturbances, and gastric rupture.

Warning Signs of Bulimia

- Evidence of binge eating, including disappearance of large amounts of food in short periods of time or finding wrappers and containers indicating the consumption of large amounts of food
- Evidence of purging behaviors, including frequent trips to the bathroom after meals, signs and/or smells of vomiting, presence of wrappers or packages of laxatives or diuretics
- Excessive, rigid exercise regimen—despite weather, fatigue, illness, or injury, the compulsive need to "burn off" calories taken in
- Unusual swelling of the cheeks or jaw area
- Calluses on the back of the hands and knuckles from self-induced vomiting
- Discoloration or staining of the teeth
- Creation of lifestyle schedules or rituals to make time for binge-and-purge sessions
- Withdrawal from usual friends and activities
- In general, behaviors and attitudes indicating that weight loss, dieting, and control of food are becoming primary concerns
- Continued exercise despite injury; overuse injuries

Reprinted by permission from the National Eating Disorders Foundation, "Warning signs of bulimia nervosa." [Online]. Available: http://www.nationaleatingdisorders.org [April 1, 2010].

Binge Eating

Binge eating (see the sidebar titled Warning Signs of Binge Eating) is a type of eating disorder characterized by recurrent episodes of eating large quantities of food without the regular use of compensatory measures to counter the binge eating. It is now recognized in the DSM-5 (the American Psychiatric Association's *Diagnostic and Statistical Manual of Mental Disorders, Fifth Edition*). According to the National Eating Disorders Association, the most significant health consequences of binge eating include the following:

- High blood pressure
- High cholesterol
- Heart disease
- Diabetes mellitus
- Gallbladder disease

Binge eating occurs in about 1 percent to 5 percent of the general population, and it affects women slightly more often than men. It is often associated with symptoms of depression. People who struggle with the disorder often express distress, shame, and guilt over their eating behaviors. They often eat unusually large amounts of food and feel out of control during the binges. Unlike individuals with bulimia or anorexia, binge eaters do not throw up their food, exercise a lot, or eat only small amounts of only certain foods. As a result, binge eaters are often overweight or obese. People with binge eating disorder may also do the following:

- Eat more quickly than usual during binge episodes.
- Eat until they are uncomfortably full.
- Eat when they are not hungry.
- Eat alone because of embarrassment.
- Feel disgusted, depressed, or guilty after overeating.

Warning Signs of Binge Eating

- Evidence of binge eating, including disappearance of large amounts of food in short periods of time or the existence of wrappers and containers indicating the consumption of large amounts of food
- Development of food rituals, such as eating only a particular food or food group (e.g., condiments), excessive chewing, not allowing foods to touch
- Stealing or hoarding food in strange places
- Hiding one's body with baggy clothes
- Creating lifestyle schedules or rituals to make time for binge sessions
- Skipping meals or taking small portions of food at regular meals
- Experiencing periods of uncontrolled, impulsive, or continuous eating beyond the point of feeling comfortably full
- Not purging
- Engaging in sporadic fasting or repetitive dieting
- Body weight that varies from normal to mild, moderate, or severe obesity

Based on National Eating Disorders Association (2003).

Underweight or Slender?

Although **underweight** (less than 90 percent of ideal body weight) is a symptom of disordered eating, some children are simply genetically thin. An eating disorder can be diagnosed only by a qualified professional.

About 2.8 percent of the U.S. adult population suffers from binge eating disorder at some point in their lifetime; up to 1.6 percent of adolescents may have the disorder (Swanson, Crow, Le Grange, Swendsen, & Merikangas, 2011).

Based on National Eating Disorders Association (2003).

Addressing the Problem

Use the following guidelines to approach the situation in a professional manner.

- Always maintain the privacy of the student and family.
- Approach the student and family diplomatically; avoid making statements that may be perceived as accusatory.
- Respect parental wishes unless you believe that the child is in danger.
- Work with other school personnel, such as the school nurse or counselor, and seek written permission to share your observations with the child's health care worker. At the same time, seek advice on how to tailor a program to meet the child's needs. School districts have access to registered dietitians who may be able to tailor a meal plan for students with weight problems or eating disorders. Eating regular, well-balanced meals throughout the day may decrease the urge to binge and may help the student lose weight, if needed, and improve body composition.
- Ensure that the physical education program is engaging and promotes physical activity as a lifestyle choice for all students. Avoid setting unreasonable expectations. For example, obese children are more likely to maintain, and therefore benefit from, mild physical activity than moderate to vigorous physical activity (U.S. Department of Health and Human Services, 1999).
- Refer students with serious problems to a professional who is qualified to treat the problem.

Summary

Although approaching body composition in the physical education setting can be a delicate matter, it is just as important as any other health-related component of physical fitness. Handle body composition instruction professionally and effectively by focusing not on assessment results but on how an active lifestyle positively affects body composition. Connect this material to the other components of health-related fitness. Make assessment voluntary and respect each student's privacy. Finally, learn to recognize when a student's body composition may pose a serious health concern and refer such children to a qualified health care professional.

Discussion Questions

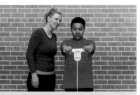

1. Why is body composition included as a component of health-related fitness?
2. What is the rationale for conducting health-related fitness testing, including body composition assessment, in schools?
3. What are the health risks associated with excess body weight? Which components of body composition confer the risks?
4. What are the limitations of body mass index as a measure of body composition? Given its limitations, why is it used so widely?
5. What is the utility of measuring waist circumference along with body mass index for risk assessment?
6. How are the cut points determined for levels of body fat that relate to health risks?
7. How does body composition relate to other components of health-related fitness?
8. Explain which measure of body composition would work best in your current or future teaching environment. Explain why it is the best choice and discuss its limitations.
9. Identify and discuss the warning signs of disordered eating.
10. Identify Physical Best activities that might help increase students' understanding of healthy nutrition and increase their physical activity levels with an eye toward the goal of meeting federal guidelines for dietary intake and regular physical activity.

CHAPTER 7

Flexibility

Elizabeth A. Burkhart
and Philip C. Dlugolecki

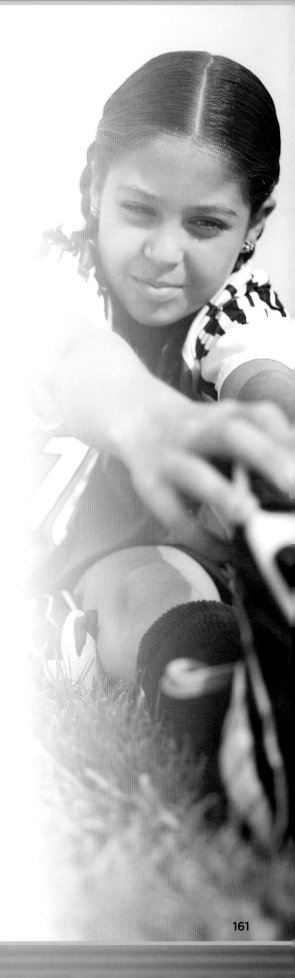

CHAPTER CONTENTS

Flexibility is a component of health-related fitness that is often misunderstood by students, teachers, trainers, and professional athletes. Adding to the misunderstanding is the conflicting research and anecdotal evidence that appears in journals and popular media. As a physical education teacher, it is vital that you understand the science of flexibility, its benefits, related research and anecdotal evidence, and safe and effective exercises. This understanding will enable you to help your students achieve physical literacy and navigate the often-conflicting information they will be exposed to as adults. Physical Best can help enhance your understanding of flexibility based on current research and give you examples of best practices for teaching flexibility in your physical education program.

Though sometimes overlooked or addressed only as an afterthought, flexibility is in fact one of the major components of health-related fitness, along with muscular strength, muscular endurance, and cardiorespiratory endurance. As such, it must be incorporated into a comprehensive health-related fitness program. Students may have little or no knowledge of safe and effective flexibility training, and much of what they do know (correctly or incorrectly) may have been picked up by mimicking role models at home or in sport or recreation settings. Therefore, your responsibility as a physical education teacher is to educate students about the importance of flexibility and guide them in doing various flexibility exercises with proper form and safe technique (see figure 7.1).

This chapter will help you identify and develop training exercises to incorporate into a well-rounded program for lifelong health-related fitness that helps students

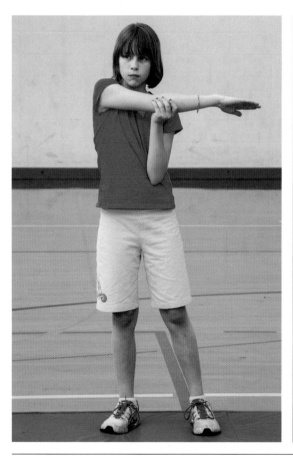
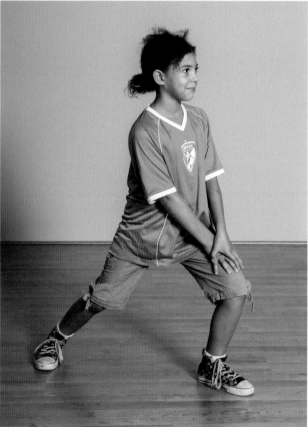

FIGURE 7.1   Sample stretches that can help students improve flexibility.

achieve and maintain a healthy level of flexibility. In addition, it will help you inform students about the many health-related benefits associated with regular flexibility training. For example, a well-designed flexibility program (which follows the principles of training described in chapter 3) aids muscle relaxation; improves overall health-related fitness, posture, and body symmetry; and reduces the risk of injury and soreness—all of which make physical activity of all types easier and safer to do. Furthermore, stretching can relieve emotional stress, increase feelings of well-being, and help prepare the body to move from resting to exercising more smoothly.

Definitions of Flexibility Concepts

Flexibility is a term used to characterize the range of motion (ROM) of a single joint or a series of joints (American College of Sports Medicine, 2014). Optimal flexibility allows a joint or group of joints to move freely and efficiently, whereas laxity or hypermobility in a joint is not healthy and may lead to injury. **Laxity** refers to abnormal motion in a given joint, which means that the ligaments connecting bone to bone do not provide the joint with sufficient stability. **Hypermobility** refers to excess ROM in a joint (Heyward & Gibson, 2014). Both conditions may predispose a person to injury. People with hypermobility should not be allowed to stretch into the extremes of ROM and should try to maintain as much joint stability as possible (American College of Sports Medicine, 2014).

Children may not understand the concept of joint movement through a full ROM, but they will understand how well they bend and twist. For younger learners, an activity such as "head, shoulders, knees, and toes" may be used to demonstrate bending and twisting at different levels. For older students, you can use bouncing putty to demonstrate flexibility by showing students that, like muscles, it does not bend or stretch well when cold but stretches and elongates easily when warm. Another analogy can be found in trees that bend in the wind and remain intact versus trees that don't bend and therefore break.

Types of Stretching

The health-related component of flexibility and the act of stretching are two related but different things. Flexibility is something you possess, whereas stretching is something you do. Specifically, stretching is a method for maintaining or increasing one's flexibility; it both lengthens the muscle and affects your mental perception of the associated discomfort. It's that perception that changes the most in the short term, thus allowing you to stretch farther. In the long term, much of our flexibility is genetic and doesn't change without months of consistent work.

Many types of stretching can be incorporated into a physical education course. The types that foster flexibility are classified as follows (American College of Sports Medicine, 2014):

- In an **active stretch** (unassisted), the person stretching provides the force of the stretch, and assistance comes only from the opposing (antagonist) muscle. For example, see the trunk lift shown in figure 7.2.

- In a **passive stretch** (assisted), the force of the stretch is provided either by the person stretching or by gravity, a partner, or an implement. See the example shown in figure 7.3.

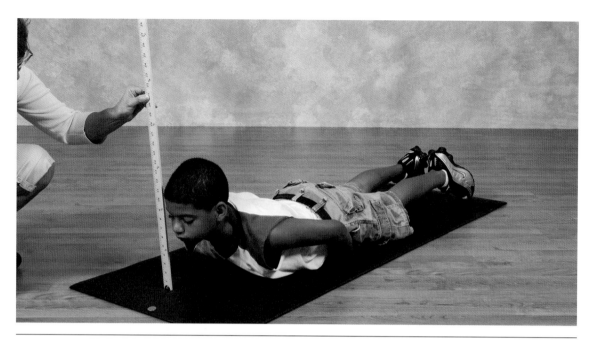

FIGURE 7.2   Example of active stretching.

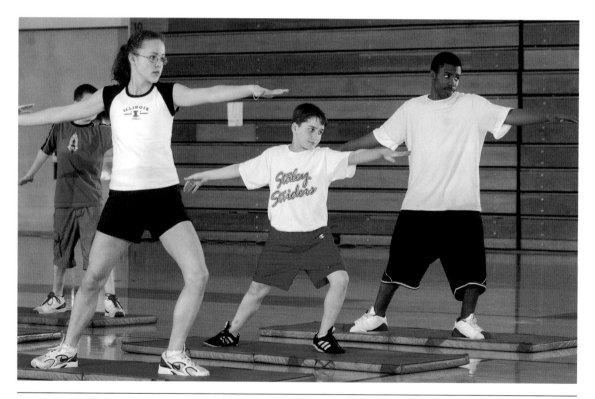

FIGURE 7.3   Example of passive stretching.

- A **static stretch** is a slow, sustained stretch. The person stretches the muscle–
  tendon unit to the point where mild discomfort is felt, then backs off slightly
  and holds the stretch at a point just before discomfort occurs. Static stretching
  is productive only if the person stretching understands the concept of mild

discomfort. During the beginning of a static stretch, muscle spindles are activated in the muscle group being worked, thus inhibiting flexibility enhancements. Individuals must achieve the feeling of mild discomfort for a substantial amount of time to gradually improve flexibility. This type of stretch is generally considered safe, and it does not rely on cooperation from a partner. Thus it is preferred in physical education classes, especially at the elementary level.

- **Dynamic stretching** involves moving parts of the body and gradually increasing ROM, speed of movement, or both. People tend to use the terms *dynamic* and *ballistic* interchangeably, but dynamic stretching differs from ballistic stretching in that it avoids bouncy, jerky movements. Dynamic stretching is an active warm-up that helps prepare the body for the training session to come while opening the joint capsules, which have the ability to shut down proper range of motion if not worked. Examples of dynamic stretches include controlled leg and arm swings that safely go through the individual's ROM. Dynamic movements also include light exercises focused on form—for example, high-knees (forward and backward and side to side), skips (forward and backward and side to side), ankle hops, and fast feet.

- **Ballistic stretching** involves moving quickly, bouncing, or using momentum to produce the stretch. It forces a limb to extend past its normal range of motion and puts pressure on the engaged muscles and joints. This type of stretch is often viewed as necessary for sport movements and should be reserved for coaching or conditioning athletes; it should *not* be used in general physical education classes. An example of ballistic stretching is to begin in standing position and put one leg on a weight bench or chair, then bend forward toward the elevated leg while repeatedly reaching forward toward the toes. Ballistic stretching should not be identified as a variation of dynamic stretching. Granted, both stretches aim at increasing flexibility through repetition. However, whereas dynamic stretching involves smooth, well-governed moves and remains close to or beneath the usual range of motion, thus posing no threat to muscle tissue, ballistic stretching uses unrestrained strikes and surpasses the usual range of motion.

- **Proprioceptive neuromuscular facilitation (PNF)** involves a static stretch using a combination of active and passive stretching. In the example shown in figure 7.4, the student pulls the towel toward herself until she feels mild tension, holds the towel in position and tries to point the toes against the towel resistance for several seconds, relaxes, and then pulls the towel toward herself again. This specialized static stretch uses a contraction–relaxation combination of movements to relax the muscles by taking advantage of reflexes and neuromuscular principles (Ciocioi & Macovei, 2016).

This type of stretch should not be performed by children younger than 10 years old, but it can be performed by pubescent or postpubescent students (Bompa & Haff, 2009) and by those who have developed a solid base of training and are undergoing formal athletic conditioning with help from a qualified coach. PNF may produce slightly larger flexibility gains in some joints than other techniques, but it is less practical because of the need for a partner (Garber et al., 2011). When performing this type of stretch, the keys are safety, proper instruction, and responsibility. Injury may result if children are not responsible, fail to listen to partners' cues (and thereby force a stretch), or perform a stretch incorrectly.

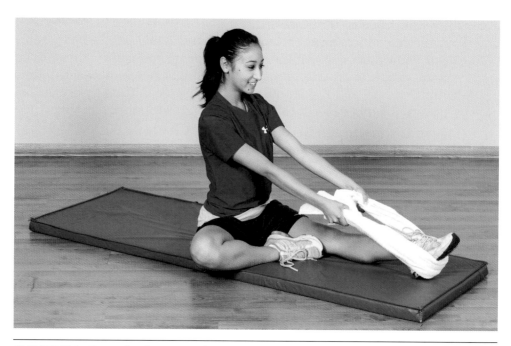

FIGURE 7.4   Example of PNF stretching.

- **Yogic stretching** involves unique stretching maneuvers that are mainly static and focus primarily on the trunk musculature (American College of Sports Medicine, 2014). Each pose requires the body to be aligned in a specific way that allows the muscles to work effectively in order to hold a position. If practiced regularly, yoga can not only help a person achieve and maintain a healthy level of flexibility but also help align the body. In addition, it can contribute to muscular strength and endurance through body-weight resistance and the holding of poses for long periods of time. This type of training also helps control breathing during exercise; specifically, as students hold poses in their proper form, they focus on lengthening and deepening their breathing. Yoga can also improve athletic performance. For example, a study of basketball athletes aged 17 to 20 years found that regular yoga exercise (four times per week for nine months) increased their vertical jump, speed, speed endurance, retention of equilibrium (balance), free-throw shooting, three-point shooting, and tactical execution (Brynzak & Burko, 2013). Yoga training can be differentiated to suit a variety of ability levels. It is crucial to understand proper alignment and technique for each pose in order to prevent injury and ensure that students move effectively and safely with attention to the body's current limitations.

- Similar to yoga, **Pilates** involves a series of organized exercises that can improve flexibility (Kloubec, 2010). Created by Joseph Pilates in the early 20th century, the system emphasizes core strength, good alignment, and good posture. This type of training improves muscle elasticity and joint mobility through muscle elongation. The foundation of Pilates training is the inclusion of movements focused on breathing, alignment, muscular control and movement, and working from the center of the body. It also aids flexibility, which facilitates daily functions such as walking up stairs and picking up objects from the ground. This practice of stretching and strengthening the muscles to function effectively is used not only as exercise but also in rehabilitation and recovery to treat imbalances and injuries.

Figure 7.5 shows an example of how one chest stretch can be varied in one of three ways: PNF, static, or ballistic.

Benefits of Flexibility

The specificity principle states that the observed range of motion at each joint is specific to the flexibility exercises performed at that joint. Therefore, the benefits that follow apply only to the muscles and joints used in a stretching program. The following benefits of increased flexibility are identified in *Foundations of Professional Personal Training* (Canadian Fitness Professionals, 2016) and by the American Council on Exercise:

CHEST STRETCH (PNF, STATIC, OR BALLISTIC)

1. Stand in a forward stride position in a doorway. Raise your arms slightly above shoulder-height. Place your hands on either side of the doorway.
2. Lean your body into the doorway. Resist by contracting your arm and chest muscles. Hold the position for 3 seconds. Relax.
3. Immediately lean further forward, letting your body weight stretch your muscles. Hold the position for 10 to 30 seconds.
4. For a ballistic stretch, gently bounce your body forward.
    Note: For a static stretch, omit steps 2 and 4.

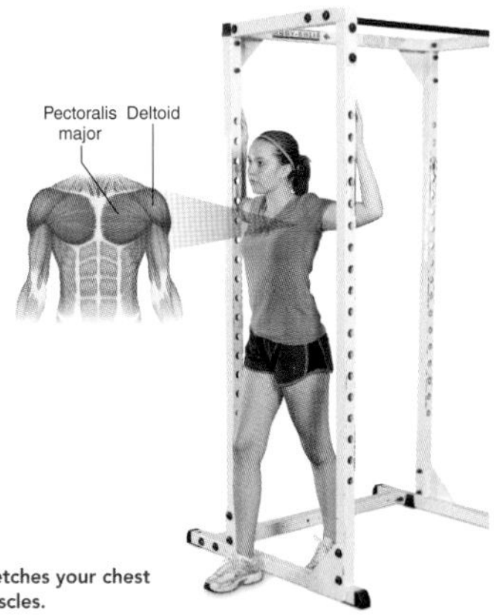

This exercise stretches your chest and shoulder muscles.

FIGURE 7.5   Stretches can be varied to use different methods and achieve different purposes.

- Reduces stress in the exercising muscles and releases tension developed during a workout.
- Helps with posture by balancing the tension placed on a joint by the muscles that cross it. Proper posture minimizes stress and maximizes the strength of all joint movements.
- Reduces the risk of injury during exercise and daily activities.
- Improves performance in everyday activities, exercise, and sport.
- Helps prevent low-back pain and injury.
- Helps relieve muscle cramps.
- Improves ease of movement.
- Facilitates relaxation and stress relief, both mental and physical.
- Improves range of motion and coordination, which may benefit athletic performance.

Flexibility is for everyone. Regardless of ability or disability, everyone can learn to stretch and benefit from improved range of motion. The benefits contribute to overall health and well-being and affirm the importance of including flexibility activities in your daily physical education lessons. For specific examples of flexibility lessons, see the web resource.

Factors Affecting Flexibility

Although flexibility may be limited by a number of factors, most people can improve their flexibility through a training program. If a student's current level of flexibility needs improvement, then the teacher should help the student implement a separate program, much like a strength program. It should be a routine that targets tight muscles caused by sedentary behaviors such as sitting. Another reason for a stretching-focused program is to improve muscles that are used in everyday activities. Remember, however, that many factors influence the amount of flexibility observed or measured at each joint. Emphasize to students that irregular participation in a flexibility program yields poor results; the old adage "use it or lose it" applies here.

Here are some factors that affect flexibility:

- *Muscle temperature.* The temperature of a muscle affects its elasticity, or ability to stretch beyond its normal resting length and then return to its prestretched length at the completion of the exercise.

- *Age and gender.* Young people tend to be more flexible than older people, and females tend to be more flexible than males. Differences in flexibility between young men and young women result in part from structural and anatomical differences, as well as type and extent of activity (Baechle & Earle, 2008).

- *Tissue interference.* Flexibility can be affected by excess body fat or well-developed musculature. For example, an athlete with large biceps and deltoids may experience difficulty in stretching the triceps (Baechle & Earle, 2008). However, you should not allow tissue interference to prevent your students from improving their flexibility. High body fat is generally a result of inactivity, and a student with well-developed musculature as a limiting factor (usually not a factor until late high school, if at all) may simply lack a flexibility exercise program. These students, if taught, can develop and maintain adequate flexibility (Heyward & Gibson, 2014).

- *Genetics.* Flexibility can be limited or excessive (i.e., hypermobile) due to a person's genetic makeup. Even so, the person must use the joints regularly and within normal means in order to develop and maintain flexibility; otherwise, the person's ROM and joint stability may be adversely affected. In addition, research shows that maintaining a good flexibility plan across the life span may limit or reduce natural changes in elasticity and compliance of muscle tissue (American College of Sports Medicine, 2014).

Other factors that may limit flexibility include pain, poor coordination and strength during active movement, and extensibility of the **muscular–tendon unit** (i.e., tension in muscles). Most of these limitations can be reversed, and those reversals constitute benefits of flexibility—that is, decreased pain after injury, improved coordination, and reduced tension. Each individual's ROM needs to be taken into account when designing flexibility programs for students.

Although most of the limitations can be overcome through a well-designed, appropriately progressive flexibility program, pain should never be ignored, and limitations caused by bone or joint structures may require special attention and individualization. Flexibility can also be limited by certain diseases (e.g., muscular dystrophy, cerebral palsy), and for many of these conditions, you should consult with an adapted physical educator or the child's physician to inquire about appropriate stretching activities.

Teaching Guidelines for Flexibility

Before beginning any health-related fitness unit, physical education teachers should have students perform flexibility assessments in order to understand their current status and establish a basis for monitoring their progress. One way to determine an individual's current state of flexibility is to use a test such as the back-saver sit-and-reach or the shoulder stretch.

Teachers should explain the relationship between flexibility exercises performed in class and the back-saver sit-and-reach assessment, the shoulder stretch assessment, and the trunk extensor strength and flexibility assessment performed during health-related fitness assessment. After engaging in a health-related fitness program that incorporates flexibility, students should be retested in each flexibility assessment in order to evaluate their progress. As with all areas of health-related fitness, conducting periodic flexibility assessments will let students measure their current status and help them set goals for improvement or maintenance.

During a physical education course, flexibility should not be merely incorporated into a warm-up or cool-down session but should be taught as a distinct aspect of health-related fitness. Flexibility training can enable rapid improvement. Anyone can learn to stretch correctly, and everyone can attain the benefits of improved flexibility.

First, select the type of stretch that meets the needs of the lesson. Allow students to participate in selecting various flexibility exercises that fit their current ROM. The exercises may be completed in a warm-up or a cool-down or incorporated throughout the lesson. After you have instructed students on a repertoire of exercises for the total body, you can use station cards, modify the warm-up or cool-down, or ask students to select an exercise that meets their individual goals.

In the physical education setting, static stretching is generally preferred and is considered among the safest methods for enhancing ROM at the end of a class period. Studies (Faigenbaum et al., 2005) also show benefits from adding controlled dynamic stretching to the curriculum. A program of planned stretches (such as those shown in figure 7.6) does not take much class time, and it is generally easy to ensure that each individual in a large group of students is performing them correctly.

Establish a regular schedule of flexibility fitness lessons and stretching activity in your classes. Include definitions and basic concepts related to the FITT guidelines and safety precautions. This approach not only teaches students the importance of stretching but also allows you to integrate flexibility concepts into all aspects of health-related fitness.

The following sequence provides an example of how to incorporate flexibility activities into a separate physical education unit:

- *Day 1.* Incorporate stretching before and after a workout (e.g., dynamic stretches, cardio workout, static stretches).
- *Day 2.* Incorporate stretching before and after a workout (e.g., dynamic stretches, mobility work for lower-body muscles, lower-body muscular strength and endurance workout, static stretches).
- *Day 3.* Focus on stretching for the entire workout (e.g., yoga, Pilates, individual stretches, partner stretches, PNF stretches).
- *Day 4.* Incorporate stretching before and after a workout (e.g., dynamic stretches, mobility work for upper-body muscles, upper-body muscular strength and endurance workout, static stretches).
- *Day 5.* Focus on stretching for two-thirds of a workout (e.g., dynamic stretches, core endurance workout, more stretching).

As in weight training, flexibility training requires proper form and technique. Students who stretch improperly put excess stress on their joints and connective tissues and increase their risk of injury during activities designed to improve health and well-being. Emphasize that flexibility training, with or without a partner, is no place for horseplay, which can result in injury. This caution is especially important when using PNF or partner stretching. Stress safety and slow, gradual, individualized progression (see the sidebar titled Partner-Resisted Hamstring Stretch, as well as figure 7.7).

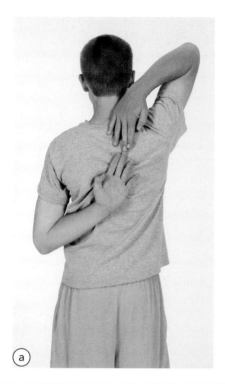
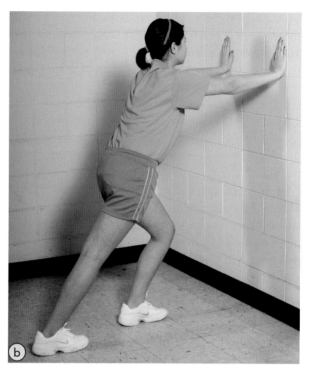
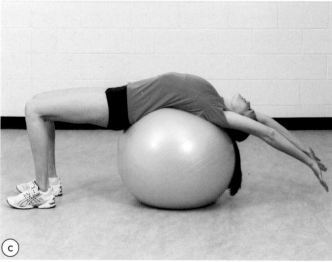
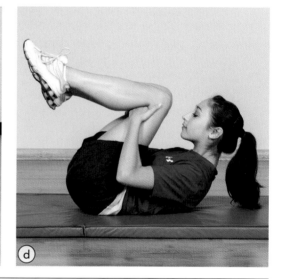

FIGURE 7.6 Examples of (*a* and *b*) static stretches and (*c* and *d*) dynamic stretches.

Incorporating Flexibility Into Physical Education

When incorporating flexibility into physical education (either as a separate unit or infused into another unit), follow these simple guidelines:

- *Foundation movements.* Perform basic fundamental movements (e.g., beginner poses in yoga, beginner modifications for stretches).
- *Expansion movements.* Expand knowledge of the muscular system used and broaden the flexibility practice of movements; expose students to options for each movement (e.g., intermediate modifications, equipment variations).
- *Progression.* Progress to body awareness and advanced movements.

Partner-Resisted Hamstring Stretch

1. The stretcher lies supine and lifts the thigh to flex the hip to 90 degrees with the knee bent.

2. The partner stabilizes the thigh in this position while the stretcher straightens the raised leg as far as possible without pain. This action lengthens the hamstrings to the pain-free end of range. The straight leg should remain flat on the mat.

3. The partner can offer resistance to the isometric contraction of the hamstrings, while at the same time ensuring that the stretcher keeps the hips flat on the mat. Before this stretch is performed, the partner may need to work with the stretcher on body awareness until the stretcher is able to stabilize the hips properly.

4. The partner directs the stretcher to begin slowly attempting to push the heel toward the floor, bending the knee, which isometrically contracts the hamstrings.

5. After the isometric push, the stretcher relaxes and inhales deeply while keeping the leg in the starting position.

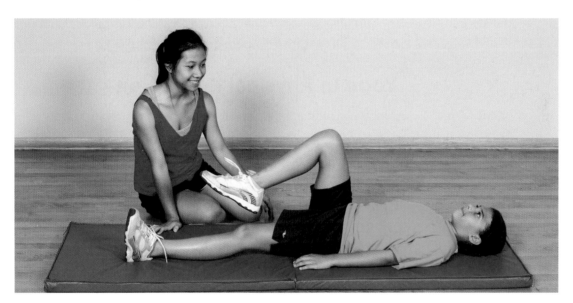

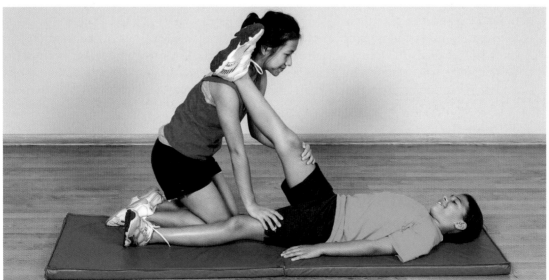

FIGURE 7.7   In order to achieve a proper partner stretch, partners must work together slowly and safely.

Adapted by permission from R.E. McAtee and J. Charland, *Facilitated Stretching* (Champaign, IL: Human Kinetics, 1999), 34.

Never make flexibility training competitive; instead, as with muscular strength training, emphasize correct technique and personal bests. Monitor students while they perform stretches and help them set effective goals. Students who are very flexible may need to be instructed to work for flexibility maintenance rather than continued improvement. Some stretches can cause injury if students continue to push beyond normal limits. As a built-in protection, FitnessGram flexibility assessments do not allow students to measure or input data above a normal limit; this restriction discourages the pursuit of hyperflexibility, which can result in injury.

Flexibility training does not require much equipment or space. For example, students can stretch in a gymnasium, on a field, on a blacktop, in a classroom, or, if traffic is sparse, in a hallway. When stretching outdoors, mats or parachutes can be placed on the ground to protect clothing. When working independently at stations, students may benefit from using visual aids, such as posters, task cards, and pictures of schoolmates performing stretches.

As a result of instructional time spent on flexibility, students should understand the definition of flexibility, ways to stretch safely, the importance of maintaining flexibility across the life span, and methods for assessing and improving flexibility.

Yoga in Physical Education

Many forms of yoga are now practiced in private studios, at health and fitness clubs, in people's homes, and in K-12 curriculums. Yoga is wonderful for children because it allows them to explore and enjoy their bodies. It also nurtures the development of strength, flexibility, and a calm mind. Yoga practice can result in a deep sense of relaxation and decreased stress and anxiety (Kraines & Sherman, 2010). At the same time, care should be used when considering yogic stretching in physical education, because some extreme asanas (postures) may lead to an increased chance of injury.

When teaching flexibility through yoga, use appropriate assessments to help your students understand this component of health-related fitness and learn ways to engage in flexibility activities safely. For assessment, have students perform health-related fitness tests (pretests and posttests), use peer checklists for form and technique, and construct portfolios of yoga poses (upper body, lower body, core, and modifications) and creation of a sequence. As with all areas of health-related fitness, conducting periodic assessments will allow your students to measure their progress and help them set goals for improvement or maintenance. Table 7.1 shows an example of a peer assessment for a yoga pose. It provides specific skill cues for students to look for when evaluating a partner's form; this type of formative assessment helps students

TABLE 7.1 Sample Peer Assessment for Tree Pose

Skill cues	Y	N	Common errors	Y	N
Lifted foot flexed and on either inner calf or thigh			Lifted foot over knee		
Working leg grounded and engaged (knee not locked)			Knee of standing leg locked		
Hips even			One hip lower than the other		
Torso lifted and core engaged			Torso sags toward the floor		
Arms lifted and extended to ceiling			Shoulders not relaxed		
Gaze directed to ceiling and not wavering			Gaze wandering		
Overall skill rating (circle one): Masterful Proficient Basic Needing improvement					

use proper form and technique. It also benefits the peer assessor, because teaching others is a great way for students to learn!

Figure 7.8 shows a rubric that can be used for a summative assessment in which high school students develop a dynamic yoga sequence to perform before moderate

Final Project: Yoga Warm-Up

Objective: Create a 6- to 10-minute yoga warm-up that includes the following elements:

- *Dynamic* lower-body yoga poses
- *Dynamic* upper-body yoga poses
- Thoughtful organization of poses to enable flow through the sequence
- Correlation of poses chosen to the physical education lesson
- Instruction and appropriate feedback provided to peers

You will lead us through each movement, describe or demonstrate how to perform it, and indicate how many sets and reps to perform.

	Advanced (4 points)	Proficient (3 points)	Basic (2 points)	Below basic (1 point)
Time (min)	6 to 10	4 to 5:59	2 to 3:59	1:59 or less
Yoga poses	Identifies a variety (3+) of dynamic yoga poses (upper and lower body). Poses are purposefully chosen to prepare for the physical activity of the lesson.	Identifies a variety (3+) of dynamic yoga poses (upper and lower body). Some poses are purposefully chosen to prepare for the physical activity of the lesson.	Identifies only 2 dynamic yoga poses (upper and lower body). Some poses are purposefully chosen to prepare for the physical activity of the lesson.	Identifies 1 or 0 dynamic yoga poses (upper and lower body) and/or the poses are not purposefully chosen to prepare for the physical activity of the lesson.
Instruction	Explains or provides images showing how to perform each yoga pose in an exemplary way.	Explains or provides images showing how to perform each yoga pose.	Somewhat explains or provides images showing how to perform each yoga pose.	Does not explain or provide images showing how to perform each yoga pose.
Sequence	All poses flow smoothly from one pose to the next.	Most poses flow smoothly from one pose to the next.	A few poses flow smoothly from one pose to the next.	There is no flow from one pose to the next.
Feedback	Common errors are explained, and appropriate individual feedback is given to peers.	Common errors are explained, and appropriate group feedback is provided.	Common errors are explained, *or* appropriate feedback is given.	No common errors are explained, and no appropriate peer feedback is given.

Overall score ____/20

FIGURE 7.8   Sample summative assessment for dynamic yoga sequence in high school.

or vigorous physical activity. Student projects can be graded on staying within the allotted time, variety of poses, instruction of poses, flow of movement from one pose to the next, and correlation of poses to the physical activity that follows. This example promotes student empowerment through their designing and presenting of their own yoga warm-up; it also reinforces the importance of a proper warm-up before engaging in physical activity.

As much as assessments are intended to showcase students' application of knowledge, class structure also plays an important role in this process. Class structure is influenced by many variables, and two of them may affect how you incorporate yoga into your physical education program—namely, time and teaching progressions. In order to maximize physical education time, remember these teaching progressions:

- *Foundation.* Gain basic knowledge and broaden exposure to the practice. For example, attend to flowing movement, deep breathing, and flexibility (e.g., yoga squats, folds, sun/moon salutation).
- *Expansion.* Progress with yoga movements; utilize skill-related components to expand your basic practice (e.g., arm balances, kneeling poses).
- *Progression.* Progress your practice; be awakened in body, mind, and spirit through innovative and versatile movements (e.g., binds, inversions, sequences, and restorative movements).

Different types of yoga to explore include Bikram (basic poses in a hot, humid environment), hatha (basic poses and relaxation techniques), vinyasa (postures and breathing), power (sequences of poses performed fast), Kundalini (focus on inner soul), Iyengar (props used for proper body alignment), Anusara (focus on inner self, mind, and soul), and restorative (simple poses with props to rest the body and cleanse the mind for rejuvenation).

Regardless of type, safety is a priority with yoga. Always offer movement modifications for students who are less flexible. For example, in the downward-facing dog movements, students may struggle to get their heels flat on the ground; if so, you can modify the movement by having them bend their knees.

Equipment options include cards with poses and techniques, mats, blocks, straps, chairs, and glow sticks. Students' textbooks can be used as yoga blocks for certain poses if students lack sufficient ROM. In addition to a regular lighted gym, examples of possible settings include the outdoors, water, and darkness (with the use of black lights and glow sticks).

To help students make the most of yoga practice, offer them the following reminders:

- There is no such thing as "being good" at yoga. It is not competitive; it is an individualized activity that can cater to different abilities.
- Correct form and alignment are necessary at all times; never force anything.
- Breath is vital in yoga. Never hold it; do stay connected to it by always trying to match the duration of the inhalation with that of the exhalation.
- Be present. Stay aware of your body and your thought process during the practice. If your mind wanders, focus on your next inhalation or exhalation to get yourself back into the present with your practice.
- Let go of expectations. Each practice is different. Expectations close the mind to possibilities.
- Relax. Yoga is a time to unwind the body. Keep yourself tension free at all times.

- Practice. The only way one becomes more flexible is through practice and repetition.
- Combine yoga training with a regular health-related fitness program that meets the FITT guidelines. Although yoga training does offer muscular strength benefits, it does not effectively improve all muscle groups in the body.

Through goal setting and regular training, students will progress in their yoga practice. Beginner students should use equipment to help control and lengthen the poses. Over time, the modifications and equipment will help with the tightness and tension in their muscles, and their flexibility will increase.

If you are interested in sharpening your training knowledge and skills, consider obtaining a group fitness certification or a specialty certification focused on yoga. Organizations that offer teacher training programs include Yoga Works, Yoga Tree, and Sun Moon Yoga Studios. These certification programs offer useful information and the opportunity to enhance your teaching ability.

Principles of Training

All students should learn how to apply the principles of training to flexibility. The principles are discussed in chapter 3 and in each chapter related to the health-related fitness components. Applying these principles will help students improve flexibility and implement the FITT guidelines (discussed later in the chapter) in their programs.

Overload, Progression, Specificity, Regularity, and Individuality

The principle of overload asserts that in order to adapt and improve flexibility, the muscle–tendon unit must be stretched until tension is felt (i.e., to the point of mild discomfort). The person then backs off slightly and holds the stretch at a point just before discomfort occurs. Next, the principle of progression calls for gradually increasing the amount of time for which the stretch is held, starting with 10 seconds and building up to at least 30 seconds. Students should not, however, use the progression principle to increase the load (tension) placed on the muscle; to the contrary, they should stretch a joint only through the limits of normal ROM (American College of Sports Medicine, 2014). If they stretch to the point of mild discomfort and then back off slightly, they will overload the muscle at the proper tension. The stretch should feel tight, but not painful. Above all, dispel the "no pain, no gain" notion. Flexibility training should not be painful (see the section titled Safety Guidelines for Flexibility Activities later in this chapter).

As with other areas of health-related fitness, the principles of specificity and regularity hold that in order to increase flexibility in a particular area, a person must perform exercises for a specific muscle or specific muscle group—and must do it on a regular basis. The American College of Sports Medicine (2014) recommends that flexibility exercises be done on at least two days per week and up to seven days per week. For lasting changes, try progressing to 60 seconds or even two minutes for each stretch! If the stretch becomes uncomfortable, take a break and repeat to achieve more consistency.

According to the regularity principle, any improvements in flexibility will be lost if the person stops performing flexibility exercises. Therefore, if flexibility training is not done on a regular basis, the body will eventually become tight and less mobile. It is far more difficult and time consuming to regain mobility than to maintain it. In order to prevent regression, move often throughout the day. For example, encourage students and teachers to get up from their desks, chairs, or couches and move all parts of the body. Encourage them also to take advantage of opportunities to work on stretching practices by performing movements when watching television and using a computer. Finally, as stated throughout this book, each student should set individual goals for flexibility based on need, physical limitations, and personal motivation.

FITT Guidelines

Table 7.2 provides information about how to manipulate time and type based on the FITT guidelines when performing stretching exercises (partner-assisted and PNF stretching). The recommended *frequency* for flexibility training calls for stretching at least two times per week but preferably daily in order to attain maximum benefit. Increasing the number of flexibility sessions per week from three to seven increases the overload placed on the muscle. As indicated earlier, the *intensity* for all flexibility exercises should be to the point just before discomfort occurs (stretch to the point of slight discomfort, then back off slightly). Intensity is an extremely important factor in a safe and effective flexibility training program. A static stretch that goes beyond the point of mild discomfort (to pain) will not only decrease a students' desire to stretch but also increase the likelihood of injury. Recommendations for the *time* of a stretch range from 10 seconds through 30 seconds. The American College of Sports Medicine (2006) proposes holding a stretch for at least 10 seconds and progressing to 30 seconds. (Note that a student should always begin by holding a stretch for a short period and gradually progress to the 30-second length.) Finally, the *type* of stretching performed may be static, PNF, partner, or dynamic.

Before students begin any flexibility exercise, provide them with proper instruction and have them perform an active warm-up. Younger or less experienced students should learn the basic static stretches that increase flexibility of major muscle groups, whereas older or more experienced students may be ready for a greater variety of sport-specific stretches and advanced stretching techniques.

TABLE 7.2 FITT Guidelines Applied to Flexibility

	Guidelines
Frequency	At least two days per week, and preferably daily, after a warm-up to raise muscle temperature
Intensity	Slow elongation of the muscle to the point of mild discomfort, then backing off slightly Modifications: • Developmental appropriateness • Equipment • Sequencing • Time that stretch is held
Time	Up to four stretches per muscle or muscle group with each stretch held for 10 to 30 seconds (always after warming up properly) Three sets of at least 10 seconds and gradually increasing the time
Type	In physical education, preferably controlled stretching for all muscles or muscle groups Principles of training applied in a health-related fitness program to improve or maintain healthy flexibility

Adapted from D.V. Knudson, P. Magnusson, and M. McHugh, Current Issues in Flexibility Fitness, in *The President's Council on Physical Fitness and Sports Digest,* 3rd ed. ser., no. 10, edited by C. Corbin and B. Pangrazi (Washington, DC: Department of Health and Human Services, 2000); American College of Sports Medicine (ACSM). *ACSM's Resource Manual for Guidelines for Exercise Testing and Prescription,* 5th ed. (Philadelphia: Lippincott, Williams, and Wilkins, 2006).

Bompa and Haff (2009) suggest laying a strong foundation of static stretches with children who are 6 to 10 years old, which they view as the initiation phase of training. They also suggest using various stages of maturation as a guide to indicate when it is appropriate to perform the three basic types of stretching (static, dynamic, and PNF). Remember that PNF and partner stretching require extensive instruction and mature, responsible students; these types of stretches may pose safety threats if not performed correctly.

Teach students to follow the FITT guidelines using controlled, steady stretching and holding each stretch only to the point of mild tension—not pain, regardless of what they have been told in the past. Students should be empowered to individualize each stretch, doing only what is comfortable for them, not necessarily what a classmate can do. Teach students that ballistic stretching is appropriate only in certain sport situations and even then only if done correctly.

If a student is too flexible (i.e., displays hypermobility), has abnormal ROM (laxity), severely lacks flexibility, or has another structural limitation—and if the anomaly seems to cause serious performance or safety concerns—meet with the student and parents. Suggest that they visit a trained health care professional for further evaluation.

Warm-Up and Cool-Down

Emphasize to your students the purpose of warming up and cooling down. A warm-up prepares muscles for flexibility by dilating blood vessels and ensuring that muscles are well-supplied with oxygen; it also raises the temperature of muscles for optimal flexibility. The ideal warm-up before a hard workout involves dynamic stretches targeting specific muscles that your students will be using, *if* they are doing something that requires range of motion. However, if students are merely going for an easy jog or workout, then they can just do so—that doesn't require a flexibility warm-up.

Static stretching is not recommended for physical educators to begin their classes. In the 1990s, problems with traditional pre-workout static stretching were examined by David Behm, an expert on stretching and a research professor at Memorial University of Newfoundland. One of the resulting studies (Behm, Button, & Butt, 2001) highlighted the fact that runners ran an uphill mile 13 seconds *slower* after performing static stretches than when they did not stretch at all. Other studies discovered drops in power and explosive force. These findings suggest that static stretching should not be done in physical education warm-ups and should be saved for the cool-down portion of the program.

Dynamic movements are the most effective techniques for warming up the body. Therefore, you should plan for and provide a dynamic warm-up that targets the specific muscles your students will be using during the class period.

Many experts caution that participants should perform at least five minutes of low-intensity cardiorespiratory endurance activity to warm muscles before performing any stretching (American College of Sports Medicine, 2014). We recommend that teachers ensure that their students take this simple precaution before beginning flexibility activities. You can help your elementary students understand this concept by making a connection to spaghetti: When cold, it snaps easily, but when warmed through cooking, it becomes pliable and bends easily. Older students may appreciate a connection to their favorite professional athletes, who warm up for an hour or more before a game. Help your students understand the difference between a warm-up to prepare for a workout or game (which includes dynamic flexibility exercises) and flexibility training (which may include a variety of types of stretching and is much more thorough).

A cool-down is designed to relax muscles that were active during the workout, thus preventing the buildup of lactic acid, which can lead to cramping and stiffness. Static stretching performed at the end of a training session is a great way to improve flexibility. When deciding what to focus on for static stretching, consider the training program for that day and your expectations about the body's response. If your students are working the lower body through exercises such as squats and lunges, then stretching should focus primarily on the hip flexors and extensors, the hamstrings, and the quadriceps.

Introduce and reinforce the importance of stretching and flexibility training for reducing students' injury risk and enhancing their quality of life. Make connections to your students' lives that will matter to them now, in addition to focusing on the long-term benefits of flexibility.

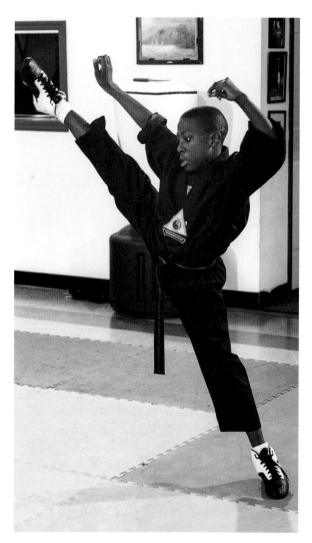

If your students want to be able to punt a football or perform a high kick in martial arts, they must have good leg flexibility in order to succeed.

Addressing Motor Skills Through Flexibility Activities

Naturally, a student who can move through a full range of motion is more likely to be ready to learn and perform motor skills correctly. Similarly, a student with limited ROM will have a more difficult time mastering the same motor skill. The specificity principle applies here: Students who want to be able to punt a football or perform a high kick in soccer must have good hip and leg flexibility in order to succeed. Good flexibility, then, enhances motor skill development. Address motor skills through flexibility activities and vice versa by pointing out the connections between the stretches and the motor skill activities that students practice in class. When students make the connection between flexibility and their physical activities, they are more likely to continue working on enhancing flexibility as a lifestyle choice.

Safety Guidelines for Flexibility Activities

Stretching in a physical education setting brings up many safety issues. For starters, be aware of the factors discussed earlier that may limit flexibility. Before stretching, students should complete a general whole-body warm-up. Students with physical disabilities may need to do a longer warm-up in order to enhance joint mobility. For static stretching, students should use slow movements, holding each stretch at the point just before mild discomfort occurs (backing off slightly when discomfort is felt) for 10 to 30 seconds. For dynamic stretching, students should mimic movement from a specific sport or exercise in an exaggerated but controlled manner (American College of Sports Medicine, 2014). By following these protocols, you can allow students to individualize their efforts.

Teach students to limit or avoid locking any joint when performing flexibility exercises. Advising students to maintain "soft knees" and "soft joints" can help them avoid any unnecessary overstretching of ligaments.

Students should also avoid forcing any stretch. Help students pay attention to their bodies, particularly any feelings of discomfort or pain. These feelings are signals that the student is forcing the stretch, going beyond the normal range of motion, and possibly damaging ligaments.

Never allow students to hyperflex (bend from the waist) or hyperextend the spine while stretching; doing so places undue stress on the spine's intervertebral discs. Bending from the hips in a forward-flexed position is okay, but bending only from the waist is not. Compression of discs in the lower back is one reason that the back-saver sit-and-reach assessment was implemented. Specifically, the forward-flexed position at the waist causes increased pressure on the discs, and stretching one leg at a time reduces the pressure.

Hyperextension also compresses the discs. Going from a flexed position to extension is okay, but going beyond normal extension into hyperextension (bending backward) is not. Be aware that in some instances a physician may prescribe hyperextension exercises to rehabilitate the lower back, but most of the population should generally avoid this motion. The undue stress on the intervertebral discs is exacerbated if twisting or rotation is combined with hyperflexion or hyperextension. Although this motion may not present an immediate concern or injury, it may contribute to chronic degeneration of discs and to low-back pain as a person ages.

Contraindicated Exercises

Contraindicated exercises are those that have been determined to be unsafe or to risk injury if a person continues to incorporate them into a physical activity program. An injury may not occur every time a contraindicated exercise is performed; even so, injury may result over weeks or years due to repeated microtrauma in the tissue. Several exercises should be avoided in order to reduce the risk of joint injury. Alternatives to these contraindicated exercises are provided in the web resource (see figure 7.9).

Safety issues related to hypermobility, joint laxity, and flexibility were discussed earlier. When a student performs an exercise that takes a joint well beyond its normal range of motion, as in some **hyperflexion** or **hyperextension** exercises, the risk increases for developing joint laxity and possible injury (Corbin, Welk, Corbin, & Welk, 2009).

For all of these reasons, provide alternatives when designing your flexibility instruction and keep in mind the specificity principle and the availability of exercise prescriptions by medical personnel. Some sports demand extreme ROM—for example, gymnastics, dancing, and certain positions in team sports (e.g., baseball catcher, which requires a full squat). In these instances, it may be necessary to follow the medically

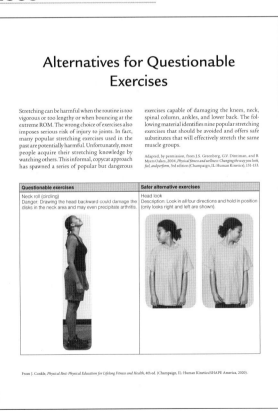

Alternatives for Questionable Exercises

Stretching can be harmful when the routine is too vigorous or too lengthy or when bouncing at the extreme ROM. The wrong choice of exercises also imposes serious risk of injury to joints. In fact, many popular stretching exercises used in the past are potentially harmful. Unfortunately, most people acquire their stretching knowledge by watching others. This informal, copycat approach has spawned a series of popular but dangerous exercises capable of damaging the knees, neck, spinal column, ankles, and lower back. The following material identifies nine popular stretching exercises that should be avoided and offers safe substitutes that will effectively stretch the same muscle groups.

Adapted, by permission, from J.S. Greenberg, G.V. Dintiman, and B. Myers Oakes, 2004, *Physical fitness and wellness: Changing the way you look, feel, and perform*, 3rd edition (Champaign, IL: Human Kinetics), 151-153.

Questionable exercises	Safer alternative exercises
Neck roll (circling) Danger: Drawing the head backward could damage the disks in the neck area and may even precipitate arthritis.	Head look Description: Look in all four directions and hold in position (only looks right and left are shown).

From J. Conkle, *Physical Best: Physical Education for Lifelong Fitness and Health*, 4th ed. (Champaign, IL: Human Kinetics/SHAPE America, 2020).

FIGURE 7.9 Alternative exercises to replace contraindicated exercises are included in the web resource.

prescribed exercise prescription and to teach dynamic, sport-specific flexibility exercises. If so, use extreme caution, active warm-ups, and static stretching after the muscles have been warmed up. In many instances, teachers do not have the time or expertise to prescribe exercises for special situations. Corbin et al. (2004) suggest that physical educators teach to the needs of the majority and include exercises with the least potential for negative effects and the most potential for benefits. When alternative exercises are available to high-risk stretches, use the alternatives for a safer, more effective program.

Summary

Flexibility is just as important to health-related fitness as other components are; therefore, we must resist the temptation to relegate it to warm-ups and cool-downs. Flexibility exercises performed during warm-ups are important to prepare the body for activity, but flexibility training also needs to be featured as the core activity of some lessons. This approach allows time to demonstrate how important, relaxing, and pleasurable flexibility exercises can be. As with all aspects of health-related fitness, students should strive to improve and maintain flexibility through regular and adequate participation. In addition, it is educational to make explicit connections for students between the stretches taught in class and the activities they perform in and outside of class.

For model flexibility-training activities, see the flexibility activities included in the web resource. Also refer to the principles of flexibility and the FITT formula to enhance students' performance in flexibility and other areas of the physical education curriculum.

Good flexibility is crucial for a healthy range of motion, which in turn improves overall health-related fitness, posture, risk of injury, and safety when engaging in physical activity. Remember that in a health-related physical fitness education program, controlled stretching is most appropriate. Moreover, static stretching offers the safest type of flexibility training for the majority of students with the least negative effect; it should be done when muscles have already been warmed up. Address the appropriate types of stretching with your students and provide them with examples and experiences of different types of stretching. By doing so, you give them a lifelong tool for safely maintaining individual flexibility. The next chapter focuses on appropriate incorporation of muscular strength and endurance into an effective physical education program.

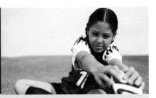

Discussion Questions

1. As a physical education teacher, compare static stretching with dynamic stretching.
2. How would you explain the difference between stretching and flexibility to a middle school student?
3. How does flexibility training affect the body?
4. Describe how flexibility can affect the following health problems: injury, soreness, and poor posture.
5. Describe how flexibility can help a person in day-to-day life.
6. Describe factors that impact flexibility and how you may address them while teaching flexibility in physical education.
7. Design a lesson for high school students to create a personal health-related fitness program based on individual performance on a flexibility assessment.
8. Choose an activity or sport that interests you and describe how flexibility training can enhance performance.
9. What important safety guidelines apply to flexibility training in physical education?
10. If a student is engaged in a contraindicated exercise during physical education, how would you handle it if the student said, "I do it all the time in practice"?

CHAPTER 8

Muscular Strength and Endurance

Patrick McHenry

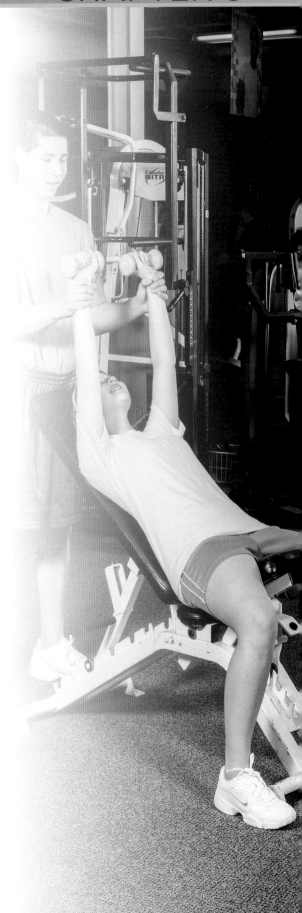

Any well-rounded program for health-related fitness must address muscular strength and muscular endurance. Research has shown that youth and adolescents can benefit from a properly designed, well-supervised resistance training program. In fact, resistance training for youth and adolescents is supported by the American College of Sports Medicine (ACSM), the National Strength and Conditioning Association (NSCA), the American Pediatrics Association (APA), the President's Council on Physical Fitness, and organizations in countries around the world (Baker et al., 2007; Behm, Faigenbaum, Falk, & Klentrou, 2008; Lloyd et al., 2012; Lloyd et al., 2013). These organizations even suggest that children who participate in youth sport programs should perform strength-developing activities before participation—much like adult preseason conditioning, albeit on a much smaller scale—in order to prevent injury and enhance skill development (Faigenbaum & Myer, 2010a, 2010b).

When developing muscular fitness programs for children and adolescents, it's crucial to recognize that young people are not little adults; therefore, adult principles of resistance training do not necessarily fit (Dahab & McCambridge, 2009). In physical education classes, training for muscular strength and endurance should focus on creating positive experiences that teach correct technique, allow for progression of fundamental movement skills, and develop physical literacy. Physical education programs that emphasize physical literacy help prepare students to be lifelong learners, which may incline them to participate in sport and other physical activities throughout their lives and try new activities as they get older.

Understanding pediatric exercise physiology will help you help your students understand the growth and maturation they will experience from childhood through adolescence; it will also help you design safe, developmentally appropriate lessons for muscular strength and endurance (Rowland, 2005). This chapter will help you develop a safe, scientifically sound program for muscular strength and endurance, teach basic movement drills to enhance your students' motor abilities, and provide activities to help them develop high-quality motor patterns. Physical Best serves as a guide for physically educating students in the area of muscular strength and endurance.

Definitions of Muscular Strength and Endurance Concepts

To administer a safe and effective resistance training program for children, teachers must understand a variety of terms related to the development of muscular strength and endurance. **Muscular strength** is the ability of a muscle or a muscle group to exert maximal force against a resistance one time through the full **range of motion** (Lloyd, Cronin, & Faigenbaum, 2016), which is the degree of movement that occurs at a joint (Baechle, Earle, & Wathen, 2008). Full range of motion must be required and strictly enforced for healthy students who do not have a physical limitation in order to help prevent injury and develop proper movement patterns. If you allow a student to perform partial movement patterns as part of a regular routine, it may lead to a shortening of the muscles, which could lead to overdevelopment of the agonist and underdevelopment of the antagonist. This condition can make the student more vulnerable to injuries.

Muscular endurance, on the other hand, is the ability of a muscle or a muscle group to exert a submaximal force repeatedly over a period of time (Lloyd, Cronin, & Faigenbaum, 2016). In Physical Best, muscular strength and muscular endurance are treated in combination as **muscular fitness** because they are difficult to separate in practical application during activities and exercises, especially at the primary grade level.

When referring to a component of fitness, **muscular power** is described as explosive strength or the ability to exert strength quickly (Corbin, Pangrazi, & Franks, 2000; Corbin, Welk, Corbin, & Welk, 2016; U.S. Department of Health and Human Services, 1996). There is a century-old concept that power also influences health; for this reason, power-enhancing activities should be included in physical education.

Resistance training, or **strength training**, consists of a systematic, planned program that uses any of various methods and types of equipment (e.g., body weight, elastic bands, sandbags, dumbbells, medicine balls, kettlebells, free weights, machines) to progressively stress the musculoskeletal system in order to improve muscular strength or endurance or both (Faigenbaum et al., 2009; Faigenbaum & Micheli, 2017; Faigenbaum & Westcott, 2007). Throughout this text, the term *resistance training* is used when referring to activities that develop muscular strength and muscular endurance because it encompasses a greater variety of activities and does not require the use of weights only. Students, even young students, can safely participate in resistance training, or strength training, when it is correctly implemented.

On the other hand, competitive muscular strength activities are not appropriate for physical education. Specifically, **weightlifting** is an Olympic sport consisting of the clean-and-jerk and the snatch (USA Weightlifting, n.d.); **powerlifting** involves the deadlift, squat, and bench press; and in **bodybuilding** the contestants are judged on muscle size, symmetry, and definition (American Academy of Pediatrics, McCambridge, & Stricker, 2008). You should not include these types of muscular strength activities in your physical education classes, but you should educate your students so that they understand the differences between these activities and appropriate resistance training and why these exercises are not safe for physical education.

Student Age and Resistance Training

When working with students of different ages, levels of physical development, maturity, and experience, it can be helpful to measure their ages in a variety of ways.

- **Chronological age** is age in years, which enables a general estimate of what type of objectives and activities are appropriate for a group of students. For the purposes of this chapter, the following terms are used to describe students in terms of chronological age:
  - *Adolescent* for girls age 12 to 18 years and boys age 14 to 18 years
  - *Youth* and *children* for girls up to age 11 and boys up to age 13
- **Biological age** is age as an indicator of a student's developmental status. Is the student a "late bloomer" or an "early bloomer"? For instance, a student may be in the 12th grade but not physically mature, and such a student should not be expected to perform the same muscular resistance training exercises as a student who has already matured.
- **Training age** is age associated with how long the student has been working out with a teacher. Starting all students at the training age of zero if they have not previously been in your class allows them to see, hear, and understand the proper technique for each exercise or activity. This experience-related factor can also be important when individualizing instruction.

Developmentally Appropriate Resistance Training

Your students' risk of injury will be increased if the resistance training part of your physical education program uses activities designed for adults (age 21 or older), asks students to lift as much weight as possible, or fails to focus on proper technique (Myer, Quatman, Khoury, Wall, & Hewett, 2009). Improper movement patterns can cause muscle imbalances, which increase the risk of injury and may adversely affect movement patterns later in life. Therefore, a sound practice in resistance training for children, adolescents, and adults is to focus on good form and multiple **repetitions** (for muscular endurance) before focusing on heavier weights with fewer repetitions (for muscular strength).

In addition, no student participant should engage in rapid repetitions in which momentum aids the lifting process. Some elite athletes may perform high-speed power training, but this method is highly specialized and would be unsafe for most participants. Therefore, it is inappropriate for use in physical education. Instead, participants should use a six-second count, taking two or three seconds to lift the weight and three or four seconds to lower it, all while focusing on proper technique. Furthermore, children should not engage in lifting heavy weights (i.e., weights with which one can perform fewer than six repetitions).

For most students, building muscle or "bulking up" is not a realistic goal, and students need to be educated about what *will* occur as they begin a resistance training program. Teach students that the first step is neuromuscular. That is, the message must get from the brain to the muscle, and students can solidify that message pathway by correctly practicing movements. Using correct technique ensures the proper firing of muscles so that movement patterns are correct. Students will see gains in strength; however, they will not see **hypertrophy** (increase in size) at this point. As a student moves from child to adolescent, the body will get taller and more mature. Strength gains will improve as long as the student continues to exercise in a correct manner. Research has shown that the greatest strength gains occur due to neural adaptations, not from hypertrophy (Faigenbaum, Lloyd, & Myer, 2013). In addition, when males reach the Tanner stage 5 of development and their long bones have stopped growing, they experience about a 33 percent increase in hormones associated with hypertrophy; this change usually occurs between 19 and 22 years of age. With this knowledge, you can help students set realistic goals depending on their development and needs.

Resistance Training for Students With Special Needs

Students with special needs can participate in a strength and conditioning program if the teacher and any student aides are aware of the student's needs and limitations and are prepared to make the correct accommodations while following the basic guidelines used with all students. Research has shown that a properly developed resistance training program can help students with special needs to develop muscular fitness (Fragla-Pinkham, Haley, & Goodgold, 2006). Students with special needs who do not have limitations in their ability to grasp or hold an implement can use sandbags, medicine balls, and bands in a manner similar to that of any other student. Students who have physical limitations or range-of-motion issues can use similar equipment as long as the teacher keeps the resistance light and monitors their movement patterns.

The safety of all exercises depends in part on the person performing the movement, the person's ability level, and any injury or condition the person may have. It also depends on the teacher's supervision and ability to create developmentally appropriate learning activities. The teacher must know the students and what is appropriate for them.

Position of the National Strength and Conditioning Association on Resistance Training in Youth

This is the 2009 position of the NSCA:

1. A properly designed and supervised resistance training program is relatively safe for youth.
2. A properly designed and supervised resistance training program can enhance the muscular strength and power of youth.
3. A properly designed and supervised resistance training program can improve the cardiovascular risk profile of youth.
4. A properly designed and supervised resistance training program can improve motor skill performance and may contribute to enhanced sports performance of youth.
5. A properly designed and supervised resistance training program can increase a young athlete's resistance to sports-related injuries.
6. A properly designed and supervised resistance training program can help improve the psychosocial well-being of youth.
7. A properly designed and supervised resistance training program can help promote and develop exercise habits during childhood and adolescence.

Reprinted by permission from A.D. Faigenbaum et al., "Youth Resistance Training: Updated Position Statement Paper From the National Strength and Conditioning Association," *Journal of Strength and Conditioning Research* 23, no. Suppl 5 (2009): S60-S76.

A word of caution for adolescent students going through puberty: As students grow, their movement patterns needs to be reeducated, or at least practiced. During these growth phases, it is good to have the student reduce the weight and concentrate on technique with supervision by a qualified instructor.

Parents may have concerns about resistance training for children and adolescents because they have not been educated about the safety and benefits of developmentally appropriate resistance training. Multiple recommendations or position statements on resistance training are available to provide guidance in developing children's resistance training programs (see the sidebar titled Position of the National Strength and Conditioning Association on Resistance Training in Youth). You can also refer parents to SHAPE America's 2012 guidance document *Instructional Framework for Fitness Education in Physical Education*, which highlights developmentally appropriate training techniques for muscular strength and endurance. In addition, you can reassure parents that proper safety guidelines will be adhered to in your classes. Their concerns should be generally allayed by learning that experts view resistance training (under the guidance of a qualified professional) as beneficial for students and that you are conscientious about students' safety. However, if necessary, schedule a parent conference or provide an open gym event in the evening so that parents can learn firsthand about their children's experiences in your physical education classes.

Benefits of Resistance Training

Muscular strength is an essential component of motor skill performance (Lloyd et al., 2013). It is also a foundational segment of health-related fitness because it is associated with a variety of benefits. Many of these benefits are age related, and greater sport-performance benefits are associated with postpubescent adolescents. Potential benefits of resistance training include the following (American Academy of Pediatrics, McCambridge, & Stricker, 2008; Baechle et al., 2008; Casa et al., 2013; Faigenbaum, Lloyd, & Myer, 2013; Faigenbaum & Myer, 2010b; Faigenbaum & Westcott, 2007; Lloyd et al., 2013; Rowland, 2005; Whitehead, 2018):

Power and Health-Related Fitness

Since the 1960s, power has been considered a part of skill-related fitness in physical education. However, long before that time, as far back as the 1880s, the health benefits of power were recognized by physical educators. Recent research (Corbin, Janz, & Baptista, 2017) supports this view and recognizes power as a "combined" component (strength × speed) of fitness. Developing muscular power in students can help optimize skeletal development and support a healthy body composition. It can be increased when students participate in physical activities that put their muscles and bones under sufficient loads (this concept of overload is discussed later in this chapter) (Corbin, Janz, & Baptista, 2017). Thus, encouraging students to become their physical best must include encouraging them to engage in physical activities for power development.

- Increased physical confidence and competence
- Development of physical literacy
- Increased muscular strength
- Increased muscular power, or ability to exert force rapidly
- Increased muscular endurance
- Improvement in cardiorespiratory endurance using circuit weight training
- Prevention of musculoskeletal injury
- Improved sport performance
- Reduced risk of fractures in adulthood
- Enhanced bone development, in both bone strength and bone growth, during the skeletal growth period

Postpubescent children achieve these benefits, as well as many of the health benefits associated with adult resistance training programs, including the following (American Academy of Pediatrics, McCambridge, & Stricker, 2008; Dahab & McCambridge, 2009; Whitehead, 2018):

- Improved blood lipid profile
- Improved body composition
- Improved mental health and well-being
- More positive attitude toward lifetime physical activity

Teaching Guidelines
for Muscular Strength and Endurance

Many children at the elementary level lack the emotional maturity to engage in formal resistance training, but they can perform developmentally appropriate activities for muscular strength and endurance (such as the Physical Best activities available in the web resource). Late elementary may be the first opportunity to introduce a more formal or comprehensive resistance training program (Faigenbaum & Micheli, 2017). Although most guidelines refer to chronological age, always take into account the participant's psychological and physical maturity when implementing resistance training programs.

Teaching About Muscular Strength

Teaching basic exercises to elementary students will help with their movement patterns and support their learning of fundamental movement skills. Good ways to introduce elementary students to resistance training include push-ups, body squats, lunges, prone pull-ups, and weight-training movements performed with little or no weight in order to understand proper technique. If you would like to develop a unit or explore the topic in more depth, consult any of the many books that include age-appropriate exercises and show proper progression; a number of such books are available from Human Kinetics (www.humankinetics.com).

A student of any age who begins a program with no experience should start at lower levels and progress to more advanced levels as permitted by exercise tolerance, skill, amount of training time, and understanding. In strength training, a beginning student should start slowly—performing a single set of 8 to 12 repetitions twice per week—in order to gain confidence. The student can then progress gradually to performing one to three sets of 6 to 12 repetitions two or three times per week. Any increases in training load should be small (5 percent to 10 percent) for most exercises.

As with all components of health-related fitness, help your students understand the health and lifestyle benefits of resistance training and how it applies to their own lives. The following suggestions may help to ensure students enjoy resistance training in your class:

- Emphasize having fun.
- Incorporate variety into your classroom activities.
- Introduce new exercises.
- Emphasize intrinsic enjoyment.
- Change the training mode.
- Vary the number of sets and repetitions.
- Use multiple goals and have students help set them.
- Do not limit the goals to increasing only muscular strength or only muscular endurance. It is appropriate to set goals for each.
- Have students use personalized logs to track individual progress.
- Share personal success stories.
- Teach students about their bodies and about safe lifting techniques; aim for development of positive attitudes toward physical activity.

Adapted by permission from A. Faigenbaum, "Youth Resistance Training," *PCPFS Research Digest* 4, no. 3 (2003): 1-8; Faigenbaum, A.D., and W.L. Westcott. *Youth Strength Training: Programs for Health, Fitness and Sport* (Champaign, IL: Human Kinetics, 2009).

If you apply these suggestions, you can motivate students to learn about and participate in muscular strength and endurance activities.

Muscular fitness concepts and resistance training sessions can be taught even if state-of-the-art equipment is not available. For instance, surgical tubing and other materials for resistance bands are inexpensive and readily available. In the primary grades, most children will be challenged by using the weight of their own body, and for some children this challenge carries through to middle school and high school. Another idea is to collect cans of food and use them as small weights (they can later be donated to a local food bank). If you or a parent is handy with a sewing machine,

Youth Resistance Training Guidelines

- Provide qualified instruction and supervision.
- Ensure that the exercise environment is safe and free of hazards.
- Begin each session with a 5- to 10-minute dynamic warm-up period.
- Start with one set of 8 to 12 repetitions with a moderate load on a variety of exercises. Progress to two or three sets of 6 to 12 repetitions depending on needs or goals.
- Increase the resistance gradually (by 5 percent to 10 percent) as strength improves.
- Focus on correct exercise technique rather than amount of weight lifted.
- Train two to three times per week on nonconsecutive days.

Adapted from A.D. Faigenbaum et al., 2009, "Youth Resistance Training: Updated Position Statement Paper From the National Strength and Conditioning Association," *Journal of Strength and Conditioning Research* 23(Suppl 5): S60-S76.

small saddlebags can be made to hold small weights, cans of food, or other items used for resistance training. The saddlebags can be draped over the extremities, and a child can individualize the program by selecting appropriate weights at each station. Balls can also be used for balance and strength activities, and partner-resistance exercises can be used if equipment is lacking.

When purchasing equipment, focus on buying items that will meet the primary needs of the students. Most machine weights are not designed for the small size of children; therefore, it may be a better choice to go with resistance bands, dumbbells, medicine balls, or free weights. This recommendation does not come without caution, because the use of free weights poses additional safety concerns related to form and spotting techniques. Most injuries in youth resistance training activities involve improper lifting, maximal lifts, or lack of qualified adult supervision; in addition, injury often occurs in exercise involving deadlifts, the bench press, or the overhead press (Myer et al., 2009).

Remember that using traditional weight-training equipment represents only a small segment of the available exercises and activities. Students should first manage their own body weight before lifting heavier weights. The Physical Best activities teach muscular strength and endurance concepts without requiring the use of a weight room.

Principles of Training

The basic training principles presented in chapter 3 apply to resistance training, and teachers may use a variety of activities to improve muscular strength or endurance as long as these training principles are followed. You can manipulate the mode of exercise, the number of sets, the number of repetitions, or the amount of resistance or weight lifted. For example, a beginning adolescent student who is participating in weightlifting should do one set of 8 to 12 repetitions with a light or moderate load; with progression, the student can move to three sets of 6 to 8 repetitions for multijoint exercises and two sets of 10 to 12 repetitions for single-joint exercises (Baker et al., 2007; Faigenbaum et al., 2009; Lloyd, Cronin, & Faigenbaum, 2016; Lloyd et al., 2013).

Overload, Progression, Specificity, Individuality, and Regularity

The **overload principle**—which calls for placing greater-than-normal demands on the musculature—indicates that people seeking to improve muscular strength or muscular endurance must increase their workload periodically. Specifically, overload requires increasing the resistance against the exercising muscles to a level greater than that used before. Increasing the number of repetitions provides another avenue to overload the muscle; this type of overload develops muscular endurance, not muscular strength. You can also decrease the rest interval between activities. Keep in mind that the increase must be appropriate for the age and health-related fitness of the student; remember also that chronological age may not always be the best indicator for determining the amount of weight or the number of repetitions. These recommendations differ slightly from exercise prescription for adults, and they yield a safe and effective method of increasing strength in children and adolescents.

The **progression principle** calls for gradual increase of resistance training exercise. It is a systematic approach to increasing the resistance and intensity of the activity. To avoid injury, however, students must understand appropriate progression and set goals accordingly. For example, as beginners, high school students may start with a body-weight squat. Once they master it, they can move to a goblet squat (i.e., holding the dumbbell in both hands against the sternum) and then to a front squat. Each time the student progresses to the next exercise, ensure that proper technique is maintained. From the front squat, the student can move to the back squat and then add weight.

Students should know that developing a good base for muscular fitness often entails using the weight of their own body first, followed by one set of 8 to 12 repetitions. Resistance begins with a weight that can be lifted 8 to 10 times (but not 11), and the number of repetitions is gradually increased to 12. Point out that each exercise is more difficult than the previous one. Weight can be added to each level if technique is maintained. Another variable that can be used to increase the difficulty of an exercise without adding weight is speed of movement. In some instances, one component can be increased while others are decreased; for example, as exercise intensity increases, load may decrease, or vice versa.

For younger students, progression may involve changing the resistance training exercise to make it more difficult. For example, some students may begin by holding a bent-knee plank for a set amount of time. While the teacher or peers provide feedback on proper form, students practice until they can achieve a desired time goal. At this point, they can move on to straight-arm planks. Other students may be ready for bent-knee push-ups; these students also need supervision and feedback to ensure proper form. Once a desired repetition goal is reached while maintaining proper form, these students can progress to regular push-ups. This approach makes it easy to see how progression allows your students to individualize their resistance training. As an example, the web resource provides a Physical Best activity named Mission Push-Up Possible that teaches progression in a fun, individualized manner.

Whether your students have achieved a health-enhancing level of muscular strength and endurance or are working their way there, you should develop a plan of health-related fitness activities that will lead them to improved levels of health-related fitness in a safe but progressive manner. The Physical Best activities have been developed with this principle in mind.

The **specificity principle** holds that the effects of training from exercise are specific to the exercise that is performed and the muscles that are engaged (Faigenbaum & Micheli, 2017). For resistance training, specificity suggests that the activities selected should provide the outcome represented by the class objectives for the day or correspond to students' resistance training goals. The Muscle FITT Bingo activity in the web resource reinforces the concept of specificity to your middle and high school students. This activity requires students to identify and perform exercises that will strengthen a targeted muscle. The foundation for specificity in the teaching plan is provided by the previously described principles of overload and progression. When teaching these concepts, it is important that students understand what muscle(s) are being trained by a particular exercise. Knowing more than one way to train each muscle will allow students to individualize their resistance training and provide options to prevent boredom and accommodate changing circumstances.

The **regularity principle** states that activity must be performed on a regular basis in order to be effective and that long periods of inactivity can lead to loss of the benefits gained during training. Engaging in muscular strength and endurance training two or three times per week is sufficient for a lifetime of good muscular health. Even so, you will likely encounter students who want to achieve higher levels of health-related fitness. In this case, you are responsible for providing accurate and helpful information to help them safely reach their goals for muscular strength and endurance.

The **individuality principle** takes into account the fact that each child has different goals for physical activity and muscular fitness, as well as different initial levels of muscular fitness. For children, the program should incorporate a variety of activities, including muscular fitness activities, in order to facilitate a broad range of skill development. This variety gives all children opportunities to succeed and provides a baseline of motor skills for future development as the child matures and shows interest in specific sport activities.

FITT Guidelines: Frequency, Intensity, Time, and Type

Guidelines for muscular fitness are based on policy or position statements from the National Strength and Conditioning Association, the UK Strength and Conditioning Association, and the American College of Sports Medicine. It is generally agreed that the *frequency* of resistance training should be two or three times per week. In examining exercise *intensity*, the recommendations are more complex and relate to stages of maturation. Table 8.1 summarizes the FITT (frequency, intensity, time, and type) guidelines based on age and current recommendations by the NSCA, the ACSM, and the American Academy of Pediatrics; these guidelines are intended for children and adolescents (Lloyd et al., 2012).

Childhood (prepubescence) is generally thought of as a period during which students should learn proper technique and use the weight of their own bodies. During and following puberty, weight should always be added in small increments—1 to 3 pounds (about 0.5 to 1.5 kg)—and a range of 8 to 12 repetitions should be performed. Students then progress to the postpubescent stage, when the adult model may be applied. Table 8.1 offers general progression guidelines based on training experience for older students (prepubescent children can progress only within the beginner column and should not move beyond that until permitted by sufficient body development).

The *time*, or duration, of resistance training should be at least 20 to 30 minutes, or the time required to lift one to three sets with rest periods based on the goal of the activity session (American Academy of Pediatrics, McCambridge, & Stricker, 2008). A rest period of 2 or 3 minutes should be used for a strength session, whereas shorter periods (90 seconds) may be used for a muscular endurance or power session. Remember that students' anaerobic systems may not be fully developed, and feelings of light-headedness or nausea may result if they are not allowed short rest periods while progressing through an endurance session.

Type refers to the kind of resistance training performed during the session, such as muscular strength, power, or endurance training (see table 8.1). It may also refer to the variety of weight-training methods available, such as tension bands, free weights, body weight, machine weights, or partner-resistance exercise.

Estimating 1RM

Extreme caution must be applied when discussing the **one-repetition maximum (1RM)**, which is the maximum amount of weight one can lift for one repetition of a movement. Children and adolescents will naturally want to know how much weight they can lift and will want to challenge classmates to determine who is the strongest. Remember that safety precautions must be taught first and that 1RM should absolutely *not* be used to determine training intensity. The risk for injury and inaccuracy is high, particularly when technique quality has not been established or the student has not fully matured physically. Students should not be exposed to loads greater than 80 percent of an estimated 1RM or to explosive lifts using free weights during prepuberty, puberty, or early postpuberty. These suggestions apply to most children and most educational programs; in some instances among late postpubescent youth, explosive lifting techniques may be taught with proper training and supervision.

A variety of methods are used to estimate 1RM, such as performing a 10RM and then using a table to extrapolate 1RM (Faigenbaum et al., 2009) or calculating 1RM from a weight lifted for no fewer than 6 and no more than 12 repetitions. Another simple approach involves doing a multi-repetition set. Ask students to do three sets

TABLE 8.1   FITT Guidelines Applied to Muscular Fitness

Training experience	Beginner or child	Intermediate	Experienced	Advanced
Frequency of training (sessions per week)	1-3	2-3	2-4	2-5
Volume (sets × reps)	1-2 × 8-12	2-3 × 6-12	2-4 × 5-8	2-5 × 2-5
Number of exercises per session	6-10	3-6	3-6	2-5
Intensity (% 1RM)	Body weight, or 50%-70% 1RM	60%-80% 1RM	70%-85% 1RM	85%-100% 1RM
Repetition velocity (speed of movement)	Slow to moderate	Slow to fast	Fast to maximal	Maximal
Rest intervals (minutes)	1	1-2	2-3	2-5
Recovery (hours between sessions)	72-48	72-48	48	48-24
Type (variety used as appropriate: body weight, resistance bands, medicine balls, kettlebells, stability balls, free weights, weight machines)	Major muscle groups (one exercise for each)	Major muscle groups (one exercise for each)	Major muscle groups (two exercises for each)	Major muscle groups (8-10 exercises selected for muscular strength, muscular endurance, or power)

Adapted by permission from R. Lloyd, et al., "UKSCA Position Statement: Youth Resistance Training," *Professional Strength and Conditioning* 26 (2012): 226-39.

of 10 repetitions of a given exercise. If they can complete all three sets with correct technique for two workouts in two consecutive weeks, then they can increase the weight in the third week. If they cannot finish the repetitions with correct technique, then they need to reduce the weight. After the fourth week, they have a light week to ensure that they do not overtrain. For children, it is much simpler to use the range of 6 to 12 repetitions to estimate the 1RM rather than determining a precise 10RM. Estimating 1RM should be reserved for postpubescent children (girls of age 13 to 18, boys of age 14 to 18) or those at the high school level.

To estimate a student's 1RM, consult table 8.2. In the column representing 10 reps and 75 percent of 1RM, find the tested 10RM load, then read across the row to the

TABLE 8.2   Estimating 1RM and Training Loads

Max reps (RM)	1	2	3	4	5	6	7	8	9	10	12	15
% 1RM	100	95	93	90	87	85	83	80	77	75	67	65
Load (lb or kg)	10	10	9	9	9	9	8	8	8	8	7	7
	20	19	19	18	17	17	17	16	15	15	13	13
	30	29	28	27	26	26	25	24	23	23	20	20
	40	38	37	36	35	34	33	32	31	30	27	26
	50	48	47	45	44	43	42	40	39	38	34	33
	60	57	56	54	52	51	50	48	46	45	40	39
	70	67	65	63	61	60	58	56	54	53	47	46
	80	76	74	72	70	68	66	64	62	60	54	52
	90	86	84	81	78	77	75	72	69	68	60	59
	100	95	93	90	87	85	83	80	77	75	67	65
	110	105	102	99	96	94	91	88	85	83	74	72
	120	114	112	108	104	102	100	96	92	90	80	78
	130	124	121	117	113	111	108	104	100	98	87	85
	140	133	130	126	122	119	116	112	108	105	94	91
	150	143	140	135	131	128	125	120	116	113	101	98
	160	152	149	144	139	136	133	128	123	120	107	104
	170	162	158	153	148	145	141	136	131	128	114	111
	180	171	167	162	157	153	149	144	139	135	121	117
	190	181	177	171	165	162	158	152	146	143	127	124
	200	190	186	180	174	170	166	160	154	150	134	130
	210	200	195	189	183	179	174	168	162	158	141	137
	220	209	205	198	191	187	183	176	169	165	147	143
	230	219	214	207	200	196	191	184	177	173	154	150
	240	228	223	216	209	204	199	192	185	180	161	156
	250	238	233	225	218	213	208	200	193	188	168	163
	260	247	242	234	226	221	206	208	200	195	174	169
	270	257	251	243	235	230	224	216	208	203	181	176
	280	266	260	252	244	238	232	224	216	210	188	182
	290	276	270	261	252	247	241	232	223	218	194	189

Reprinted by permission from NSCA, Program Design for Resistance Training, by J.M. Sheppard and T. Triplett, in *Essentials of Strength Training and Conditioning*, 4th ed., edited by T.R. Baechle and R.W. Earle (Champaign, IL: Human Kinetics, 2008), 455.

column representing 1 rep and 100 percent of 1RM to find the student's projected 1RM. For example, if a student's 10RM is 75 pounds (34 kg), the estimated 1RM is 100 pounds (45 kg) (Baechle, Earle, & Wathen, 2008). You can also obtain an estimated max by means of a simple math formula: (weight lifted $\times$ 0.03 $\times$ repetitions) + weight lifted. For example, here is the calculation for a student who performs a bench press at 135 pounds for 5 repetitions: (135 $\times$ 0.03 $\times$ 5) +135 = (4.05 $\times$ 5) + 135 = 20.25 + 135 = 155.25.

Manipulating the Intensity of the Workout

A person can develop either muscular strength or muscular endurance with the same total load by manipulating the intensity of the workout. To develop muscular strength, increase intensity by increasing the weight lifted and reducing the number of reps; for example, a student might leg-press 100 pounds (45 kg) for 6 reps, thus making a total load of 600 pounds (270 kg). To develop muscular endurance, on the other hand, increase intensity by decreasing the weight lifted and increasing the number of reps; in this case, the student might leg-press 50 pounds (23 kg) for 12 reps, thus making the same total load of 600 pounds (270 kg).

Intensity is also influenced by speed of lifting, but this variable should be introduced only when the student can perform the movement with proper technique. Circuit training that involves multiple repetitions in a specified period should include activities that use the weight of the body, such as push-ups, curl-ups, and other activities not performed with machine or free weights. It is better to specify the number of repetitions to perform slowly and with correct form than to specify how many repetitions to complete in, say, a 30-second time span. Also be aware that, especially with weight machines, lifting too fast creates momentum that aids the lifting, thereby reducing intensity. For these reasons, resistance training for children should focus on developing proper form and technique, not on changing the intensity by varying the speed at which the weight is lifted. Lifting too fast (4 seconds or faster per rep) also increases the likelihood of injury. Teach students to use 6-second reps (2 seconds of lifting and 4 seconds of lowering) but also let them know that 8-second reps (4 seconds lifting and 4 lowering) or even up to 14-second reps (10 lifting and 4 lowering) are also effective. Moderate to slow exercise speeds are recommended over fast lifting speeds for a variety of reasons, including longer periods of muscle tension, higher levels of muscle force, decreased levels of momentum, and decreased risk of injury (Faigenbaum & Westcott, 2000).

Training Methods
for Muscular Strength and Endurance

According to the National Strength and Conditioning Association, when guiding a student to progress from base development to intermediate to advanced development, an increase of 5 percent to 10 percent in overall load is appropriate for most children. Beginning students, especially elementary students, should engage primarily in circuit training using their own body weight, a partner, or light medicine balls; in addition, the **volume** should be low and the intensity very low (Dahab & McCambridge, 2009). Regardless of age, help each student begin slowly and gradually increase frequency, intensity, or time according to individual needs and goals. A training log can help a student see individual progress and feel a sense of accomplishment; the web resource for this chapter includes a sample log you can use (figure 8.1).

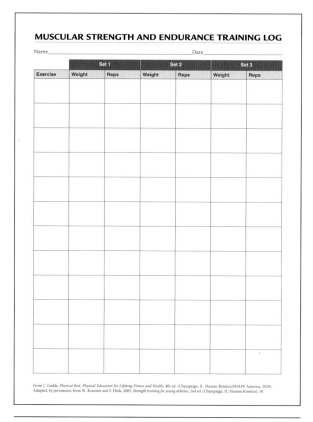

FIGURE 8.1 Sample training log.

Body-Weight Training

Although it is difficult to quantify intensity, curl-ups, push-ups, and other body-weight exercises all help build muscular strength and endurance with little or no equipment. This type of resistance training is appropriate for very young students (K-4) and those who are just beginning resistance training activity. Primary-grade students and those who have difficulty with the curl-up or push-up should do reverse curl-ups or simply perform the lowering phase of the push-up, holding this position. These activities can be presented in a fun and safe way, and they provide students with health-related benefits. You can add interest to the activities by playing music or incorporating fun equipment, such as beanbags. For example, in pairs, your students might play "plank hockey," in which each pair faces one another in plank position and tries to slide a beanbag between one another's hands to score a goal.

Around the World

Build upper-body strength and reinforce math skills with this activity. Divide students into groups of four to six. Have them each get into push-up position and form a circle with their feet in the center and their heads facing outward. Direct the students in each group to pass a beanbag from one person to the next around the circle. Have each group count the number of passes they can make in 30 seconds and then rest for 30 seconds. Conduct up to three 30-second rounds.

Reprinted by permission from J. Hichwa, *Right Fielders are People Too* (Champaign, IL: Human Kinetics, 1998), 106.

Body-weight training is useful not only for young children. Because it requires no equipment, it can form an inexpensive part of a muscular fitness training program throughout adulthood. It is also less likely to cause injury, and it is the easiest program to take on vacation! Thus it is recommended that you teach proper form for a variety of body-weight alternatives to students of all ages, even if your high school is lucky enough to have a state-of-the-art weight room (Baker et al., 2007; Behm et al., 2008; Faigenbaum et al., 2009).

Ultimately, the goal is for students to take personal responsibility for their health-related fitness. In order to do so, they need to be provided with opportunities to plan and implement their personally designed programs.

Partner-Resisted Training

This training method is an extension of basic body-weight exercises. Although it is difficult to gauge the intensity of this type of training, it is helpful when starting a program or working within a tight budget. Using either no equipment or simple equipment (e.g., towels, cords, elastic bands), partner-resistance exercises isolate individual muscles or muscle groups better than solo body-weight exercises do. Partner-resisted exercises are useful for all age groups from the upper elementary grades through adulthood; they are especially useful for individuals who are too small to fit standard weight machines (for examples, see figures 8.2 and 8.3 in the sidebars titled Partners as Resistance). When selecting partners, match height, weight, and strength

Partners as Resistance: Elbow Flex and Extension

- *Position.* Partners stand facing each other with arms at sides, elbows bent at right angles, and palms down.

- *Part 1.* Partner B places hands on top of partner A's hands and presses down. Partner A resists but allows elbows to extend until arm is straight. Rest for 10 seconds.

- *Return motion.* Partner A flexes elbows while partner B resists but allows elbows to bend to right angles in 10 counts. Rest for 10 seconds.

- *Reverse.* Partner B flexes elbows while partner A's hands are on top. Repeat the exercise.

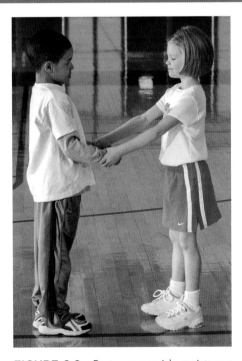

FIGURE 8.2 Partners provide resistance in the elbow flex-and-extend exercise.

Reprinted by permission from K. McConnell, C.B. Corbin, and D. Dale, *Fitness for Life Activity and Vocabulary Cards,* 5th ed. (Champaign, IL: Human Kinetics, 2005).

Partners as Resistance: Knee Flex

- *Position.* Partner B lies facedown on a bench or mat with knees hanging over the edge. If on a mat, partner B's left knee should be bent at a 45-degree angle. Partner A kneels at partner B's feet and loops a towel over partner B's left ankle with the ends downward. Partner B keeps the towel pulled perpendicular to the leg.
- *Part 1.* Partner A maintains resistance on the towel as partner B flexes the left knee as far as possible. Rest for 10 seconds and lower the leg.
- *Part 2.* Repeat with the right leg. Repeat again with each leg and rest again.
- *Reverse.* Change places and repeat all knee exercises.

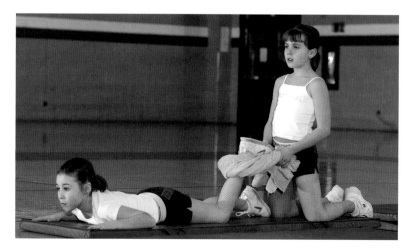

FIGURE 8.3   Partners provide resistance in the knee-flex exercise.

Reprinted by permission from K. McConnell, C.B. Corbin, and D. Dale, *Fitness for Life Activity and Vocabulary Cards,* 5th ed. (Champaign, IL: Human Kinetics, 2005).

levels as closely as possible to ensure safety and ease of working together. Encourage good communication and demand mature, safe behavior. Partners should also help each other maintain correct technique and provide motivation by monitoring and encouraging each other.

Alternative Methods of Training

Resistance band training is appropriate for upper elementary and older students. Band training involves using surgical tubing, rubber cords, or bands manufactured specifically for muscular strength and endurance training (e.g., ExerTube, Dyna-Band, Flexi-Cord, or TheraBand). Use thicker tubing for greater resistance and thinner tubing for less; resistance can also be adjusted by prestretching the cord more or less. Although students cannot measure intensity precisely with this method, it provides an inexpensive yet effective way to expand their resistance training program. An added advantage is that spotting is rarely required for such exercises. An example of resistance-band exercise is shown in figure 8.4 in the sidebar titled Rubber Cord Standing Chest Press.

Medicine ball training can be adapted for all ages, including primary-grade children, by using a variety of ball weights and sizes. Faigenbaum and Westcott (2007)

Rubber Cord Standing Chest Press

Muscles

Pectoralis major, anterior deltoid, triceps

Procedure

1. Stand with your feet about shoulder-width apart and the rubber cord wrapped around the back of your shoulders.

2. Grasp the ends of the cord firmly and place both hands (with palms facing the floor) in front of your shoulders with your elbows flexed.

3. Slowly straighten your elbows until you fully extend both arms. Return to the starting position, then repeat.

Technique Tips

- Exhale during the pushing phase of the exercise and inhale during the return phase.

- Do not twist or arch your body.

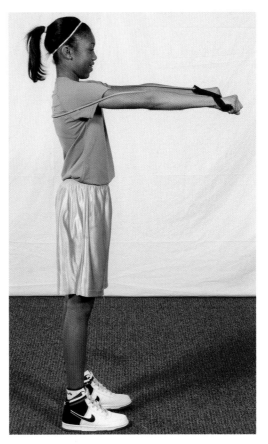

FIGURE 8.4   A student performs a chest press using a resistance band.

Reprinted by permission from A. Faigenbaum and W. Westcott, *Youth Strength Training: Programs for Health, Fitness, and Sport* (Champaign, IL: Human Kinetics, 2009), 97.

suggest three benefits of using medicine balls in your program. First, this type of training uses dynamic movements that can be performed either slowly or rapidly. Second, the balls can be used to develop the upper body, the lower body, and the trunk by using catching and throwing movements. But the third and most important reason is to develop the core, which includes the abdominal muscles and the hip and lower-back musculature (see figure 8.5). Besides offering an effective way to increase muscular fitness in children, this conditioning method is relatively inexpensive and involves multiple students participating simultaneously (Faigenbaum & Westcott, 2000). An example of an exercise that can be performed with a medicine ball is shown in figure 8.6 in the sidebar titled Medicine Ball Chest Pass.

Kettlebells have been around for decades and have regained popularity in recent years. These ball-shaped objects range in size and weight. The reason for their recent rise in popularity is that they enable whole-body conditioning. Lifting and controlling a kettlebell forces the muscles in the entire body (especially the core) to contract together, thus building strength and stability at the same time. You must train your students to use kettlebells correctly; otherwise, serious injury could occur.

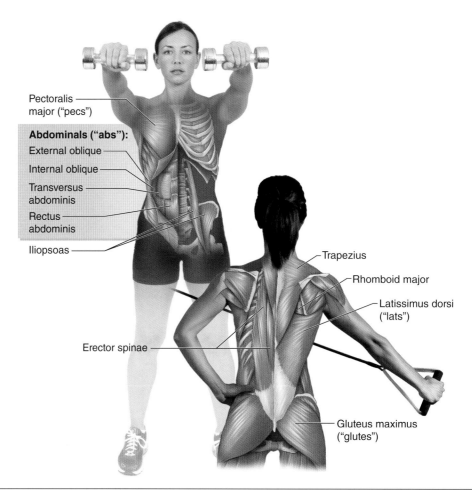

Pectoralis major ("pecs")

Abdominals ("abs"):

External oblique

Internal oblique

Transversus abdominis

Rectus abdominis

Iliopsoas

Trapezius

Rhomboid major

Latissimus dorsi ("lats")

Erector spinae

Gluteus maximus ("glutes")

FIGURE 8.5   The core muscles.

Stability balls offer another way for students to develop muscular strength, endurance, and balance. An 18-inch (45 cm) ball accommodates prepubescent children's height and allows them to use the ball constructively. One exercise for each body part and three or four core stability exercises are considered appropriate for children between 8 and 12 years of age (Goldberg & Twist, 2007). Stability balls can be fun for your students to try moving in different ways; in addition, by adjusting placement during some exercises, students can individualize the intensity of the exercise. You might also consider reaching out to classroom teachers about how to use stability balls in the classroom. For instance, using a stability ball instead of a chair might be offered as a classroom reward that students will enjoy even as it engages their core muscles while they work at their desks.

Weight Training

A weight training program may use free or machine weights or both, depending on goals, available equipment, and available space. Introduce exercises one at a time by discussing the purpose of each one; demonstrating correct technique; and outlining ranges of appropriate weight loads, repetitions, and speed. In addition, relate these

Medicine Ball Chest Pass

Muscles

Chest, arms

Procedure

1. Stand erect while holding a medicine ball at chest level with both hands.
2. Step forward and press the ball away from your chest.

Technique Tips

- Exhale as you push the ball away from your chest.
- Keep your torso erect after you release the ball; do not lean forward.
- A partner can stand about 10 feet (3 m) away and catch the ball. Over time, students can increase the distance between partners—the greater the distance, the more effort required.
- For variety, you can perform this exercise while kneeling on the floor; keep your body straight as you push the ball away from your chest.

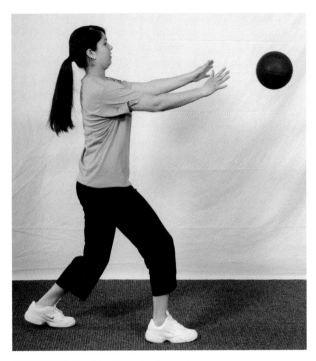

FIGURE 8.6 Medicine ball chest pass.

Reprinted by permission from A. Faigenbaum and W. Westcott, *Youth Strength Training: Programs for Health, Fitness, and Sport* (Champaign, IL: Human Kinetics, 2009), 117.

factors to intensity, program goals, and individual goals. For ideas about appropriate weights for your students to lift, see the sidebar titled Lifting the Correct Amount of Weight.

Follow the safety and health guidelines provided in this chapter to ensure a safe and effective weight training program. If weight training is done in addition to or in place of other forms of training, teach students alternative exercises that target the same muscle or group of muscles. Likewise, if a program relies heavily on machine use, demonstrate the corresponding free-weight exercises to increase the chance that students will use the exercises outside of and after their school program. Figure 8.7*a* shows the biceps curl as performed on a machine, and figure 8.7*b* shows its free-weight alternative. Most weight training done with machine weights and barbells should be reserved for postpubescent children. Table 8.3 indicates some suggested alternatives for prepubescent children (Bompa, 2000), and illustrations of these exercises are provided in the web resource (see figure 8.8).

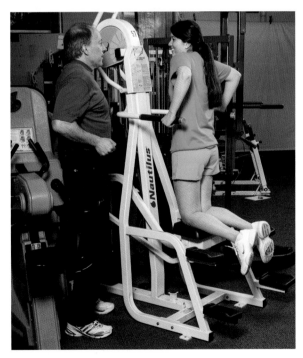

Discuss the purpose of exercises with your students and make sure they are using correct technique.

Lifting the Correct Amount of Weight

Often, an inexperienced lifter will not put enough weight on the bar to elicit a training effect. Over time, lifting with a load that is too light can even lead to a detraining effect; at the other extreme, lifting with a load that is too heavy can lead to an overuse injury. One way to avoid these pitfalls is to specify for each older student a weight that should be lifted on the bar based on his or her personalized goals. Choosing the correct amount of weight will help the student achieve the desired effect. A student who is working on power should stay in the range of 3 to 5 reps at 75 percent to 85 percent of 1RM, a student who is working on muscular endurance should perform 15 to 20 reps at 60 percent or less of 1RM, a strength-focused student should complete 2 to 4 reps at 85 percent or more of 1RM, and a student working on hypertrophy should execute 6 to 12 reps at 65 percent to 85 percent of 1RM. Charts are available to help students determine which weight to use (e.g., https://www.nsca.com/contentassets/116c55d64e1343d2b264e05aaf158a91/basics_of_strength_and_conditioning_manual.pdf).

Another option is to ask students to periodically check the load lifted against their predicted 1RM (see table 8.2). If students are setting their own weight when they lift, an easy way to determine the percentage of their workout weight is to divide the weight they lifted for each set by their predicted 1RM. The result gives the student the percentage for each set. The student can then check the workout against the intensity chart to see if the workout weight is at the correct percentage.

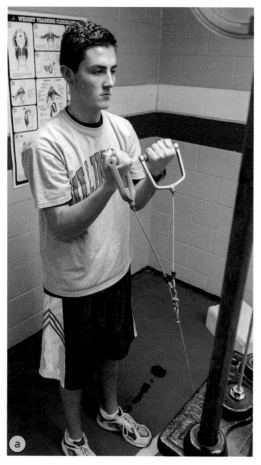 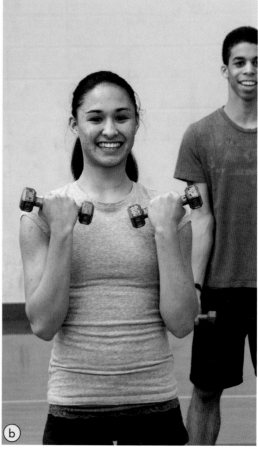

FIGURE 8.7   Biceps curl performed (a) on a machine and (b) with free weights.

TABLE 8.3 Muscular Fitness Exercises*

Exercise	Body area worked
Dumbbell side raise	Shoulder
Dumbbell curl	Biceps
Dumbbell shoulder press	Shoulder, trapezius
Dumbbell fly	Chest, shoulder
Medicine ball chest throw	Shoulder, triceps
Medicine ball zigzag throw	Arms, shoulders
Medicine ball twist throw	Arms, trunk, oblique abdominals
Medicine ball forward overhead throw	Chest, shoulders, arms, abdominals
Medicine ball scoop throw	Ankles, knees, hip extensors, arms, shoulders, back
Abdominal crunch	Abdominals, hip flexors
Medicine ball back roll	Abdominals, hip flexors
Medicine ball side-pass relay	Oblique abdominals, shoulders
Trunk twist	Oblique abdominals
Single-leg back raise	Hip extensors, spine
Chest raise and clap	Lower back
Seated back extension	Back, shoulders
Dodge-the-rope	Calves, knee extensors

*See the web resource for descriptions and photos of these exercises.

Bompa & Carerra, (2005, p.115-123).

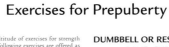

Exercises for Prepuberty

From the multitude of exercises for strength training, the following exercises are offered as guidelines only. You can use other exercises, depending on the environment and facilities.

Adapted, by permission, from T.O. Bompa, 2000, *Total training for young champions* (Champaign, IL: Human Kinetics), 115-123.

DUMBBELL OR RESISTANCE BAND SIDE RAISE

Area worked: deltoids (shoulders)

1. The student stands with the feet apart and the arms at the side.
2. He or she lifts the dumbbells or resistance band parallel to the floor and then returns to the starting position.

DUMBBELL OR RESISTANCE BAND CURL

Area worked: biceps (front of upper arm)

1. The student stands with the arms extended down in front of the hips and the palms facing upward.
2. He or she flexes the right elbow, lifting the dumbbell or resistance band toward the right shoulder.
3. The student returns to the starting position and then repeats with the left arm.

*Note: Can be done with both arms at the same time.

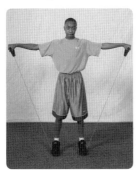 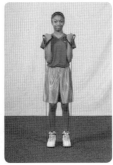

From J. Conkle, *Physical Best: Physical Education for Lifelong Fitness and Health*, 4th ed. (Champaign, IL: Human Kinetics/SHAPE America, 2020).

FIGURE 8.8 The web resource includes illustrations of exercises appropriate for prepubescent children.

Technology in Physical Education

Technology can be used in the weight room in many ways, ranging from simple video analysis with a phone to monitoring eating habits and ensuring that your students are not overtraining. Easy-to-use apps for monitoring students' movement patterns include Coach's Eye, Dartfish, BarSense, and Iron Path. Such apps allow the teacher and students to video-record exercise performance and track bar movement or joint angle during a lift. Thus it allows students to compare their movement patterns with correct form and identify needed corrections.

Addressing Motor Skills Through Muscular Strength and Endurance Activities

Simply put, a strong, more enduring muscle can do what it's called on to do reliably and accurately. Therefore, increasing muscular strength and endurance can enhance motor skill performance. Children cannot "play themselves into shape," and that preseason and in-season training time should be supplemented by a resistance training program to enhance performance in sport and recreational activities (Faigenbaum, 2001). Most research in this area indicates that training adaptations are specific to a given movement pattern, velocity of movement, contraction type, and contraction force (Faigenbaum et al., 2009; Lloyd et al., 2012; Lloyd et al., 2013). Fast movements (power movements) are generally contraindicated when weightlifting, but children can engage in plyometric exercises, or **plyometrics**, such as hops, jumps, and throws, if intensity and volume are carefully monitored. Chu, Faigenbaum, and Falkel (2006) also suggest exercising caution when using plyometric training. Specifically, they strongly suggest developing a solid base of strength training before engaging in plyometric training; they also suggest beginning plyometrics with low-intensity drills.

You can have students perform motor skills to increase muscular strength and endurance. For example, young children enjoy playing tag games using various locomotor skills, and these games increase the muscular endurance of the leg muscles. Students in the fourth grade and beyond may enjoy team-building activities that require arm strength. One example is the circle of teamwork, in which students stand in a circle, interlock their arms, and stretch the circle by each walking backward; at the tightest point, the students simultaneously lean backward. Such activities help students see how specific strength-building activities (e.g., calisthenics, weightlifting) can help a person enjoy life. They also see the practical ways in which enjoyable activities can build muscular strength and endurance. Students should be helped to see the connections among the many physical activities in their school program, as well as community-based physical activities.

Safety Guidelines for Muscular Strength and Endurance Activities

In the past, many health fitness experts, as well as parents, have feared that resistance training is dangerous for children; specifically, they have pointed to the possibility of harming bone development or stunting growth. Research does not support these fears, as long as the child strength-trains in a developmentally appropriate program that emphasizes safe limits and includes adequate adult supervision. Accordingly, both the American College of Sports Medicine (2002) and the National Strength and Conditioning Association (Faigenbaum et al., 2009) have taken the position that weight training can benefit children if it is properly prescribed by a qualified professional and supervised.

In order to be qualified to run such a program, a professional should be certified through an accredited organization (Casa et al., 2013), have a strong background in child and youth exercise physiology, possess the ability to teach age-specific exercises with a wide variety of equipment and activities, and be able to identify technique variables to ensure proper movement patterns. Furthermore, the person should be able to use common sense when designing and implementing curriculum and activities while attending carefully to students' ages, developmental readiness, abilities, maturity, experience, and health-related fitness.

If you are not comfortable with strength training techniques, you can take classes offered by the NSCA that address how to teach and what to look for when a student is participating in muscular strength and endurance activities. Such training includes using the child's body weight in calisthenics (e.g., curl-ups, push-ups) and performing high repetitions with light weights or resistance bands. Lifting maximal weights, however, should be delayed until all of the long bones have finished growing, which occurs at about 17 years of age (or older in boys). Because cartilage is not as strong as bone, the **growth plates** (sections of cartilage at the ends of long bones in children) can be highly susceptible to injury. However, the risk appears to be minimal if children are taught how to strength-train properly and use appropriate training loads (American Academy of Pediatrics, McCambridge, & Stricker, 2008; Baechle et al., 2008; Dahab & McCambridge, 2009; Faigenbaum, Lloyd, & Myer, 2013).

As previously stated, elementary prepubescent children should engage in circuit training using their own body weight, a partner, or light medicine balls; in addition, the volume should be low and the intensity very low. If properly instructed and supervised, older elementary-level children can safely use resistance bands and light free weights. Examples of exercises using free weights and medicine balls are shown in figure 8.9, *a* through *c*. Make sure that students understand the safety issues involved in partner exercises and that no horseplay will be tolerated.

Students must also understand that they will not build the large muscles that some older, postpubescent students and adults are capable of building. Physiologically speaking, this goal is simply not realistic for younger students. Middle school and high school students can and should participate in resistive muscular strength and endurance activities that involve the use of free weights if they are able to do so. Activities do not need to be limited to weight-room use of dumbbells and barbells. Moreover, resistance bands, body-weight exercises, use of homemade equipment (e.g., plastic milk jugs filled with sand), and so on may provide more opportunities for greater simultaneous participation.

One of the most important safety practices is to individualize the resistance training program. Encourage children to compete against themselves, not against each other, in terms of how much they can lift; furthermore, the emphasis should be on the amount of weight lifted 6 to 12 times, not on how much weight can be lifted in a single lift. In addition, all children—kindergarten through high school seniors—should set realistic goals and focus on using correct technique. To satisfy the competitive spirit in some children, Kraemer and Fleck (2005) suggest holding correct technique contests in which weight load plays no role in the final evaluation.

Safety matters in any aspect of physical education and health-related physical fitness, but it is especially critical to follow the safety guidelines outlined in this chapter.

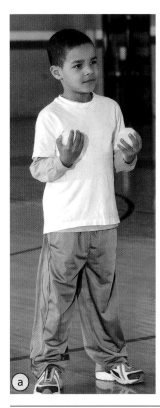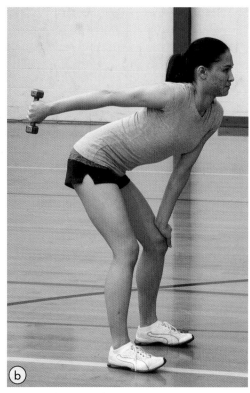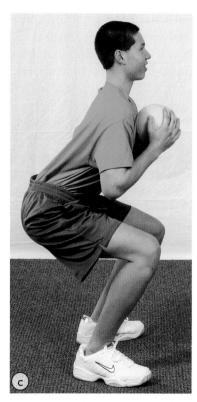

FIGURE 8.9   *(a)* Biceps curl using light free weights (tennis balls), *(b)* triceps extension using a free weight, and *(c)* front squat using a medicine ball.

Before making decisions about equipment and teaching ideas, consider the following cautions related to resistance training, especially for youth:

- The child must be psychologically and physically ready to accept teaching or coaching instruction.
- Adequate supervision must be provided by instructors who understand resistance training for children, as well as the special concerns related to prepubescent children. The teacher–student ratio should be 1:5 (or 1:10 with experienced teenage participants).
- Proper technique and safety must be emphasized for each lift.
- Caution must be used with machines that are not designed to fit children.
- Resistance training should not be an isolated activity; instead, it should be one component of a comprehensive program to increase both motor skills and health-related fitness.
- Resistance training activity should be preceded by a warm-up and followed by a cool-down.
- The program should include both **concentric contractions** (in which muscle shortens) and **eccentric contractions** (dynamic contractions in which muscle lengthens).
- Full range of motion must be emphasized.

Besides these program considerations, the American Academy of Pediatrics, the National Strength and Conditioning Association, and the National Athletic Trainers' Association also recommend that children and adolescents receive a medical evaluation in order to identify any underlying medical condition or orthopedic problem that might limit or prohibit their participation in resistance training.

These cautions should not deter teachers from incorporating resistance training into physical education. With proper instruction and supervision, resistance training can be a fun and safe activity for all ages (Lloyd et al., 2013; Myer et al., 2009).

Although most programs use age-specific criteria for applying the FITT guidelines, your program should accommodate the training ages *and* biological ages of the students in your classes when developing resistance activities (see the sidebar Student Age and Resistance Training earlier in this chapter). This approach will allow younger, more experienced children to challenge themselves safely with proper instruction and supervision (using the progression and overload principles) while also providing necessary support for older students whose bodies are maturing more slowly or whose experience with resistance training is limited.

Appropriate training guidelines, program variations, and competent supervision will make resistance training programs safe, effective, and fun for children. As a physical education teacher, you understand the physical and emotional uniqueness of children and, in turn, must teach children to appreciate the potential benefits and risks associated with resistance training. Although the needs, goals, and interests of children will continually change, resistance training should be considered a safe and effective component of youth health-related fitness programs (Lloyd et al., 2013; Myer et al., 2009).

Finally, if the school has a weight room, ensure that it is set up so that traffic flows through it efficiently and that the space between stations is sufficient. Kraemer and Fleck (2005) recommend a minimum of 5 feet (1.5 m) between machines and adequate room for free weights to be dropped suddenly if need be. If possible, use machines instead of free weights for overhead movements, such as those required in the bench press; furthermore, reserve the bench press for older high school students. Always use spotters for free-weight exercises, even though some light exercises may not seem to require one. Using a spotter for all exercises is a good habit for students to develop, and it leaves no room for incorrect decisions regarding whether to use one. Students can work in pairs, spotting each other and monitoring correct technique.

Above all, in order to provide a safe and beneficial muscular fitness program for children, do *not* use a program designed for adults, even with adolescents. *Do* individualize the program, modify progress slowly, and reassess the safety and effectiveness of the program frequently.

Training a Student to Spot a Partner

The **spotting** techniques recommended by experts vary, but everyone in the weight training community agrees on one important point: Proper spotting is vital to the overall safety of the person lifting the weight and to the effectiveness of incorporating the FITT guidelines. This chapter is not geared specifically to weight training, but rather to health-related physical activity that suggests weight training as one of many methods. Still, when your students train with resistive weights, proper spotting must be used.

Summary

By following the guidelines outlined in this chapter, you can teach your students the importance of muscular strength and endurance training in safe and effective ways. The best way to keep each child safe is to teach safety rules, closely monitor behavior and technique, incorporate individual choice, and help each child set realistic goals. Never push a child to lift a heavier weight than he or she has trained for or to perform "just one more rep." Instead, motivate children to participate and progress by creating an enjoyable and supportive class atmosphere and by rewarding effort and correct technique rather than physical prowess. Resistance training can be extremely interesting and rewarding. When selecting activities for students, hold in mind that the ultimate goal of health-related fitness education is to produce graduates who take personal responsibility for each area of health-related fitness as a way of life. Consult the web resource for a variety of age-appropriate Physical Best activities related to muscular strength and endurance. The next chapter offers help for integrating health-related fitness into a physical education curriculum.

Discussion Questions

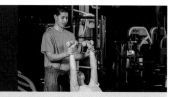

1. Why should muscular fitness be included as part of a well-rounded, health-related fitness program?

2. Why should teachers avoid using a one-repetition maximum with their students?

3. What are the differences between training age, chronological age, and biological age? Explain why these distinctions are important to physical educators.

4. Name four resistance training exercises that help elementary students with movement patterns and support their learning of fundamental movement skills. Describe an activity or lesson that can incorporate all four.

5. Define resistance training. How would you explain it to an elementary student? How can you add relevance to this definition for a high school student?

6. Describe three benefits of resistance training in adolescence.

7. Describe the importance of three cautions when teaching resistance training in physical education.

8. Give an example of how the overload principle can be applied to strength training in adolescence.

9. Give an example of how the progression principle can be applied to weight training in physical education.

10. Describe how to apply the FITT guidelines for resistance training with elementary students.

PART III

Curriculum and Teaching Methods

Part III provides an overview of curriculum development and teaching methods relevant to health-related fitness education. It also covers ways to include children of all abilities and backgrounds in health-related fitness education. Chapter 9 addresses basic program design principles and recommendations for core content. Chapter 10 explores teaching styles, cooperative learning, teaching strategies, the teaching environment, and teaching tools. Part III concludes with chapter 11, which focuses on inclusion and offers practical tips for including students with special needs; along the way, it addresses gender, culture, and ability.

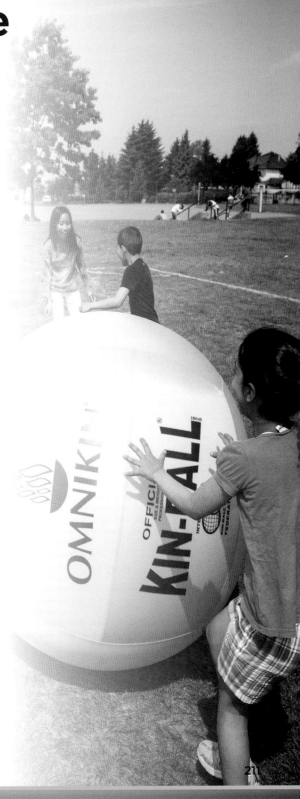

CHAPTER 9

Integrating Health-Related Fitness Education Into the Curriculum

Bane McCracken

CHAPTER CONTENTS

Physical education teaches skills that make physical activity enjoyable over a lifetime. It is not recess, it is not a recreation period, it is not where students go to get fit, and it should not be viewed as the student's physical activity opportunity. *Physical education is where students go to learn.* Students should be physically active because of what they learn in their physical education classes. In order for physical education teachers to most effectively enhance students' learning, they need a well-developed, comprehensive curriculum based on the National Standards for K-12 Physical Education (SHAPE America, 2014) and the National Health Education Standards (Joint Committee on National Health Education Standards, 2007). This chapter will help you develop curriculum that includes health-related fitness instruction and promotes developmentally appropriate, physically active lifestyles among your students (SHAPE America Standard 3).

Curriculum Development

SHAPE America's National Standards for K-12 Physical Education and the accompanying Grade-Level Outcomes define what a physically literate individual should know and be able to do (SHAPE America, 2014). Thus they provide clear direction for how to develop robust and effective physical education programs. Such physical education programs have a written curriculum that guides teachers by acting as a road map to accomplish specific outcomes and provide evidence of student progress (SHAPE America, 2015). For more guidance in the area of setting the framework for physical education curriculum, you can read SHAPE America's 2015 guidance document, "The Essential Components of Physical Education."

For the purpose of this chapter, then, an effective curriculum is a written document that helps teachers meet the standards of learning for a specific subject area. A well-written curriculum includes the following elements:

- An overview describing the goals of the program in general terms
- A scope and sequence of instruction indicating what is to be included in the curriculum (The scope could be a specific grade level, one middle school, an entire school system for grades K through 12, or even a state-level curriculum. The sequence details when the specific parts of a curriculum are taught.)
- Learning objectives aligned with national, state, or local standards
- Assessment tools for every objective to provide evidence of student progress

Physical Best is not a complete physical education curriculum. Rather, it is a curriculum supplement that helps incorporate the teaching of health-related fitness into a standards-based physical education curriculum. The Physical Best materials, philosophy, and resources can be used to create a complete fitness curriculum model for a school or system. A curriculum model is a method used to develop a curriculum, such as movement education, fitness education, sports education, wilderness sports education, and Understanding by Design. Each model uses patterns based on a theme for developing curriculum. A fitness model focuses, of course, on fitness and helps students learn to recognize fitness benefits and fitness requirements for the activities included in the curriculum. When discussing various curriculum models, Physical Best is many times used as an example of a fitness education model. In this chapter, however, it is considered a curriculum supplement.

Discussion of curriculum development in this chapter may include other components of the physical education curriculum, but the focus is on developing objectives for physical activity and health-related fitness. As previously indicated, this focus comes from alignment with the National Standards for K-12 Physical Education and the National Health Education Standards (SHAPE America, 2014; Joint Committee on National Health Education Standards, 2007).

National Standards

A physical education curriculum that focuses only on skill development and teaches only competitive team sports is no longer appropriate. Today's physical education curriculum must focus on health-related fitness, teach authentic lifetime skills, and be standards based. Physical education programs that teach students the skills needed to make physical activity enjoyable over a lifetime include specific objectives that help students learn to be physically active and develop a health-enhancing level of fitness. Tables 9.1 and 9.2 list the standards set by the national governing bodies for physical education and health. These standards are included in the Physical Best activities (see the web resource) to demonstrate the connection of each activity to the applicable standards.

TABLE 9.1   National Standards for Physical Education

Standard 1	The physically literate individual demonstrates competency in a variety of motor skills and movement patterns.
Standard 2	The physically literate individual applies knowledge of concepts, principles, strategies and tactics related to movement and performance.
Standard 3	The physically literate individual demonstrates the knowledge and skills to achieve and maintain a health-enhancing level of physical activity and fitness.
Standard 4	The physically literate individual exhibits responsible personal and social behavior that respects self and others.
Standard 5	The physically literate individual recognizes the value of physical activity for health, enjoyment, challenge, self-expression and/or social interaction.

Reprinted from SHAPE America, *National Standards & Grade-Level Outcomes for K-12 Physical Education* (Champaign, IL: Human Kinetics, 2014), 12.

TABLE 9.2   National Health Education Standards

Standard 1	Students will comprehend concepts related to health promotion and disease prevention to enhance health.
Standard 2	Students will analyze the influence of family, peers, culture, media, technology, and other factors on health behaviors.
Standard 3	Students will demonstrate the ability to access valid information and products and services to enhance health.
Standard 4	Students will demonstrate the ability to use interpersonal communication skills to enhance health and avoid or reduce health risks.
Standard 5	Students will demonstrate the ability to use decision-making skills to enhance health.
Standard 6	Students will demonstrate the ability to use goal-setting skills to enhance health.
Standard 7	Students will demonstrate the ability to practice health-enhancing behaviors and avoid or reduce health risks.
Standard 8	Students will demonstrate the ability to advocate for personal, family, and community health.

Reprinted with permission from the American Cancer Society, Inc. *National Health Education Standards: Achieving Excellence, Second Edition.* (Atlanta, GA: American Cancer Society, 2007), cancer.org/bookstore.

Writing Curriculum

In an ideal situation, a local school agency has a coordinator of physical education who is in charge of curriculum development. To develop a physical education curriculum, or refine an existing curriculum so that it includes health-related fitness education, the coordinator assembles a team to write the curriculum. It is reviewed by all teachers in the system, their input is evaluated, and amendments are made. The curriculum is coordinated and sequenced for all grades, K through 12. If the school system does not have such a coordinator, then individual teachers may be delegated to handle curriculum development. Regardless of the situation, the initial considerations for writing a curriculum are scope and sequence, requirements and policies, appropriate movement skills or forms, assessment tools, and user-friendliness.

Scope and Sequence

Program scope identifies the number and types of schools for which the curriculum is to be developed. The curriculum's programs may be designed for a single elementary school or for all schools in a city, county, or district-level system. It is advantageous for the scope to carry across all programmatic levels, because it is difficult to develop physically literate students without coordinating the teaching of skills from one grade level to the next. However, though the curriculum should be written for all schools in the system, sufficient flexibility should be allowed for schools to take advantage of local physical activity opportunities, especially in larger systems.

The curriculum sequence indicates the order in which skills will be presented and coordinates skill development from one grade level or programmatic level to the next. As a result, it is helpful to include a representative from each grade level in the writing of the curriculum to enable smooth transition of skill development from one level or school to the next. It is especially important to make smooth transitions from one programmatic level to the next—that is, from K-2 to 3-5, from 3-5 to middle school, and from middle school to high school. Specifically, proper sequencing of standards, assessment of individual skills, and record keeping all help teachers know where to start at the beginning of the year, how to individualize instruction, and how to document improvement.

Local and State Requirements and Policies

According to *Shape of the Nation Report: Status of Physical Education in the USA* (SHAPE America, 2016), nearly all states have adopted standards for physical education based on SHAPE America's National Standards. These state standards, along with state and local requirements and policies, should be used as the basis for developing a local curriculum. Some school districts provide excellent facilities and equipment for physical education and require daily classes taught by a certified professional. In other areas, the physical education program may share a facility with the food service program and require only 30 minutes of class per week. Although setting high standards may be good practice, writing an impractical curriculum is not a good idea, and educators must be realistic about working with the resources and limitations of their location.

In most programs, time is a limiting factor to one degree or another. The amount of time that students spend with their teachers determines what and how much can be accomplished. For example, a curriculum with delivery on only one day per week will necessarily be sequenced differently than a daily program. Few school systems provide adequate time during the school day for the students to practice and learn the skills taught in their classes. Programs in which teachers have particularly limited time with their students must use creative means to help students achieve desired outcomes. For instance, providing equipment during recess, lunch, and before and after school allows students to practice the skills taught during physical education class. Another means is to assign regularly scheduled homework that requires students to practice skills outside of the school day, thus providing them with additional learning opportunities, encouraging them to break the habit of inactivity, and teaching them to take responsibility for their own learning.

Effective homework assignment for physical education starts by spending more time providing quality instruction and less time playing games. After providing instruction, challenge your students to practice at home and outside of class in order to be prepared to demonstrate improvement during the next scheduled class. You can also involve parents and siblings by having students create activity logs that require a responsible adult's signature and by scheduling parent and family fun nights that address the importance of physical activity and how to monitor a child's progress. You can also get classroom teachers and support staff involved to provide opportunities for students to practice outside of physical education. In addition, the school may be able to offer after-school activity time to give students a safe place and equipment to practice their skills.

A well-written curriculum includes lessons that teach students how to monitor and change their physical activity outside of physical education class. For example, elementary curricula should include specific lessons that help students distinguish between moderate and vigorous physical activity, choose specific forms of physical activity outside of class, monitor the intensity of physical activity, and document outside-of-class physical activity.

Middle school and high school students can demonstrate progress by using digital cameras and other multimedia tools. For instance, during a high school golf unit, students could be filmed while hitting golf balls during the first week, then use multimedia tools to identify flaws in technique. During the last week of the unit, students could again film themselves and make comparisons with the earlier footage to demonstrate how their practice resulted in better form. A variety of apps are available to help students see and analyze their skill performance as compared with that of a professional or an earlier recording of themselves. These apps allow students to analyze performance, demonstrate improvement, and use technology in a meaningful way to support learning, which can continue beyond physical education—all the while reserving precious class time for instruction. Students who do not have access to these types of technology can use self-assessment checklists to document progress via pre- and posttesting.

Middle school students should be taught to document outside-of-class physical activity and develop physical activity plans based on the results of health-related fitness assessment. High school students should document outside-of-class participation as part of a unit of study, research equipment sources, and develop budgets for physical activity pursuits. For instance, students might be encouraged to play a round of golf during a golf unit or participate in a local tournament during a tennis unit; similarly, a bicycle unit might include after-school group rides.

Appropriate Movement Skills or Forms

For any curriculum to be sound, a physical educator must consider the developmental appropriateness of the selected content. **Developmentally appropriate physical activities** are based on a student's developmental level, age, ability level, interests, experience, knowledge, and opportunities for participation. Appropriateness for grade level should be the initial focus. First, study the guidelines set by experts in the field, such as those developed by SHAPE America. Then use experience as the best teacher and learn by trial and error what each particular group of students can handle. But remember that although developmental appropriateness is important, you must not overlook the age of the student for whom the content is being developed. For example, if a high school student lacks cardiorespiratory endurance, then tag is not an appropriate activity to offer as a choice. Instead, riding a stationary bike while reading a favorite magazine would be a good alternative based on the student's age and ability. Both activities will accomplish the basic goal.

Select content along a continuum ranging from completely childlike to as nearly adultlike as possible. Figure 9.1 shows a sample continuum for cardiorespiratory endurance activities that proceed from childlike activities in the early grades to adultlike activities in high school.

Assessment

Many people view assessment as the most important component of a curriculum, and some even recommend that developing assessment tools should be the first step in writing a curriculum. As Lewis Carroll said, "If you don't know where you are going, any road will get you there." No curriculum is complete without assessment. Every objective in the curriculum needs to be associated with an assessment tool that directs the teaching and guides the students' learning. More information about assessment in physical education is provided in chapters 12 and 13.

User-Friendliness

A curriculum is meant to be used. Too many times, however, a curriculum (whether purchased or created) is stuck in a desk drawer and never seen again. To make sure that teachers use curriculum documents, keep them simple and easy to understand.

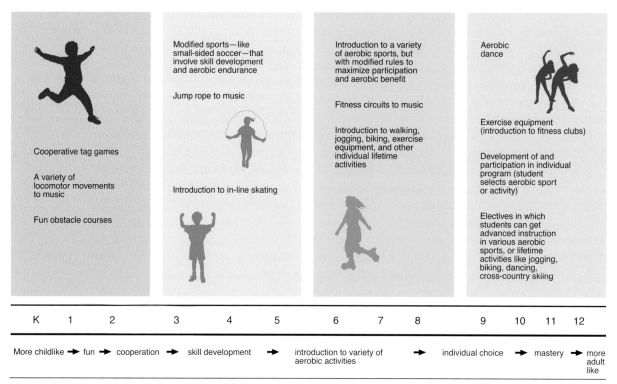

Cooperative tag games	Modified sports—like small-sided soccer—that involve skill development and aerobic endurance	Introduction to a variety of aerobic sports, but with modified rules to maximize participation and aerobic benefit	Aerobic dance
	Jump rope to music	Fitness circuits to music	Exercise equipment (introduction to fitness clubs)
A variety of locomotor movements to music	Introduction to in-line skating	Introduction to walking, jogging, biking, exercise equipment, and other individual lifetime activities	Development of and participation in individual program (student selects aerobic sport or activity)
Fun obstacle courses			Electives in which students can get advanced instruction in various aerobic sports, or lifetime activities like jogging, biking, dancing, cross-country skiing

| K | 1 | 2 | 3 | 4 | 5 | 6 | 7 | 8 | 9 | 10 | 11 | 12 |

More childlike → fun → cooperation → skill development → introduction to variety of aerobic activities → individual choice → mastery → more adult like

FIGURE 9.1 Your activity selection should occur along a continuum that moves students from childlike activities to adultlike ones. This example describes a possible continuum for teaching cardiorespiratory endurance.

A committee should develop the curriculum, and members of the physical education teaching staff should make up the majority of the group and do most of the writing.

Physical Education Curriculum Analysis Tool (PECAT)

The Centers for Disease Control and Prevention (CDC) has used physical education experts to develop the Physical Education Curriculum Analysis Tool (PECAT). The purpose of the PECAT is to help school districts conduct a clear, complete, and consistent analysis of physical education curriculum. The results can help school districts enhance and develop effective physical education curriculum and refine existing curriculum to include health-related fitness education. The PECAT is available at no cost, and copies and further information can be obtained in several ways:

- Searching for "PECAT" on the web
- Downloading from the CDC website: www.cdc.gov/HealthyYouth/PECAT
- Requesting information from the CDC: www.cdc.gov/cdc-info/requestform. html
- Requesting information via toll-free phone call: 800-CDC-INFO

Several trainings for using the PECAT have been conducted nationally, and more are scheduled. The PECAT is designed to analyze an existing curriculum, but it can also be used as a guide when developing a new curriculum. It includes specific examples of lesson outcomes for all grade levels and all standards. Here are some examples of PECAT recommendations for meeting SHAPE America Standard 3 (Centers for Disease Control and Prevention, 2006):

Elementary: K-2
- Specific lessons about the response of the body to physical activity (e.g., increased heart rate, faster breathing, sweating)
- Specific lessons about developing basic knowledge of the components of health-related fitness (e.g., cardiorespiratory endurance, muscular endurance, muscular strength, flexibility, body composition)
- Specific lessons that allow students to participate in vigorous, intermittent physical activity for short periods during physical education class
- Specific lessons about the concept of personal choices in physical activity and ways in which those choices contribute to health-related fitness
- Specific instructions that clearly indicate the appropriate grade level at which each concept and activity related to health-related fitness should be introduced and subsequently taught

Elementary: 3-5
- Specific lessons on self-assessment of health-related fitness (e.g., teaching activity using a criterion-referenced standard fitness test such as FitnessGram for self-assessment of health-related fitness)
- Specific lessons on the definition of the components of health-related fitness and appropriate use of tools for assessing each component (e.g., flexibility, body composition, muscular strength and endurance, cardiorespiratory endurance)
- Specific lessons that allow students to participate in moderate to vigorous physical activity for longer periods without tiring

- Specific lessons that teach how to interpret health-related fitness test results and choose appropriate activities to improve each component of health-related fitness
- Specific instructions that clearly indicate the appropriate grade level at which each concept and activity related to health-related fitness should be introduced and subsequently taught

Middle School: 6-8

- Specific lessons on how to assess personal health-related fitness status for each health-related fitness component and use this information to develop individualized health-related fitness goals with little help from the teacher
- Specific lessons on basic principles of training (e.g., overload, specificity) and how these principles can be used to improve a student's level of health-related fitness
- Specific lessons that provide opportunities for students to participate in and effectively monitor physical activities that improve each component of health-related fitness
- Specific lessons that identify how each component of health-related fitness relates to overall fitness
- Specific instructions that clearly indicate the appropriate grade level at which each concept and activity related to health-related fitness should be introduced and subsequently taught

High School: 9-12

- Specific lessons on appropriate activities for each health-related fitness component, as well as activities that help students meet their personal health-related fitness goals
- Specific lessons on basic exercise physiology concepts, such as the brain's ability to send signals and receive them from muscles, the cardiorespiratory system's ability to adapt to varying levels of intense physical activity, and the principles of training for competitive sports and recreational activities
- Specific lessons on age- and gender-appropriate standards for health-related fitness and ways to monitor and interpret personal health-related fitness data
- Specific lessons that allow students to develop a personal health-related fitness program based on goals that are specific and individualized
- Specific instructions that clearly indicate the appropriate grade level at which each concept and activity related to health-related fitness should be introduced and subsequently applied to the development of a personalized health-related fitness program

Note that the examples provided of the PECAT lesson outcome recommendations are for SHAPE Standard 3 only and relate to developing a health-enhancing level of fitness. To find recommended lesson outcomes for all other standards, refer to the PECAT.

Program Design

Health-enhancing physical activity and health-related fitness education focus on helping students assume progressively more responsibility for their own physical activity, health-related fitness, and well-being. Overall, a K-12 physical education program should build toward the ultimate goal: producing members of society who take lifelong personal responsibility for engaging in health-enhancing physical activity.

One way to think about designing developmentally appropriate content is to consider a diamond-shaped curriculum framework, such as that shown in figure 9.2.

National Standards and Guidelines

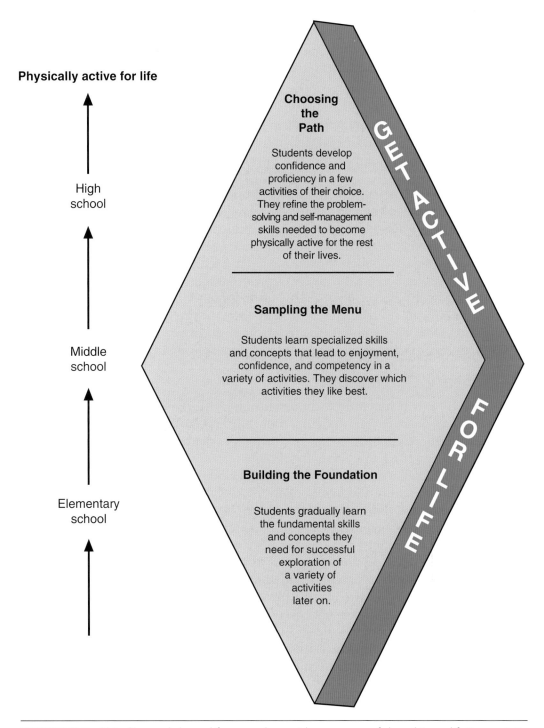

FIGURE 9.2   This diamond-shaped framework provides one way of describing a lifetime activity continuum.

Reprinted by permission from C. Himberg, *Teaching Secondary Physical Education in the 21st Century* (Champaign, IL: Human Kinetics, 2003), 19.

In the diamond framework, elementary-level students develop the basic skills and knowledge (for both movement and health-related fitness) that they will ultimately need in order to enjoy lifetime activities. In middle school, students use these skills to sample a variety of physical activities. This approach gives students the opportunity to form personal opinions about various activities and sports. Then, in high school, students select a few physical activities in which to specialize and use them to build personal physical activity plans. Building a foundation of basic skills in elementary school and developing proficiency in self-selected areas in high school forms a continuum that is likely to lead to positive health-related fitness behaviors in adulthood.

Sequencing of Health-Related Fitness

Proper sequencing of health-related fitness in a physical education curriculum allows students to progressively develop the knowledge and skills that enable them to achieve the ultimate goal of becoming physically literate individuals. Such a sequence should incorporate health-related fitness education and physical activity in two ways: as a stand-alone unit and by embedding health-related fitness objectives into the teaching of movement skills. The objectives of a separate unit on health-related fitness should require students to assess their personal health-related fitness and make lifetime plans for developing and maintaining a health-enhancing level of fitness. In this unit, students learn to exercise. In other units, they learn to use various training techniques to enhance performance and maintain a level of health-related fitness that allows continued participation. For instance, in a tennis unit, students might learn to use dumbbells to increase the power of their tennis strokes and reduce the chance of developing tennis elbow. Similarly, a volleyball unit might include plyometrics to improve jumping, or stretching to address specific muscle groups used in volleyball. During a ballroom dance unit, students might be surprised to learn that dancing is an excellent way to improve cardiorespiratory fitness and burn a lot of calories.

Elementary Curriculum

An elementary curriculum must focus on teaching basic movement skills (e.g., throwing, catching, striking, fleeing, dodging, volleying) and health-related fitness concepts (e.g., recognizing physiological changes during physical activity). At the elementary level, students first learn to identify the physiological changes that occur in response to physical activity. Later, they learn to distinguish between moderate and vigorous activities and to identify the components of health-related fitness while learning basic movement skills. For instance, they might learn to compare the relative intensity levels of walking, skipping, jogging, and running while also learning locomotor skills. Similarly, connecting push-ups, modified pull-ups, and curl-ups with muscular strength and endurance teaches students the components of health-related fitness in a physically active way. For example, you might have first graders put their hands on their chests to feel their hearts beating fast and talk about how that speed is caused by being active. Third graders might practice counting how many times they feel their heart beat and discuss more specifically how heartbeat relates to physical activity. Fifth graders can be taught to find their pulse in two ways (at the wrist and at the carotid artery) or use a heart rate monitor and then graph their rates for various activities.

Middle School Curriculum

During the middle school years, the curriculum should offer the chance for students to learn basic skills and comparative health-related fitness benefits in a variety of activities that take advantage of local opportunities. These activities might include team sports, individual and dual competitive sports, individual noncompetitive activities, outdoor adventure activities, and rhythmic activities. Spend most of your class time teaching skills; play games only when they match students' skill levels and have been modified as necessary to allow maximum participation.

As middle school students learn to apply the movement skills learned in elementary school to specific movement forms, they also learn the relative health-related fitness benefits of these activities. For example, you might ask students to rank a variety of activities based on their value for health-related fitness or to identify the health-related fitness component best associated with a specific sport. Middle school students can also begin to experience the FITT guidelines and the principles of progression and overload. By the end of middle school, students should understand that a brisk 30-minute walk may benefit health-related fitness more than two hours of softball. Seventh graders might be asked to monitor their heart rate while doing different activities over the course of a week, graph the results, and write a paper comparing the various rates and offering reasons for the differences.

High School Curriculum

The high school years should allow students to choose from activities that they have found enjoyable during middle school and in which they wish to refine their skills for lifetime participation. They should also learn how their chosen activities can contribute to a health-enhancing level of physical activity. High school students might be asked to develop an exercise plan based on their target heart rates, carry out the plan, and record the results (which requires knowing how to take their own pulse). They might also create a class blog for sharing research about the heart's response to stress on the body.

The high school curriculum should include specific objectives that require students to demonstrate the skills, knowledge, and understandings needed for participation in a lifetime of physical activity. Students' knowledge of health-related fitness should progress so that they understand how the activities they take part in affect their health. Golf is an excellent example of a lifetime sport that can be appropriate to include in many middle school and high school curriculums, but it may not be feasible in economically depressed areas where many residents cannot afford it. Volleyball is a popular activity found in many middle school and high school curriculums, but many students may dislike it by the time they get to high school because their middle school instruction was ineffective, the curriculum was not properly sequenced, or too much time was spent on playing the game and not enough on teaching the necessary skills to make it enjoyable.

Often the biggest restricting factors are found in local and state policies. If policies related to physical education do not require all students to participate, only provide minimal time for participation, or allow waivers, exemptions, or substitutions, opportunities for physical education learning may be eliminated. Other restricting policies may include the absence of full inclusion in physical education, class sizes that are larger than those for other content areas, physical education being withheld as punishment, or allowing physical education to be taught by non-state certified instructors (SHAPE America, 2015). Policies such as these will require physical education teachers to absolutely maximize learning opportunities during physical education, and it will be especially important to coordinate middle school and high school curriculums.

Developing Objectives and Outcomes

The next step in writing a curriculum is to develop objectives that specifically describe the knowledge, skills, and understanding needed to accomplish performance tasks. You can achieve this goal by referring to the National Standards for K-12 Physical Education and listing specific objectives for each standard. Objectives should be measurable, observable (when possible), and written in terms of what students will be able to know and do. They should also be written for all three domains of learning: cognitive, affective, and psychomotor. For example, objectives for a middle school tennis unit aligned with national standards might include the following elements:

- *Standard 1.* The physically literate individual demonstrates competency in a variety of motor skills and movement patterns.
  - Uses mature form when hitting forehands and backhands.
- *Standard 2.* The physically literate individual applies knowledge of concepts, principles, strategies and tactics related to movement and performance.
  - Identifies, describes, and analyzes tennis skills; recognizes mistakes and flaws in techniques; and creates a plan for correcting errors.
  - Incorporates the use of appropriate game tactics, such as hitting to an opponent's backhand.
- *Standard 3.* The physically literate individual demonstrates the knowledge and skills to achieve and maintain a health-enhancing level of physical activity and fitness.
  - Recognizes health-related fitness benefits of tennis and develops and participates in a plan to enhance health-related fitness for tennis using local and regional tennis facilities, off-site training, or both.
- *Standard 4.* The physically literate individual exhibits responsible personal and social behavior that respects self and others.
  - Understands, describes, analyzes, and applies rules of tennis (e.g., for serving, keeping score).
- *Standard 5.* The physically literate individual recognizes the value of physical activity for health, enjoyment, challenge, self-expression and/or social interaction.
  - Demonstrates and practices appropriate behavior while playing tennis, such as complimenting an opponent on an excellent play and participating in tennis matches outside of physical education class.

A well-written physical education curriculum must include objectives that encourage students to develop and maintain a healthy, physically active lifestyle. Participating in an activity only during class time does not meet this objective. In fact, students should participate in activities outside of class because of what they learn in class. If your students are not participating outside of class in an activity included in the curriculum, then you must ask yourself why. To find the answer, analyze course content, instructional practices, and local policies.

When we write objectives that allow students to demonstrate their ability to meet national standards, we create sequential learning opportunities and lend credibility to the physical education program. Properly written objectives also guide physical education teachers in student assessment and program evaluation and revision.

A good way to begin developing unit outcomes is to create a performance task that describes what a student should be able to do at the conclusion of the unit and details how the task will be assessed. When designing a curriculum, it can be useful to start at the end and work backward. What should students know and be able to do when they graduate from high school? For example, a high school curriculum outcome might call for students to be able to use cycling, tennis, volleyball, personal fitness, and golf as means of establishing a physically active lifestyle. Such movement activities should be separated into units, and for each activity a performance task should be developed. A **performance task** describes in a general way what students should know and be able to do at the end of the unit. For example, a performance task for a tennis unit might require students to demonstrate the ability to participate in a local tennis event. A performance task for a cycling unit might require students to demonstrate the knowledge, skills, and understanding necessary to participate in a local cycling event. And a performance task for a hiking and backpacking unit might require students to be able to hike the Appalachian Trail. This does not mean that the students must actually hike the trail; rather, it means that they must demonstrate that they possess the skills, knowledge, and understanding necessary to complete the task if they so choose.

Each performance task should also include the form of assessment that will be used to measure student performance. Without an assessment, neither you nor the student will know whether the student has achieved the desired outcome. As described in chapters 12 and 13, assessment can take many forms, including written work, teacher observation of performance, and an activity log. For example, in a hiking and backpacking unit, physical activity outcomes and performance tasks for Standard 3 might include locating the Appalachian Trail and other National Scenic and Historic Trails, planning and participating in a local hike or overnight camp-out, developing a budget, researching local regulations, applying for permits, and so on. To demonstrate their content knowledge, students could create a brochure to entice other hikers to use the trail and highlight the health-related fitness benefits associated with participation. Health-related fitness outcomes and performance tasks for Standard 3 might include developing a training program to hike 20 miles (32 km) per day while carrying a 60-pound (27 kg) backpack, analyzing diet, and calculating and comparing calories burned while hiking with and without a backpack.

Developing performance tasks for each grade level also helps to maintain appropriate sequencing of objectives from one grade level to another and provides a means of documenting student progress. Table 9.3 presents an example of sequential performance tasks, as well as grade-level objectives for Standard 3, for volleyball. After the performance task has been established, objectives for each standard and grade level are written to guide student learning.

Developing a Curriculum to Promote Lifetime Health-Related Fitness

During the first part of the 20th century, farmers lifted bales of hay, coal miners used picks and shovels, and factory workers manually produced their products. Housework was done by hand, lawns were mowed with push mowers, most children walked to school, and families played together instead of watching television. Many people naturally developed a health-enhancing level of fitness simply by means of the regular physical labor that was required in everyday life.

TABLE 9.3   Sample Volleyball Performance Objectives

Grade level	Performance task	Standard 3 objectives
K-2	Students will volley a balloon over an obstacle with a partner.	Students will describe physiological changes while volleying with a partner.
3-5	Students will use a forearm pass to volley a light-weight volleyball over an object with a partner.	Students will compare physiological changes while participating in volleyball activities to changes during other forms of physical activity.
6	Students will participate in modified volleyball games (e.g., with smaller numbers, lightweight balls, smaller court, lower net) during physical education class.	Students will identify ways in which participating in volleyball activities can contribute to a health-enhancing level of physical activity.
7	Students will participate in modified volleyball games (e.g., with smaller numbers, lightweight balls, smaller court, lower net) during physical education class and in other opportunities during the school day (e.g., at recess, before and after school).	Students will participate in volleyball activities that include methods of improving strength and muscular endurance for volleyball.
8	Students will participate in modified volleyball games (e.g., with smaller numbers, lightweight balls, smaller court, lower net) during physical education class and in other opportunities during the school day (e.g., at recess, before and after school), and document participation in volleyball activities outside of the school environment.	Students will design and implement a program that includes volleyball to improve levels of health-related fitness and nutrition.
9-12	Students will participate in semi-competitive volleyball games during physical education class and during other school-sponsored volleyball activities and will organize and participate in volleyball activities outside of the school community (neighborhood, churches, friends).	Students will design and implement a strength and conditioning program to enhance volleyball performance and allow for continued participation in volleyball for a lifetime.

During the second half of the 20th century, however, lifestyles became sedentary. When the *Surgeon General's Report on Physical Activity and Health* was published in 1996, it told us what physical educators already knew: Physical activity is good for your health, and everyone can develop a health-enhancing level of fitness by participating regularly in moderate to vigorous physical activity (U.S. Department of Health and Human Services, 1996). In order to do so, students need to be able to recognize the health-related fitness benefits of physical activity, understand the health-related fitness requirements of specific activities, and learn to develop a plan to achieve and maintain a health-enhancing level of fitness. Physical education had already begun to change, and physical education programs now began to focus on health-related fitness. Many teachers, however, were unprepared for the change, because traditional preparation did not include health-related fitness. Therefore, many teachers needed to find a resource that could help them develop programs to teach students about health-related fitness.

Now that there has been sufficient time to adapt to the necessary changes in physical education, many resources are available to help you teach students to become active throughout their lives. One way to do so is to use SHAPE America's physical education standards when developing your curriculum. For example, the Stairway to Lifetime Fitness (Corbin & Le Masurier, 2014) succinctly outlines the process through which teachers must guide students (see figure 9.3). Younger students are

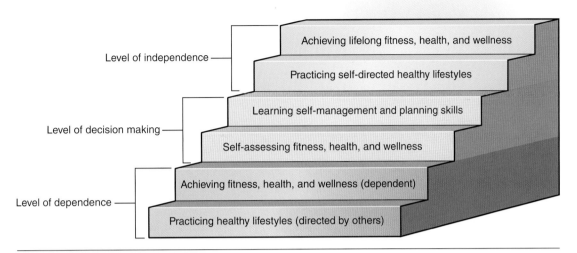

FIGURE 9.3 The Stairway to Lifetime Fitness outlines the steps that teachers can use to guide students toward a lifetime of fitness.

Reprinted by permission from C.B. Corbin and G.C. Le Masurier, *Fitness for Life*, 6th ed. (Champaign, IL: Human Kinetics, 2014), 34.

more likely to be on a lower, more dependent step, whereas older students need to be operating on a higher step (see table 9.4).

Teaching for Lifelong Fitness

Exercise becomes drudgery when done with poor technique or without understanding of health-related fitness concepts. People often begin the New Year by making a resolution to start exercising and get back in shape, and these intentions cause a January surge in membership at fitness centers. Unfortunately, many people fail to make immediate progress; instead, they fall prey to fatigue and injury, and fitness center participation returns to normal within a few weeks as people become discouraged and stop exercising. As this pattern indicates, a physical education curriculum should help students develop understanding of exercise skills, principles, and strategies. A physically literate person should be able to exercise efficiently and use exercise as a means of maintaining a health-enhancing level of physical activity and fitness.

The object of health-related physical activity and fitness education is to teach students how to achieve and maintain a health-enhancing level of physical activity and fitness throughout their lives. To do so, students need to understand the health-related fitness benefits of physical activity, identify the fitness requirements of selected movement forms, and develop health-related fitness plans to improve performance ability and allow for continued participation.

The sport activities typically taught in physical education take time and effort to continue when a person is outside of the school system. Often, the responsibilities that come with maturity do not allow for frequent trips to the golf course, tennis court, or bike path. Participation opportunities can also be reduced by poor weather. When opportunities for enjoyable recreation are limited, other measures need to be used to maintain a health-enhancing level of fitness. To help students prepare for this reality, you must incorporate activities and health lessons into your curriculum that

TABLE 9.4   Sample Activity Progressions by Topic

Topic	Primary (K-2)	Intermediate (3-5)	Middle school (6-8)	High school (9-12)
Corbin and Lindsey's Stairway to Lifetime Fitness (2014)	Step 1—Doing regular exercise	Step 2—Achieving physical fitness	Step 3—Establishing personal exercise patterns	Step 4—Self-evaluating Step 5—Solving problems and making decisions
Heart rate	Place hand on heart before and after vigorous activity and compare the two rates.	Count pulse; learn math to find heart rate (HR) based on partial count.	Practice math to find HR based on partial count; graph HR to monitor data; assess effort based on graphed data.	Design workouts based on knowledge of HR and target heart rate zone.
Running	Learn correct stride; run in low-organization games.	Analyze running strides of peers using rubric; design low-organization games that incorporate a high amount of running.	Teach peers to run more efficiently; report on how running efficiently helps a person succeed in a favorite sport.	Design interval workouts that alternate high- and low-intensity effort as determined by HR; make the workout fun for a friend to do.
Upper-body strength training	Play on the monkey bars on the playground.	Play fun push-up games (see Hichwa, 1998); learn tubing exercises.	Learn more tubing exercises; design games that increase muscular strength without equipment.	Learn how to lift weights safely; design a personal weight-training program; explore community options for weight training and do cost analysis.

help students continue to pursue their goals for lifelong health-related fitness after they are out of school.

As students move from middle school to high school, you should select activities with relevance to their lives both now and in the future. Show students what is available for young adults in their community. Are there bike paths, volleyball leagues, cross-country skiing areas, walking paths, and health clubs? Take field trips to introduce students to the available options. Invite community members (e.g., health fitness instructors, league directors, running club leaders, sport facility owners) to come to class to demonstrate new activities and tell students how they can get involved. Assign homework that relates to the real world—for example, consumer education assignments. Ask students to select a health club that they might join as an adult and create a flyer promoting that facility or write an online journal to express why that club would be their choice. In short, the older the students are, the more authentic and connected to their personal lives the activities should be.

Most forms of physical activity offer some health-related fitness benefits. Identifying the health-related fitness requirements of specific movement forms can help students learn how to continue participation throughout their life span and make physical activity more enjoyable. Some activities—for instance, playing a round of golf while riding in a golf cart—offer only limited benefits for health-related fitness. Riding rather than walking does not raise one's pulse rate and does little to improve cardiorespiratory endurance or maintain a health-enhancing level of fitness. Similarly, yoga and tai chi are great for developing flexibility but provide limited cardiorespiratory benefit. Walking, on the other hand, provides excellent cardiorespiratory benefits but may not develop sufficient muscular strength to prevent injury or enhance enjoyment of other activities. Therefore, students should be able to identify forms of cardiorespiratory activity, such as swimming, that can help improve their readiness for other cardiorespiratory activities, such as hiking.

Beyond being introduced to activities and community-based opportunities for lifelong activity, students must learn what benefits come from various activities. Understanding the relative health-related fitness benefits of specific physical activities helps students realize that they must participate in a variety of movement forms in order to develop and maintain a health-enhancing level of fitness. For instance, a golf enthusiast needs to know that walking instead of riding in a cart will greatly improve the health-related fitness benefits of golf and that participating in yoga may enhance one's golf game by improving flexibility. Similarly, hikers will find that weight training increases their enjoyment by making it easier to carry a backpack and thus reducing fatigue.

Understanding the relative health-related fitness benefits of selected movement forms helps students realize that no single activity can develop and maintain all components of health-related fitness. Participation in a variety of activities is necessary in order to address all components of health-related fitness and develop and maintain a balanced, health-enhancing level of fitness. Students should learn how to improve performance by developing and participating in activity-specific training programs. For role models, they can turn to the many top professional athletes who participate in training programs to lengthen their careers and improve their performance. When students research successful professional athletes, they see the importance of sport-specific training and can use those examples to develop their own programs; however, they should also learn how these athletes balance their training to create a well-rounded health-related fitness plan.

Fitness Education Cycle

Before students can plan for lifetime fitness, they need to know how to assess, and if necessary, improve their health-related fitness. They can be prepared to do so by an effective physical education program. One tool for creating a program that focuses on health-related fitness is the fitness education cycle (figure 9.4), a concept that helps students progress through fitness education in a systematic and cyclical manner. The eight steps of the fitness education cycle represent a progression for teaching health-related fitness concepts. The concepts and activities that must be taught *before* a health-related fitness assessment are fitness concepts, student preparation, and practice procedures; those that should come *after* a health-related fitness assessment are program planning and goal setting, promoting and tracking physical activity, reassessment, and revising and refining goals. The conclusion of one cycle leads directly into the beginning of another cycle as students are developmentally ready to move to the next level of knowledge and skill development. If students are to be active, fit, and capable of leading an active lifestyle in the future, they must take responsibility for their own health and personal health-related fitness. Therefore, you must teach them this process, as well as the content and skills that go with it. Fitness education is integrated and clearly addressed in a curriculum that is aligned with all national standards for physical education.

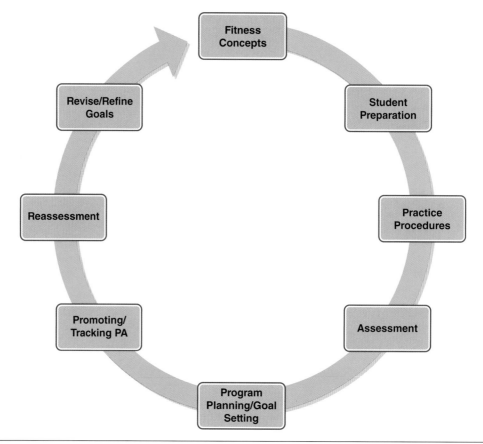

FIGURE 9.4   Fitness education cycle.

Reprinted by permission of The Cooper Institute.

Student Choice

Providing students with choices of activities in physical education takes cooperation among programmatic levels and the members of each department. For instance, the curriculum of the feeder middle schools must be coordinated with that of the high school that their students will all attend. Begin with the curriculum diamond, which exposes middle school students to a variety of activities in which they apply the movement skills learned in elementary school to specific movement forms. The activities could be categorized into the following groups:

- Traditional competitive team sports (e.g., basketball, volleyball, softball)
- Individual and dual competitive sports (e.g., golf, tennis, bowling)
- Individual noncompetitive activities (e.g., yoga, Pilates, tai chi, swimming)
- Fitness, personal fitness, and conditioning activities (e.g., weight training, aerobics)
- Rhythmic activities (e.g., aerobics, ballroom dance, line and country dance, hip-hop dance)
- Outdoor adventure (e.g., hunting, fishing, cycling, canoeing, hiking, camping)

We hope that middle school students will find activities that they enjoy and wish to pursue and that high school students will develop more competent skills related to those activities.

A high school curriculum depends on the physical education requirements of the school district. For instance, a school that requires only one year or one credit of physical education will of course have a more limited curriculum than one that requires two or more credits. More specifically, a high school that requires only one year or credit may offer one semester (and one-half of a credit) of introductory physical education that is similar to middle school classes and provides the opportunity for students to develop higher skill levels and finalize their activity choices. The second semester (and second half-credit) may allow students to choose from one of the activity categories discussed a moment ago. The class will focus the entire semester on one or two activities—for instance, golf and tennis—and allow students to become proficient in them. Teachers can work together to offer more choices overall, and students can then choose their preferred activities or students can be offered high school physical education electives in addition to regular physical education classes.

This approach provides a unique opportunity for students to self-select in order to enhance their physical learning. Students can be assigned to research physical activity resources to make connections between what they learn in class and the opportunities available outside of the school environment. They might do research, for example, on clubs and organizations such as the League of American Bicyclists, Trout Unlimited, the YMCA, and the United States Golf and Tennis Associations. Local chapters of these organizations hold regularly scheduled meetings, and many of the organizations offer youth development programs to recruit new members. For instance, attending a local chapter meeting of Trout Unlimited may result in a lifetime interest in fishing.

Fitness for Life

The most widely used program for lifetime health-related fitness in the United States is Fitness for Life, created by Charles Corbin and Ruth Lindsey. Fitness for Life courses and programs complement Physical Best, are fully integrated with both Physical Best and FitnessGram, and share the same HELP philosophy (see the sidebar titled

HELP Philosophy

The HELP philosophy is shared by SHAPE America, FitnessGram, ActivityGram, and Corbin and Lindsey's Fitness for Life.

H stands for *health* and health-related fitness. The primary goal of the program is to promote regular physical activity among all youth. Of particular importance is promoting activity patterns that lead to reduced health risk and improved health-related physical fitness.

E stands for *everyone*. FitnessGram program is designed for all people, regardless of physical ability. Used together, FitnessGram and ActivityGram assessments are designed to help all youth find some form of activity in which they can participate for a lifetime. Too often, activity programs are perceived to be only for those who are "good," rather than for all people. Physical activity and fitness are for everyone, regardless of age, gender, or ability.

L stands for *lifetime*. FitnessGram and ActivityGram share the goal of helping young people to be active now, but a long-term goal is to help them learn to do activities that they will continue to perform throughout their lives.

P stands for *personal*. No two people are exactly the same. No two people enjoy exactly the same activities. FitnessGram and ActivityGram are designed to personalize physical activity to meet personal or individual needs.

Reprinted by permission from C.B. Corbin and R. Lindsey, *Fitness for life*, 5th ed. (Champaign, IL: Human Kinetics, 2005), 5.

HELP Philosophy). Physical Best sets the foundation leading up to such courses and programs; then, once they are completed, it reinforces the skills and concepts needed for lifetime health-related fitness.

Fitness for Life is a comprehensive K-12 program designed to help students take responsibility for their own activity, fitness, and health and to prepare them to be physically active and healthy throughout their adult lives. This standards-based program offers a variety of resources and has been carefully articulated following a pedagogically sound scope and sequence to enhance student learning and progress. For more information, visit www.fitnessforlife.org or www.HumanKinetics.com or call 800-747-4457.

Summary

Effective physical education curriculums provide a framework for students to learn necessary concepts of health-related fitness education. They integrate motor skills and physical activity in a developmentally appropriate K-12 progression, as well as other subject areas, to create a well-balanced, meaningful approach. Such programs produce students who view physical activity as a worthwhile, pleasurable, and lifelong endeavor. You can help your students discover where their physical activity interests lie and learn how to design and implement a personal health-related fitness plan that suits their individual needs and situations. A well-designed and expertly implemented curriculum can inspire and empower students to lead physically active lives.

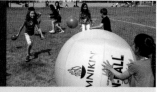

Discussion Questions

1. Compare a curriculum to a road map.
2. Define *curriculum* and describe the major components.
3. In order to be effective, what does a physical education program need to provide for students?
4. Discuss ways to overcome limiting factors in physical education (e.g., time).
5. Discuss technology applications for physical education and how they can help meet curricular requirements.
6. Explain the curriculum diamond and its importance in curriculum development for physical education.
7. Select one of the national physical education standards and develop an example of how it might be addressed in elementary school through high school.
8. Analyze the scope and sequence of a physical education curriculum that you are familiar with as a student or teacher.
9. Select a unit of instruction and a grade level, then create a performance measure that could be used as part of a health-related fitness curriculum.
10. Explain the parts and importance of the fitness education cycle.

CHAPTER 10

Employing Best Practices for Teaching

Betsy Gunther

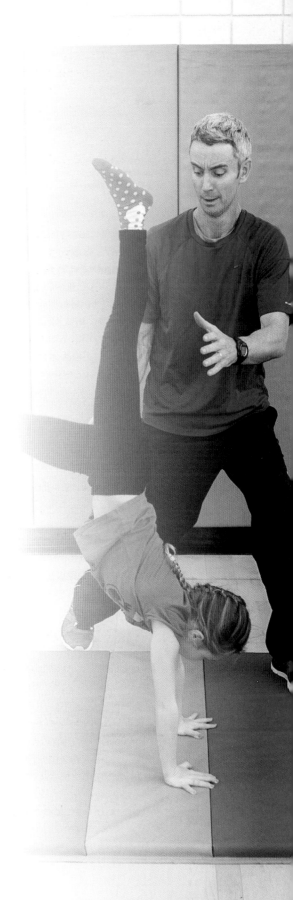

Meeting students' varied learning objectives is one of the greatest challenges that teachers face every day. Teaching strategies have less to do with your personal philosophy or style and more to do with your ability to comfortably shift from one teaching style to another in order to match the ever-changing needs of your students. Many teachers think of teaching style as a behavior that occurs naturally or as something to be taken for granted. However, the most effective teachers spend more hours planning than they do in front of the class.

Furthermore, teaching style is only one element in the formula for a successful educator. Any overall teaching strategy must consider not only teaching style but also the content to be taught, the suitability of the physical environment for certain styles, the time allotted or necessary to implement the style, the amount of class time allocated, the teacher's strengths and skills, and, most important, the students themselves. Across the nation, school demographics are changing, and instructional practices must be modified to meet the challenges of a more diverse population.

Consider these factors as you read about teaching styles and strategies throughout this chapter; more specifically, think about whether a particular style matches certain program objectives, areas of content, and developmental levels among students. Consider also what modifications might be made to allow a match between teaching style and each lesson. No single teaching style has been demonstrated to enhance learning for all students, and each style can produce unique outcomes. Using a variety of teaching strategies appropriately will help ensure that you meet the needs of all of your students. The main goal is for all students to experience success in physical education and in their lifetime physical activity pursuits. As you seek to accomplish this goal, Physical Best is one tool that can help you succeed.

Preparing the Environment

The physical education learning environment plays an important role in establishing the tone for student development. Although some environmental factors cannot be modified—for instance, the size of playing fields—teachers can design a learning arena that is inviting, encouraging, and safe. The key is to enhance the environment that you are given and to maximize your use of equipment and time. A well-prepared environment enhances learning opportunities for all students, accounts for the individual needs of each participant, and leads all students toward achievement.

Aesthetic Appeal

Pay attention to the look of your learning environment. Does it invite students to learn and inspire them to embrace healthy living? Craft bright and engaging bulletin boards and other wall displays that draw students in and help them learn. Integrate work and action pictures of your students. Set up visual aids as attractive focal points during a lesson—for example, a model of the human heart, a skeleton, an oversized rubber band to represent a muscle stretching, or attractive posters highlighting the bones or muscles that you are studying that week. For younger students, you might obtain a cardboard skeleton and put it together as you study the anatomy of the human body. You can also motivate students in new and exciting ways by using technology to enhance learning through interactive visuals, movement activities, games, and the use of music.

Displays enhance student learning, especially if the materials are available for them to see up close or examine personally during a lesson. For help in generating such displays, you can seek help from students, parents, and other volunteers. You might also consider asking an art teacher to integrate this work as a special project in an art class.

Music

Music provides an excellent way to enhance the learning environment. It can be used to welcome students, signal station changes, offer cultural stimulation, and provide a background that invites participation. You can also incorporate music with a good beat and tempo to help students develop spatial awareness, as well as kinesthetic awareness of the body in motion. Music helps students integrate multisensory skills that are necessary for accomplishing all physical activities. Allow students to bring music from home (screen their choices to ensure they're within the bounds of good taste before using them in class).

Safety

A safe environment provides a foundation for learning. No one can learn about or enjoy physical activity if he or she is afraid. Thus, it is crucial for students to know that they are in an emotionally safe environment where they can interact without judgment or criticism. Physical safety requires an environment free of debris, hazards, and other unsafe situations. Make sure that activity areas, locker rooms, and classrooms are clean and safe. Teach students specific safety information. Remind them often about safety concerns and practice emergency procedures.

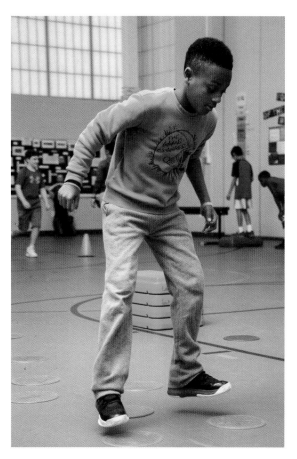

An attractive learning environment helps students engage with the topics you're teaching.

Another best practice is to position yourself strategically in the environment so that you can see the entire class at all times. Having a clear view of students as they perform activities helps you monitor their compliance with directives and with safety procedures.

Equipment Considerations

Another key for promoting student learning is to use available equipment to maximize physical activity. No one improves health-related fitness while waiting in a line to be active. Here are some effective practices:

- Set up equipment, and test audiovisual and computer equipment, before class begins.
- Ensure that equipment is in good working order by inspecting it at least once a month. Worn-out or broken equipment increases the risk of accidents.
- Secure exercise equipment, such as treadmills and stationary bikes, so that it cannot be used without adult supervision.
- Design a procedure for transporting and sharing equipment, such as rotating CPR manikins to various buildings where they will be used. Doing so promotes efficiency and maximizes storage space.
- Design a routine for distributing and collecting equipment. For example, assign squad leaders, specific students, or student assistants to pass out and return equipment.

Here are some ideas that might help eliminate or reduce equipment shortages:

- Contact community members for donations of high-quality used equipment (as a tax deduction, of course). Local health and fitness clubs may be willing to donate a portion of their retired equipment to enhance a school's fitness room.
- Scour garage sales and classified ads to purchase high-quality used treadmills, elliptical machines, rowing machines, weight benches, dumbbells, stability balls, and stationary bikes for a fraction of the original cost. Just be sure to perform thorough safety checks on this used equipment.
- Parents may be willing to donate used equipment.
- Consider having the school or a qualified individual make some equipment. For example, dot agility mats are easy to replicate at about a third of the cost of a manufactured mat. They are constructed of heavy nonslip rubber that comes in various sizes, often 24 inches or 36 inches (60 or 90 cm) square (size is based on the age of the student), with five dots marked in permanent marker (see figure 10.1).
- Pool resources (financial and equipment) with other schools. Several schools can collaborate to buy equipment and then design a rotation system for usage.
- Host fundraising projects to help purchase equipment (if the school allows such activity).
- Apply for grants. Money is available at the state and federal levels, and SHAPE America's website includes a section about grant writing and the availability of grant money.

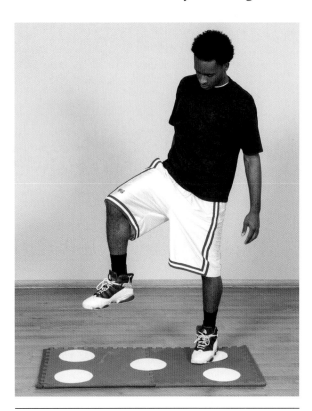

FIGURE 10.1 Dot agility mat.

Keeping Students Involved

No matter how upbeat and attractive the classroom environment is, students play a big part in creating a successful learning environment. Here are some tips for keeping students involved.

- Establish rules and procedures when the class begins. Doing so sets the tone for efficient use of time and reduces the chance of hassles caused by unclear expectations. Physical Best activities such as On Your Spot, Get Set, Go! use this concept and can increase the time that students spend on moderate to vigorous physical activity in each class.
- At the beginning of each semester or year, dedicate several days to team-building or cooperative activities to help increase student involvement. Design activities that provide opportunities for students to work with their classmates to attain

particular outcomes, learn leadership skills, and practice cooperation. For an example, see Project ACES on the web resource.

- Students live in the here and now, and relevant tasks and activities can provide the connection between learning in the movement setting and application in the world outside of school. To this end, you can encourage student participation by inviting students to make choices about what they want to learn. In the same vein, Physical Best is designed to help students move from dependence to independence and assume responsibility for their own health-related fitness. Letting students take ownership of their learning by becoming involved in decision making helps them see the value in activities.

- To enhance students' learning about developing an active lifestyle, ask them to locate services or opportunities in the community where they can participate outside of the school environment. For an example, see the Summer Fun–Summer Shape-Up Challenge in the web resource.

- Communicate by interacting with as many students as possible during each class session. In addition, be positive and constructive in both verbal and non-verbal communication. Students are acutely aware of body language and the tone of statements. By showing genuine interest in your students, you increase their inclination to work a little harder, which results in greater participation. If a student does not understand a task, go over the basic steps in a nonthreatening manner. For example, you might say, "Serena, let's try that skill again, only this time concentrate on keeping your elbows straight instead of bent," instead of saying, "Serena, why can't you remember that I said to keep your elbows straight!"

- Involve yourself in the lesson. The goal is to integrate various teaching styles in order to reach as many students as possible, and motivation is the key to long-term success. Don't be the teacher who just tells students what to do; instead, when appropriate, get involved by joining in the activity. Demonstrate skills and play a few minutes with each group; show them how it is done while maintaining your role as educator.

- Design or modify activities to suit the ages, experiences, and abilities of the participating students. For instance, if the class is practicing push-ups and several students have insufficient upper-body strength to perform a full-body push-up, allow them to perform a modified push-up or a wall push-up. At the other end of the spectrum, provide enhanced activities for students who are ready to move forward. For instance, students who can easily perform full-body push-ups could attempt to perform triceps push-ups (positioning the arms close to the body instead of shoulder-width apart) or clap hands between push-ups. For an example, see Mission Push-Up Possible in the web resource. This activity demonstrates how to modify a skill to meet individual needs while also working on teamwork and allowing students to use their knowledge of health-related fitness.

- When teaching new activities, some students may be reluctant to participate for any of various reasons. They may perceive themselves as less skilled and feel afraid of failure and embarrassment, or they may have had negative experiences with learning new skills. Give students the opportunity to watch before participating. Remember also that your reassurance and belief that they can succeed may help them overcome their apprehension. Establish a growth mind-set in your class by making it a safe place to try and fail in an effort to learn.

Teaching Styles

Once the learning environment has been prepared, the next step is to create lessons (following the established curriculum) that promote student learning. Students learn in a variety of ways, and an effective physical educator will plan lessons that incorporate a variety of teaching styles to address the unique learning needs of the students in their classes. Thus it is necessary to understand how students learn.

Teaching style can greatly affect students' interest and enjoyment of—and therefore their attitudes toward—physical activity. Exceptional teachers use various styles and strategies to enhance student learning. Depending on the style or strategy chosen, passive learning can be turned into active learning, and unmotivated students can become motivated, which is crucial for lifelong participation. The various teaching styles and strategies form a continuum from basic, direct instruction to student-initiated learning. In the latter approach, the teacher serves as a facilitator, and the student takes on increased responsibility for learning.

A Continuum of Teaching

Mosston and Ashworth (2010) have defined 11 teaching styles that lie along a continuum from direct (teacher-initiated) instruction to indirect (self-taught) instruction. These styles are summarized in table 10.1. Each style can enhance health-related fitness education, and the continuum approach is an excellent way to help students gain knowledge. During the initial phase of teaching about health-related fitness, students benefit from a direct approach. As they mature and gain knowledge, skills, and experience, a more student-centered approach supports their independent learning and allows them to assume more personal responsibility for their own physical activity choices.

Student Learning

In addition to considering the suitability of a teaching style to the content and purpose of a lesson, teachers must be aware of differences in how students learn. If you are using an array of teaching styles, you will automatically provide many different opportunities for students to learn. Even so, if you understand the types of learners in your classes, you will be even more able to provide high-quality, individualized programming in physical education. Acknowledging and addressing students' learning styles provides you with another strategy to help them learn effectively.

People use three basic senses in learning how to perform physical activity: auditory (hearing), visual (seeing), and kinesthetic (doing). When teachers prepare lessons that incorporate strategies for addressing individual learning styles, they enhance student learning. **Gardner's theory of multiple intelligences** (Gardner, 1983, 1993) asserts that because each person learns and produces best through various avenues, students need to have opportunities to develop weak avenues and excel in strong ones.

One example of developing a lesson using multiple intelligences involves using concept mapping to incorporate the different intelligences into a health-related fitness plan. This approach tends to increase students' involvement and thereby improve their learning. Table 10.2 details how Gardner's theory of multiple intelligences can be useful for engaging all students in active movement and active learning in physical education.

Physical Best activities address health-related fitness concepts through a variety of instructional styles and strategies in activities that are fun and physically challenging.

TABLE 10.1　Teaching Styles in Physical Education

Style	Description	Examples
Command (direct)	Teacher makes all decisions.	Students engage in motor and skill development with a high degree of classroom management by the teacher. Teaching tumbling skills is one area where safety and direct instruction are particularly important.
Practice	Students practice teacher-prescribed tasks.	Teacher demonstrates (e.g., a new skill), and students determine the amount of practice (e.g., for skill refinement).
Reciprocal	Students work in pairs with one acting as teacher and the other as learner.	This style is used for skill refinement (e.g., practicing for a FitnessGram assessment). Teacher monitors interaction and encourages observers to give positive, high-quality feedback to performers.
Self-check	Students evaluate their own performance against a set of criteria.	Teacher determines task to be completed. Students select appropriate activities and monitor their own progress. Criteria sheet is used to assess quality of performance (e.g., to log cardiorespiratory endurance activity).
Inclusion	Teacher provides alternative levels of difficulty for pupils.	Students choose a particular difficulty level within a teacher-designed task. For example, when helping students develop muscular endurance, teacher sets up three different heights to practice skier jumps. Expectations must clearly indicate that students should progress in terms of task difficulty.
Guided discovery	Teacher determines the task, then designs a sequence of questions or problems that lead students to the correct solution.	Teacher guides but does not give answer. Example: Which activity makes your heart beat faster—rope jumping, skipping around the gym, or jogging?
Convergent discovery	Teacher presents a problem that has one answer, and students find their own solution.	Teacher helps students become independent, critical thinkers by using trial and error. Example: What effect does gaining or losing weight (body fat) have on your heart rate?
Divergent discovery	Teacher presents a problem, and students find their own solution.	Teacher poses an open-ended problem for students to solve. Example: Design a good cardiorespiratory endurance program for someone who has a cast on a broken ankle.
Learner-designed individual program	Teacher decides content, and student designs the program.	Teacher asks students to design an individual health-related fitness plan to help them reach their goals for health-related fitness.
Learner-initiated	Students take full responsibility for the entire learning process.	Students show interest in a topic, seek answers to a question, or choose to engage in an activity. Teacher asks students to choose any topic related to health or physical education to research and present to the class.
Self-teaching	Student initiates an inquiry and takes full responsibility for learning.	Students suggest an activity, such as starting a club or mentoring or coaching a younger student.

Based on S. Ashworth and M. Mosston. (2010). *Teaching Physical Education*. (Old Tappan, NJ: Pearson Education, 2010). Retrieved from www.spectrumofteachingstyles.org/pdfs/ebook/Teaching_Physical_Edu_1st_Online_old.pdf

TABLE 10.2   Teaching to Different Learning Styles in Physical Education

Intelligence type	Description	Examples in physical education
Verbal-linguistic	Word smart	Create a written description of a popular dance.
Logical-mathematical	Numbers expert	Calculate target heart rate for the aerobic training zone during dance.
Musical	Relating to music, beat, and rhythmic movement	Create a dance routine that paces movement to the musical beat.
Visual/spatial	Pictures	Design a poster or video illustrating each movement of a dance.
Bodily-kinesthetic	Learning by doing; physical learning	Create a dance that tells a story through movement.
Interpersonal	Understanding through interaction with others	Mirror one another in dance while providing and receiving interactive feedback.
Intrapersonal	Self-learning or individual reflection	Find a popular movement or cultural dance to share with peers.
Naturalistic	Environmentalist	Practice dance at a park, in the pool, or at another outdoor venue.
Existential	Focused on causes, charity work	Design a dance-a-thon that raises money for a local charity.

For example, What's the Mix? combines mathematical, spatial, and kinesthetic intelligence, whereas Maintaining Balance incorporates the linguistic, cooperative, kinesthetic, and guided-discovery types. In general, station activities provide an effective way to incorporate the practice instructional style, linguistic intelligence, and health-related fitness concepts. As students move from station to station to perform the designated activities, they can refer to task cards that address relevant concepts. Students must read and accomplish the task with their groups. At the end of class, they can write in their journals or discuss the concept presented.

Incorporating a variety of styles and intelligences may strengthen a student's understanding of a concept or activity, thus increasing learning. Remember the old proverb that says, "I hear and I forget. I see and I remember. I do and I understand."

Cooperative Learning

Cooperative learning occurs when students work together to complete a specified task or achieve a certain goal. It places the responsibility for learning on students and promotes a more active learning environment. The versatility of this style allows it to integrate multiple intelligences, and it has the potential to incorporate all three learning domains (affective, cognitive, and psychomotor). The physical education environment is an ideal setting for cooperative learning to take place because students must work in teams or small groups to perform many of the traditional physical education activities. Cooperative learning is also an excellent way to help students become more involved in health-related activities because peers can encourage each other to work harder or provide leadership to help those who are struggling.

One example of cooperative learning is jigsawing, in which each member of a team is given a particular assignment to complete. Each team member then brings back her product and places her piece of the puzzle with other team members' pieces to form a complete picture. The sidebar titled Jigsawing Assignment provides an example of how students can use the jigsaw strategy in a physical education environment.

Jigsawing Assignment

Unit: Health-Related Fitness Components

Jigsawing Instructions

1. Divide the class into groups of four and either assign each member a health-related fitness component or allow students to assign themselves a component. Make sure that each group has each component.

2. Give team members three to five activities that will enhance specific health-related fitness components. If time allows, ask students to design or locate the activities themselves.

3. Ask all members to form a new group and design three or four warm-up routines that include all four components of health-related fitness.

4. Be sure to have a multitude of materials on hand to encourage creativity in design.

5. Another approach is to assign the first part of this activity as homework and then devote one class period to the group portion.

6. Now, ask each group to lead the class in the warm-up routines for the next couple of weeks.

Sample Jigsawing Activity: Move, Move, Move

For this activity, select music with a good four-count rhythm; step aerobics music will generally work well.

1. Divide the class into groups of four or fewer.

2. Give each group a particular movement to perform and have them practice it for a short while to the beat of the music. Here are a few examples.

   o Group 1: Jump in one spot eight times.

   o Group 2: Hop on the left foot four times, then hop on the right foot four times.

   o Group 3: Do feet-only jumping jacks four times (each jack counts as two).

3. Form new groups so that each new group has one person from each of the original groups representing a different movement.

4. Then ask the new groups to combine their movements to form a new routine or movement sequence.

5. Allow the groups to practice their routines.

6. Ask each group to perform its routine for the entire class.

Make the movement developmentally appropriate for the age level. For younger students, use pictures with words to describe their movement; with older elementary students, words alone should suffice. You could also allow students to design their own four- to eight-count movements.

Sample Jigsawing Activity: Aerobic Routine

After students have had several days to perform aerobics or step aerobics, let them design their own routines to teach to the class. This activity could also provide an opportunity to incorporate technology by using apps that help students design routines. Incorporating technology can appeal to different types of learners and help motivate students. Always remember, however, that not all students have access to apps.

Place students into groups of three to five members and assign each student to design a particular component of an aerobics routine. Specifically, one student designs the warm-up segment, two or three others design the aerobics segment, and another designs the cool-down segment. Then have each group come together and put the routine to music.

Adapted from J.E. Rink, *Teaching Physical Education for Learning*, 3rd ed. (New York, NY: McGraw-Hill Companies, 1998): 89-94.

This activity gives students a chance to be responsible for their own learning, while teachers serve as facilitators and provide students with instructional feedback. The activity addresses the cognitive, psychomotor, and affective learning domains through cooperative learning strategies.

Cooperative learning also enhances students' motivation by freeing students to work with friends, solve problems, and interact with a variety of people. This process naturally lends itself to the concept of team sport participation, which is arguably an extension of the classroom environment and supports the goal of lifetime fitness.

Enhancing Health-Related Fitness Education in the Classroom

Although the teaching of health-related fitness need not be relegated to the classroom setting, the classroom can be an opportune place to discuss a wide range of content, including physiology, psychology, exercise principles, and goal-setting techniques. Developing cognitive understanding helps ensure that students will receive a comprehensive health-related fitness education. Strive to create classroom lessons that complement the existing curriculum and organize lessons according to health-related fitness concepts. Teach health-related fitness lessons that reinforce concepts learned during participation in physical activity; in this way, you link what students learn in the classroom with the physical environment.

Students should be actively engaged in programs that create opportunities to develop responsibility for their own learning. To this end, the learning and teaching styles presented earlier in this chapter can, of course, be used in the classroom setting. Review the important developmental steps outlined in Bloom's taxonomy and incorporate them into your lesson plans; students should progress in their ability to remember, understand, apply, analyze, evaluate, and create. To see a visual version of Bloom's taxonomy, do a web search for "Bloom's taxonomy for physical education."

Here are some examples of content that can be used in the classroom setting:

- *Healthy heart statement.* Younger students can create several model hearts accompanied by a specific statement highlighting ways to stay heart healthy. Give several laminated heart pieces to a group of three to five students. Each piece represents part of a complete heart that the students will piece together. After completing the model, the students can discuss their statements.

- *Interpretation of heart rate data.* Middle school and high school students can calculate their resting heart rate and target heart rate zones (see chapter 5), chart the heart rates in graph form, log workout results, and calculate averages.

- *Health-related fitness plans.* Older students can take on the role of health-related fitness expert for a newspaper or magazine. Give students several hypothetical letters sent to them for advice. After students have written their responses, ask them to post their responses or read them aloud in class and discuss them. Here are some examples: (1) I am a pitcher for my team, and I want to make my arms stronger so that I can throw harder. What can I do? (2) I want to make my varsity sport team next year, but I am not very strong. What exercises or activities can I do to help me gain overall strength and run faster?

- *Treatment of injuries.* Students need to understand that injuries can occur even when they are careful. The teacher may contact the American Red Cross or the

National Safety Council for information about basic first aid and cardiopulmonary resuscitation (CPR). Several good apps are also available to provide instruction and quiz students on a variety of first aid situations. Recommended injury treatment topics to cover include heat- and cold-related problems (e.g., heat stress, heat exhaustion, hyperthermia, hypothermia), sprains and strains, fluid intake (dehydration), sunburn and skin protection, and the role of nutrition in reducing injuries and improving overall health-related fitness (see chapter 4).

- *Becoming a savvy health-related fitness consumer.* In this age of advertising blitzes, cable shopping networks, and web surfing, it is essential to be a well-informed consumer of health-related fitness information and products. Students need to know how to comparison-shop in order to get the most for their money when paying for equipment, supplies, and services. They also need to learn how to discern when a product isn't worth the container it comes in. Here are some suggestions for consumer education activities that can be adapted to fit students' ages and abilities:

  ○ Direct students to bring in an advertisement for a fad diet or a piece of exercise equipment that promises miracle results. Have them report (orally or in writing) on whether the claim is true and why or why not.

  ○ Discuss what might make an advertisement effective (e.g., flashy, quick bites of information; enthusiastic claims). Ask small groups of students to develop magazine ads or act out TV commercials that advertise the benefits of a health-related fitness activity or practice (e.g., drinking plenty of water before, during, and after exercise; playing an active game instead of watching TV).

  ○ Help students conduct a video phone call with a staff member at a local sports equipment store. Ask students to prepare specific questions about equipment that interests them. Ask the salespeople to help the students compare the features of similar products. Then, for homework, ask each student to choose one of the products and explain in writing why it was the best buy for the student's needs.

  ○ Use Nearpod to engage and assess students by means of mobile devices. Ask students to create an individual health-related fitness plan for after-school hours or blog with others about their progress, ideas, and challenges.

- *Physical activity data logging.* The classroom is an ideal setting for teaching students how to develop appropriate goals and physical activity logs. Emphasis can be placed on accurately recording data. If students have access to a computer lab, they can record their health-related fitness scores using FitnessGram and their activity logs using ActivityGram. Other phone-compatible options include apps such as MyFitnessPal and Fitbit. You can also show students how to use generic programs such as Microsoft Excel to keep physical activity logs or design a physical activity calendar. Calendars can also include goals and specific activities that use the overload principle. Help students understand the connections between their recorded results and any changes in their physical activity, nutrition, and health-related fitness scores. Students can use their written records to create new goals based on their successes.

- *Goal setting.* The classroom setting provides opportunities to explain the purpose and mechanisms of goal setting (chapter 2). Sample class activities include the following:

○ Help a fictional person set appropriate goals (e.g., help a teenager build upper-body strength for wall climbing; help a peer improve body composition).

○ Work with a friend and help each other set realistic goals and plan activities to reach those goals in a chosen area of health-related fitness. Instruct students to think of incentives that they can offer each other: "If we both follow our plan, we'll buy those new outfits." "We'll walk to the mall together so that we can talk while we exercise."

○ Brainstorm reasons that people might not stick to their physical activity plans long enough to reach their goals. Then choose one problem and list ways to overcome it.

Give younger students a handout to work on that includes a list of specific activities. Ask them how many of each activity they think they can do in a certain time (15 seconds, 30 seconds, and so on). Then ask them to perform the activity and write down the number completed. Next, ask them to circle the final number if they accomplished their initial goal or place an X over the final number if they did not. Conclude by discussing goal expectations. Recording sheets can be used during the year to help students see their progress; this activity also serves as good lead-up practice for designing personal fitness plans.

- *Designing a personal health-related fitness plan.* Primary-grade students can begin to make choices about how they will reach personal goals in each component of health-related fitness. The amount of information to present depends on students' developmental level; divide the material into small pieces so that students can understand and apply what they have learned. The Physical Best activities included in the web resource provide examples of developmentally appropriate activities that focus on specific components of health-related fitness.

In order to be effective, personal plans for health-related fitness must change as students change. Illustrate this point through examples of personal health-related fitness plans. Show students how goals are set and then reset after they are achieved; in this way, students can begin to understand the process of tailoring a program to fit their current needs.

The Concept of Homework

Many states have established physical education standards that include specific outcomes in the cognitive, psychomotor, and affective domains. To achieve these standards, teachers include homework that moves physical activity and development of health-related fitness outside the gymnasium and into the home and community. This homework prompts students to explore and personalize a topic; enables a cross-curricular approach; incorporates a variety of strategies; and can increase communication between parents, students, and the school. Keep in mind the following considerations:

- Homework assignments should be purposeful and should extend opportunities for learning or practice.

- Homework can provide an additional opportunity for lesson content to be individualized and personalized for each student.

- Incorporate actual physical activity as a homework assignment or a portion of the assignment. If students design a health and physical activity calendar, ensure that they include activity as part of it (see figure 10.2).

- Ensure that homework assignments are connected to current lessons so that students can apply what they have learned in the classroom to the real world. Students live in the here and now, and keeping homework connected to current lessons keeps their experiences relevant.
- Homework can increase family involvement. Opportunities to link families and schools together can benefit all involved by increasing physical activity participation, opening avenues for communication, and developing stronger family relationships.

The possibilities for effective homework assignments cover a wide range. Assignments can be as simple as completing a worksheet or as comprehensive as developing a portfolio; the key is to incorporate as much movement and physical activity as possible. This type of homework can be done by all students, from kindergartners through high school seniors, as long as it is designed appropriately. Much of the information described in the preceding section (as topics for the classroom setting) can be modified for use in homework assignments, thus leaving more class time available for physical activity.

Sample Homework Assignments

These are examples of either a reflection or closure activity or a simple homework assignment for your students to complete.

Sports Reporting

Students attend a sporting event at their school. As they watch the event, they attend to the health- and skill-related fitness components that the athletes need in order to perform the activity effectively. After the event, students identify the components they observed during the game and cite examples.

Interview

Students interview a family member about personal physical activity habits and write a summary of the interview. Students can be asked to engage in the physical activities with their family member and describe this experience as part of the summary.

Brain Power

Students design crossword puzzles or word-finds for their peers using health-related fitness terms. As a follow-up, during a lesson, students can engage in activities that relate to these terms.

Question for the Day

Craft a question that prompts students to reflect on the day's lesson. For example, when teaching a unit on golf, you might ask, "Which of the health-related fitness components can you maintain or improve through regular participation in golf?"

Event Participation

Students can prepare for and participate in a local activity, such as a community golf fundraiser. Students should describe their current level of skill and participation in the activity (in this case, golf). Then they detail how they are preparing for the event, describe the steps involved in taking part (e.g., registration), and record their practice activity. Finally, they can journal about their experience.

Research Paper

Students pick a successful athlete and find information about the workout regimen used by the athlete to stay sharp both physically and emotionally. Perhaps some local athletes would be willing to come to class and lead students through an appropriate workout. Even older student-athletes (carefully chosen) might serve as the "celebrity athlete" for a lesson.

(continued)

Technology Connection

Students design a web page, create a video, or create a blog with peers to highlight one of the components of health-related fitness.

Active Andy and Suzy Slug

As an example, an assignment for primary students might begin by having a discussion about what it means to be active and what activities they can do at home or after school to stay active. Reproduce pictures of children being either active or not active and send them home with the students. Ask them to draw a happy face beside the pictures that show kids being active and a sad face beside those being inactive, then try one of the activity pictures with family members.

Health Calendar

Ask students to design a calendar that celebrates physical education, health-related fitness, and being healthy. The calendar can cover a week, two weeks, or a month (teacher's choice). Students should plan activities to do during that time and log their success. Figure 10.2 presents such a calendar that was designed to celebrate National Physical Education Week, which is always the first week of May.

			MAY			
Sunday	**Monday**	**Tuesday**	**Wednesday**	**Thursday**	**Friday**	**Saturday**
1	2	3	4	5	6	7
	No television or video games today. Go outside and do something physical.	Jump rope for at least 15 minutes today.	Take a 20- to 30-minute walk around the park or neighborhood today; go with a friend or walk the dog.	While watching your favorite television program, do sitting exercises such as crunches, push-ups, stretching, leg raises, biceps curls, and so on.	Ride your bike for 30 minutes. Tell a parent where you are going. Follow the laws of the road. Be safe!	

FIGURE 10.2 Keeping a calendar is a motivating way to help students track and plan the frequency of their participation in physical activity.

Extending Physical Activity Time

The amount of time that physical educators have with their students varies widely from state to state, school to school, and level to level. Regardless of how frequently you see your students, take advantage of strategies that can extend physical activity time beyond the walls of the gymnasium. The goal is to get students into the habit of being physically active on their own and to make activities personally enjoyable so that students don't view them as drudgery. Adapt the following suggestions to fit students' age ranges and school facilities. These ideas should serve not as replacements of physical education but as extensions of it. In other words, they are meant to enhance what is taught during physical education class. Administrators and colleagues must understand this perspective and not use physical activity outside of class as a reason to reduce physical education programs. We must distinguish between what is purposeful and deliverable instruction and what is just physical activity. Both are important, but they are not the same thing.

- *Health-related fitness breaks.* Physical activity can be accumulated throughout the day in short bouts, and this approach is an increasingly popular option. It also means that classroom teachers can be asked to support increases in physical activity time once they are trained by a qualified physical educator to conduct effective activity breaks. Provide teachers with information about the value of physical activity for students' classroom behavior; for example, exercise increases blood flow to the brain and thus helps people think better. You might also offer a 5-minute summary of possible activities at each staff meeting—for instance, asking students to take a 5- to 10-minute dance break during which lively music is played and students continually move. Changing the music to a slower tempo can quiet the students; another idea is to have students cool down through a meditation-type activity. If weather permits, students can be taken to the playground to perform a variety of locomotor movements in a designated space for at least 10 minutes. For more ideas, many resources on the web describe simple break activities that require no specialized equipment. Teachers can even build activity into classroom answering procedures. For example, during a review of multiple choice answers, students can indicate their selection through movement—doing jumping jacks to indicate choice A, push-ups to indicate choice B, and so on. This approach enables effective review of the answers while also providing an opportunity for physical activity—and the students will enjoy it!

- *Recess.* Ensure that students have ample equipment for physical activity. Student input is beneficial here; in addition, activities taught during physical education can often be used during recess.

- *Lunchtime.* Lunchtime free play is simply a longer recess in most schools, but it can be much more. The physical education teacher can be available as a personal health-related fitness consultant or can train student volunteers to conduct fun activities that support health-related fitness.

- *Intramurals.* These physical activity programs are conducted between students or teams of students from the same school. You can adapt such a program to augment the health-related fitness curriculum. Ensure that the program is fun and welcoming to all who wish to participate. Consider asking students to track their minutes of activity or calculate calories burned as a way to keep the focus on physical activity and health-related fitness. Consider also allowing students to add points for using encouraging words to classmates in order to facilitate social development and fun.

- *Programs before, during, and after school.* Create a new program or enhance an existing program. To obtain help with these programs, train others, such as parents, senior volunteers, and child care workers. Start a health-related fitness club and offer incentives for participating.

- *Home-based activities.* Send home assignments in which the entire family can participate. For example, for the Family Health Minute activity, present a specific health topic to your students and then ask them to discuss it with (or explain it to) their families. Ask them to set aside a few minutes for this activity two or three times per week. Provide new information each time, or offer one topic with various subtopics. You can also ask students to create ways to be physically active while watching television. For instance, during a commercial break, a family could participate in an activity challenge in which each member performs 5 curl-ups, hops on one foot 10 times, or performs stretches. (Commercials tend to run in 15- and 30-second slots, which is an appropriate duration for a stretch). Families could also keep hand weights close by and perform various upper-body movements (e.g., lateral raises, front raises, biceps curls) during commercials.

- *Community events.* Families and community members can be involved by staging family nights, health fairs, and other events. Such events not only help students become fitter and more healthy but also provide publicity for your program.

Technology

Given that technological advances continue to occur at a rapid pace, we must consider the implications for health-related fitness education programs. Using technology in the classroom is a strategy that can enhance teaching about health-related fitness by increasing students' motivation, morale, and confidence. Moreover, because today's students far surpass many teachers in their knowledge and ingrained use of technology (from text messaging to video productions), it is helpful to incorporate technology into learning about health-related fitness in order to appeal to students' familiar modes of learning and communication. The key is to select the correct technology and use it only in ways that are purposeful—not merely for the sake of using technology.

- *Hardware.* Phones, tablets, computers, and video equipment can greatly enhance the teaching of health-related fitness concepts. Videos can be used to enhance students' understanding of health-related fitness topics as diverse as training principles, false advertising, and the functioning of the cardiorespiratory system. Students can use computers to download, analyze, graph, and store data from a heart rate monitor. They can use the web to research health-related fitness topics or encourage "fitness pals" in other schools through e-mail or social media. Students can also work in small groups to develop health-related fitness reports and then create a newscast to share with peers or younger students (some schools are even equipped with in-house television and radio stations).

  Smaller devices, such as tablets and phones, allow easier recording of data and decrease the need for pen and pencil. For instance, teachers can use handheld devices to conduct health-related fitness testing, record the results, and, later, download them to a departmental or school computer for single-student analysis or report generation. LCD projectors can be used to enlarge objectives, daily activities, and closure questions to poster size, thereby helping to ensure that instruction is focused and intentional.

- *Software.* FitnessGram software provides teachers not only with key functionality (e.g., printing reports, organizing information) but also with a means for individual students (using passwords) to track their own progress in health-related fitness. Another feature is the ActivityGram, which allows teachers and students to monitor activity levels. Electronic portfolios provide an excellent way to track student progress throughout their school years and to enable students to design their own portfolios and track their progress.

  Video games have been around for a long time and have been deemed a significant factor in causing youth to have a more sedentary lifestyle. More recently, computer companies have introduced interactive video games designed to engage players physically. These games can offer more than just animated exercise; many include built-in assessments and scoring systems based on skill performance, as well as heart rate monitors. Several sport-product companies are now marketing dance or agility programs that allow students to improve health-related fitness by watching a video and replicating the moves on specially designed electronic carpets. Wii Fit is an example of a program that includes activities to

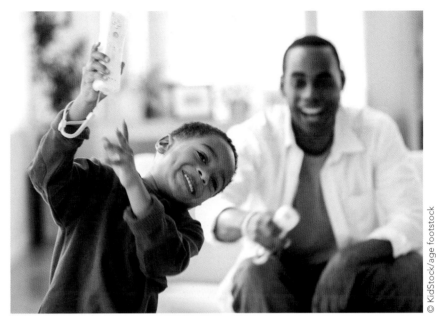

Some video games incorporate physical movement.

help improve health-related fitness (Sheehan, Katz & Koorman, 2015).

Educators and students can also choose from a multitude of apps that address health-related fitness and physical activity. Many of these apps can be used to count steps, track physical activity, plan diets, individualize exercise plans, and self-assess skill performance. Best of all, many of them are cost free. You can introduce these apps to students and encourage students to use them in their own lives and with family members. Just remember to thoroughly check out any apps before using them in class or recommending them to students.

- *Equipment.* Heart rate monitors can provide valuable information to both teachers and students. Students can learn how to monitor their heart rates during aerobic workouts and obtain information about exercise heart rate zones, recovery heart rates, and resting heart rates. Simple one- and two-function monitors can provide useful feedback to students, and sophisticated multifunction models are capable of programming individual heart rate information that can be downloaded to a computer.

Pedometers are another form of technology that students can use to monitor their physical activity levels both inside and outside of the physical education setting. Pedometers vary from simple, one-function varieties to multifunction models.

A number of products are also available to help conduct body composition evaluations. Some work like a handheld device that allows the user to download the results. Others require the user to record the information on paper and transfer it to a computer.

Even older kinds of exercise equipment such as treadmills, elliptical machines, stair steppers, and weight machines have evolved within the last few years to include recording mechanisms for heart rate and heart rate target zones.

Ever-evolving new technologies can provide you with new opportunities to engage students in a way that appeals to them. Virtual headsets are an excellent example of a way to make lessons come "alive" for students. Work with your technology department to learn about available resources that could enhance the learning environment and appeal to various learning styles.

- *World Wide Web.* Delivery of instruction can be enhanced through the use of resources housed on the web, such as video clips, webcasts, geocaching, and many other applications. A teacher can design web quests that require students to locate information from a variety of educational websites—for example, Choose MyPlate (www.choosemyplate.gov), which is an excellent site for information about a variety of health-related fitness activities. You can also consider the following websites when searching for inventive ways to use online resources with your students or to enhance your teaching:
  - The PE Geek: https://thepegeek.com/
  - SPARK PE: https://sparkpe.org/
  - support REAL teachers: https://www.supportrealteachers.org/
  - iPhys-Ed: https://www.iphys-ed.com/
  - CSPAP Comprehensive School Physical Activity Program: www.shapeamerica.org/cspap

- *Technology for inclusion.* Technology can be used to help all students, with and without disabilities, be more physically active and learn about health-related fitness. It has also provided new ways to promote the inclusion of students with a variety of disabilities (see chapter 11).

As these examples illustrate, the use of technology in a physical education curriculum can help students learn to monitor their physical activity and apply it to their activity outside of the classroom. Before deciding to purchase new technology, consider the following points:

- Remember the population you are teaching. Can your students afford to bring their own devices (e.g., iPad, Fitbit, or mobile phone for apps such as MyFitnessPal). If you use resources that your students have available on a daily basis, you can save resources and motivate students to use them more often because of their ready accessibility.

- Resist the impulse to go out and buy immediately. Instead, try to borrow the item from a colleague or conduct some research to determine whether it would be a good fit for your student population. Consider asking a sales representative to loan the equipment for a short while.

- Would this software or piece of technology help students achieve program outcomes? For the answer, do not always rely on a company's brochure and demonstration. Instead, search the web for reviews of the equipment and try to find out how sustainable it is. Will it be outdated within a couple of years? What does it cost to sustain?

- Grants can be used to help purchase health-related fitness technology. SHAPE America provides a web page identifying funding sources for physical education and related programs (www.shapeamerica.org/grants).

- Technology can help you teach, but it is no substitute for teaching and it can easily become just an expensive toy. Make sure that each item is educationally sound for your students and your program.

Keeping Up With Technology

Technology changes so rapidly that many resources are constantly being invented and can be found online. It can be challenging to stay up to date, but doing so will enhance your overall use of these tools. Participate in online physical education forums and chat groups, follow blogs, attend conventions, and use web searches to discover current ways to use technology to enhance your teaching and your students' learning.

Summary

A successful program for health-related fitness education must develop a fun and active learning environment, use appropriate teaching styles, and apply strategies that individualize programs to meet students' needs. Effective differentiation depends on selecting a variety of developmentally appropriate learning experiences and ensuring that each one is sequential, fun, safe, and inclusive. In addition, incorporating the best practices described in this chapter encourages students to pursue lifelong health-related fitness activities and develop physical literacy. The next chapter provides practical suggestions for including all students, particularly those who have special needs.

Discussion Questions

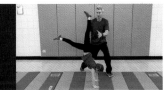

1. What does using best practices in physical education mean to you?
2. What cooperative learning activities do you currently use in your lesson plans?
3. How can you incorporate technology into physical education to enhance students' learning?
4. Explain how a student with a logical-mathematical learning style might be motivated to participate in a health-related fitness program.
5. Which of the 11 teaching styles in physical education would you use to teach a new skill? Why? Provide an example.
6. Design a lesson plan to illustrate one of the 11 teaching styles.
7. How are the best practices for lesson design presented in this chapter preferable to the "roll the ball out and let them play" philosophy? Provide specific examples.
8. Describe how you would teach a health-related fitness concept individually by using each of the 11 teaching styles.
9. Discuss your favorite teaching style. Contrast it with your least favorite teaching style.
10. Select a Physical Best activity from the web resource, then identify ways to use it to meet the needs of individual learners and learning styles.

CHAPTER 11

Including Everyone

Keith Johannes, Brian Culp, and David Lorenzi

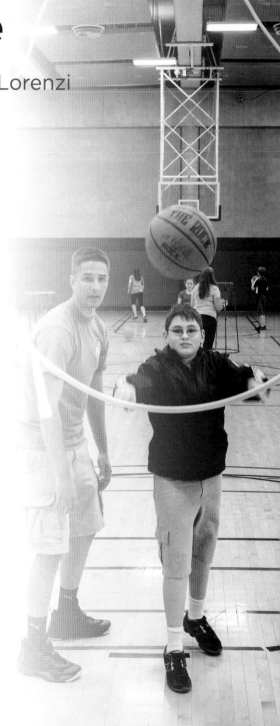

Effective health-related fitness education benefits *all* students regardless of individual or group differences. The term *inclusion* refers to the process of teaching students with disabilities together with their typically developing peers and using appropriate support systems that they otherwise would have received in a segregated setting. Although this chapter explores that concept in depth, it also looks at how to meet the needs of every student, regardless of gender, cultural or ethnic background, or ability level (whether or not a student has been identified as having a disability). In Physical Best, **inclusion** refers to the process of creating a learning environment that is open to and effective for all students whose needs and abilities fall outside the general range of those for children of similar age or whose cultural or religious beliefs differ from those of the majority group.

Relevant Laws

In short, inclusion means that all students are included in an appropriate manner and respected as individuals so that all can reach their maximum potential. This process requires physical education teachers to expand their repertoire of teaching styles and strategies (see chapter 10). To be inclusive, you should expand your approach from the perspective not of how smart or skilled a student is but *in what ways* the student is smart or skilled. Physical Best seeks to provide high-quality learning opportunities that allow all students to use their fullest abilities—not simply focus on making adaptations for disabilities.

Inclusion is the general trend in education and society; more important, it is the ethical philosophy to adopt. The Individuals with Disabilities Education Act (IDEA) mandates that students with disabilities be educated with their nondisabled peers in the least restrictive environment possible. The regulations for implementing IDEA (2004) indicate that every student with a disability who receives a free and appropriate public education must receive physical education services, and that these services may be specially designed if necessary. These regulations view disability in terms of any individual characteristic that impairs any major life activity.

IDEA was an extension of enacting Title IX of the Education Amendments of 1972, which prohibited discrimination based on gender and spelled out how public institutions should ensure an individual's civil rights regardless of gender. In response, more educators began learning to focus first on what a person *could* do, rather than on what the person *could not* do.

As the U.S. Department of Education's Office of Special Education and Rehabilitative Services says in its bulletin, *Thirty-Five Years of Progress in Educating Children With Disabilities Through IDEA*, "We cannot afford to leave anyone out of our efforts. . . . Every child is a precious resource whose full potential must be tapped" (U.S. Department of Education, 2010, p. 12). With this approach in mind, IDEA will likely continue to be redefined and to influence physical education.

With the adoption of the Every Student Succeeds Act (ESSA) in 2015, physical education is now considered part of a well-rounded education, meaning that every student should have an equal opportunity to participate in a physical education curriculum alongside peers. ESSA permits most of the decision making on education-related issues to be done at the state level, and many states have passed that responsibility on to local education agencies and school districts. As a result, physical education teachers now have the opportunity to advocate for physical education in their own school districts.

Thus it is important for you to take an active leadership role in your district to ensure that effective physical education is provided to all students. For your students with disabilities, you should be part of the process of creating an individualized education plan (IEP) through involvement with the physical education integration team. The IEP team, including the physical education teacher, should work together in a decision-making partnership that focuses on sharing information, sharing decision making, and sharing implementation (Martin, 2005).

Figure 11.1 shows a continuum of alternative instructional placements in physical education that are available to students with disabilities. Students with disabilities can move up and down the continuum based on their individual needs. Although some would advocate for total inclusion at all times, the law clearly indicates a need for determination of the least restrictive environment for each individual student based on the unique needs of the student. Other factors to be considered when determining the most appropriate placement for students with disabilities in physical education may include teacher training, staff support, class size, and available resources.

These laws have created an acute awareness of the rights and needs of the individual. Aside from legal issues, however, offering a learning environment in which all students feel welcome and successful, achieve to the best of their abilities, and learn from diversity is simply the ethical action to take. Diversity is part of our society, and you should simulate the society in which students will function as adults as closely as possible—and model appropriate behavior toward those who appear, at least on the surface, to be unlike oneself.

Benefits of Inclusion

All students can benefit from inclusion by experiencing some of the diversity that typifies society, learning from peers who appear to be unlike themselves, and pursuing opportunities to find common ground despite differences. More specifically, students with disabilities obtain many benefits from inclusion, such as opportunities to learn social skills in an integrated, natural environment with natural cues and consequences; the availability of age-appropriate role models without disabilities; participation in a variety of school activities suited to chronological age; and the potential for new

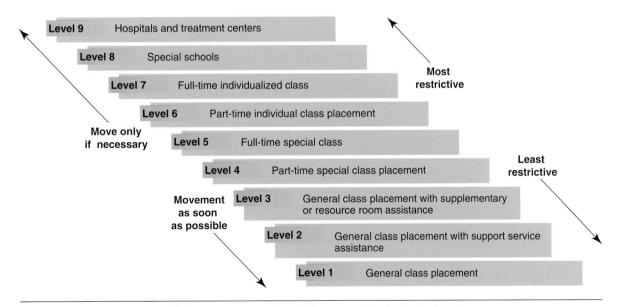

FIGURE 11.1 A continuum of alternative instructional placements in physical education.

Adapted by permission from J. Winnick, 2017, *Adapted Physical Education and Sport*, 6th ed. (Champaign, IL: Human Kinetics), 26.

friendships with peers who do not have disabilities (Downing, 2002; Snell & Eichner, 1989; Stainback & Stainback, 1990). All students benefit from being part of and creating a learning environment where all individuals are appropriately challenged while being sensitive to the needs of others. Moreover, all students need to learn to participate together in physical activities no matter their ability level. Adults work, recreate, and exercise side by side with people of varying abilities. Learning together at an early age prepares students to be more cooperative later in life.

You can implement numerous strategies to facilitate inclusion in physical education. One strategy is to use peer tutors. Peer tutoring is beneficial because it creates a setting in which students with disabilities receive one-on-one instruction, assistance, increased practice, and reinforcement (Lieberman & Houston-Wilson, 2018). Types of peer tutoring include one to one, small group, and class-wide. In addition to peer tutoring, inclusion in physical education can be facilitated by the use of paraprofessionals or teacher aides. Paraprofessionals generally spend more time with students in the classroom setting and can provide you with assistance, especially in the area of behavior management.

Another strategy to make inclusion more successful is differentiated instruction, which provides all students in a class with different options for how information is presented and how they demonstrate understanding of content (Tomlinson, 2001). Differentiated instruction provides multiple choices in three specific areas related to instruction and learning: content, process, and product. To determine how to best meet a student's needs through differentiated instruction, use your knowledge of that student. Differentiated instruction benefits all students by engaging them in creating their learning environment and allowing them to use their strengths to demonstrate learning.

Inclusion in physical education also involves considering differences related to culture, gender, and gender identity. In this regard, inclusion is beneficial because it allows students of various cultures or with gender differences to see models of cultural inclusiveness and diversity acceptance. This experience may positively influence their reactions to others in the future, validate their own culture or beliefs, and facilitate their own learning within a diverse culture. These interactions can help break down barriers and lead to acceptance and friendships between students of differing abilities and beliefs. Ultimately, inclusive physical education programs are beneficial because they are more effective at helping all students become physically literate individuals.

Methods of Inclusion

What does all this mean for a comprehensive program of health-related physical fitness education? When a program includes all students—some of whom fall outside the expected range for health-related fitness measures—then the answers include further individualizing the activity based on each student's needs; modifying the activity for all students; and collaborating with peer tutors, parents, other volunteers, and colleagues. The expectation is that all students, at their personal levels of performance, will progress in their health-related fitness programs.

One example of modifying an activity for all students is to allow them to choose which assessment of cardiorespiratory endurance they prefer to practice and perform. This approach allows students with disabilities to choose the assessment that enables them to use their abilities to their fullest. For instance, a student who is blind might choose to perform the step test independently instead of the mile run, which would require the help of an assistant (American Alliance for Health, Physical Education, Recreation and Dance, 1995). Or, a student with lower-body paralysis might use an arm ergometer for accurate assessment of cardiorespiratory endurance. Another student might use an adaptation in another component of health-related fitness, such as muscular strength or muscular endurance.

Take care to provide students with developmentally appropriate descriptions of the assessment options, including, when possible, demonstrations or practices. If students understand the testing options available to them, then they can select the assessment that will work best for them and help them feel empowered. Emphasize to students that all of the testing options are valid for assessing health-related fitness. Performing a different test does not mean that a student with a disability is getting something less or more than any other student. If possible, allow all students to select the testing option that works best for them. This approach maintains test validity while further individualizing instruction for each student and freeing students who need a different option from the potential stigma of being viewed negatively as "different."

If you are interested in an assessment tool that can be used for children with varying disabilities, consider the Brockport Physical Fitness Test (BPFT). This assessment offers 27 test items that address aerobic function, body composition, and musculoskeletal function (muscular strength, muscular endurance, and flexibility or range of motion). The results of the assessment can give instructors key information for addressing students' specific instructional needs.

Considerations for Meeting Unique Needs

Modifying or adapting an activity to include everyone means that more students will be able to engage in it. The extent to which you already are adapting lessons and activities to include all students will determine how to appropriately meet the needs of a student whose abilities lie further outside the expected range of performance. When preparing to adapt a physical activity, take care to address the following considerations for safety and best practices:

- Review of the student's records
- Conference with parents
- Review of possible contraindications for inclusion (e.g., repeated bending for students with scoliosis; large, noisy areas for students with autism)
- Appropriate class size and instructional support
- Instructional environment (e.g., noise level)
- Instructional strategies (use a variety of strategies that account for individualized learning needs: e.g., demonstration, physical guidance, peer assistance)
- Appropriate equipment

As you prepare to evaluate students with special needs, seek assistance. For example, the school nurse can provide information about any health concerns, and a parent conference can provide pertinent information about a student's individual needs. After collecting the information about safety and health concerns, organize it into an inclusion profile sheet (see figure 11.2).

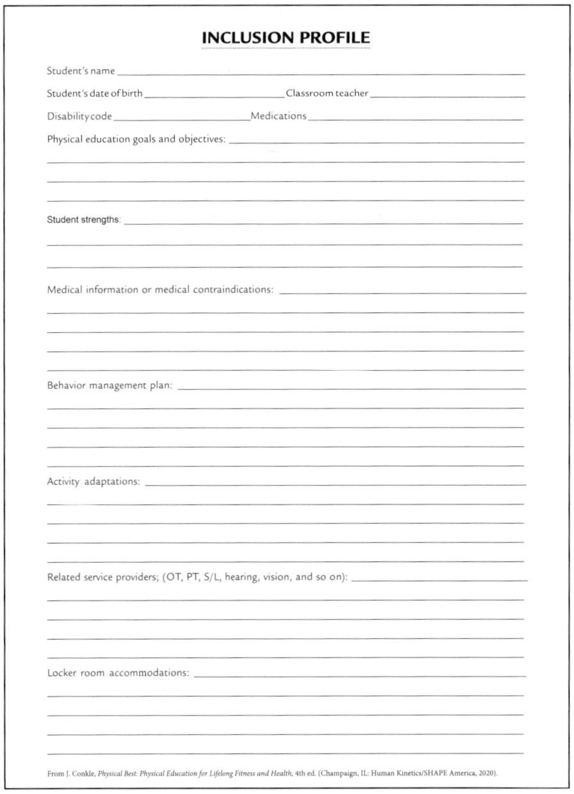
INCLUSION PROFILE

Student's name ____

Student's date of birth ____ Classroom teacher ____

Disability code ____ Medications ____

Physical education goals and objectives: ____

Student strengths: ____

Medical information or medical contraindications: ____

Behavior management plan: ____

Activity adaptations: ____

Related service providers; (OT, PT, S/L, hearing, vision, and so on): ____

Locker room accommodations: ____

From J. Conkle, *Physical Best: Physical Education for Lifelong Fitness and Health*, 4th ed. (Champaign, IL: Human Kinetics/SHAPE America, 2020).

FIGURE 11.2 Organize and store information about students in a record such as the inclusion profile sheet shown here. A reproducible version is available in the web resource for this text.

Next, turn your attention to the considerations that relate to various attributes of the teaching and learning environment: class size and instructional support, instructional environment, teaching strategies, and equipment. For a list of some specific considerations to address in these areas, see table 11.1.

Next, begin to develop specific instructional modifications based on curricular needs. Some examples of modifications based on instructional themes are presented in table 11.2. You can use many of these modifications throughout the instructional day. In addition, the adjustments you make in instruction for children with disabilities can often be used for children both with and without disabilities at all grade levels.

The sidebar titled Including Pablo (which appears a bit later in this chapter) shows some creative ways to adapt a high school weight-training class to be more inclusive. Use questioning strategies and provide opportunities in class for students to modify the games, drills, and activities to meet the needs of everyone. These kinds of lesson extensions and refinements will help you develop a positive classroom environment. The Physical Best activities presented in the web resource offer inclusion tips for each activity. The tips engage a variety of student needs that physical educators may encounter, and many of the ideas can be easily transferred from one activity to another.

Disabilities Awareness Field Days

Teachers at Western Union Elementary School (Waxhaw, North Carolina) wanted to increase students' understanding and acceptance of children with disabilities. The children began learning about various disabilities at the beginning of the school year to prepare them to get the most out of a two-day field event. Just before the field days, students were briefed about the activities and their purpose, and they were reminded that they would be hosting special guests. This meeting helped students understand that the events were for understanding what persons with disabilities *can* do, not to make fun of them. Students also raised money for the Special Olympics in a "Run for the Gold" event held the day before the main event began.

On the first day of the main event, third through fifth graders participated in six indoor activities: An Easter Seals Society representative explained the proper etiquette and preferred language to use when speaking to or about persons with disabilities; a teacher with a hearing impairment shared her daily life experiences; students taped their fingers together, splinted their arms, and so on, to simulate physical impairment; students wore glasses covered to varying degrees to simulate visual impairments; students wore socks on their hands and tried to perform fine motor tasks to simulate learning difficulties of people with intellectual disabilities; and students tried to speak with a marshmallow in their mouth to simulate speech impairment. Students were also encouraged to process what they had learned through various art and writing activities.

Meanwhile, preschool through second graders enjoyed six outdoor activities (what was simulated appears in parentheses): charades (nonverbal communication); sit-down basketball (wheelchair basketball); non-dominant-hand beanbag throw (physical impairments such as cerebral palsy); floor volleyball (physical impairments experienced by persons with amputations and paralysis); and silent 100-yard (m) dash (hearing impairment). A member of the Tarwheels (a North Carolina wheelchair basketball team) also displayed his talents and spoke of never giving up. A parent of a child with a visual impairment shared the child's successes in judo and track and field. On the second day, the two age groups followed the reverse schedule.

Reprinted by permission from M. Jobe, "Disabilities Awareness Field Days," *Journal of Teaching Elementary Physical Education* 9, no. 1 (1998), 10-11.

TABLE 11.1   Teaching Considerations for Meeting Unique Needs

Teaching area	Question	Possible answer
Instruction	What teaching style is best for maximizing this student's comprehension?	A student might benefit from visual demonstration while receiving written or spoken directions.
	What supports (e.g., communication system, additional staff) need to be put in place to assist with instruction?	Consider the need for supports such as adapted equipment, technology, communication systems, and additional staff.
Rules	Do the rules allow everyone to participate and maintain the integrity of the game?	During a basketball game, a student with special needs might be allowed to take three steps without dribbling before being called for a violation.
	Can everyone understand the rules?	Complicated rules (e.g., offsides) might be omitted or simplified to aid comprehension.
	Do the rules provide a safe environment for everyone?	A student who uses a wheelchair might be paired with a buddy to aid in throwing and catching and to create a safety circle around the wheelchair.
Environment	Is the size of the area appropriate for the students and the activity?	A large multipurpose gymnasium might have a line of cones along midcourt to create a smaller area in which to work (e.g., when teaching a small first-grade class that includes a child with autism).
	Are areas of instruction delineated clearly?	An inclusive second-grade class might be taught in a fenced area because one child has a tendency to run off.
	Is students' ability to participate compromised by noise, temperature, poor air quality, or poor lighting?	The custodian at the school might cut the grass at night so that students with allergies and asthma can participate in outdoor physical education classes.
Equipment	Can all students use the equipment, or are modifications needed to ensure total participation?	Jump ropes might be cut in half to accommodate students who aren't able to jump off the ground. They will still do the arm motions, bend their knees, and make an attempt to jump but won't have to worry about constantly being tangled in the jump rope. An activity might use beeper balls or hook-and-loop balls and mitts.
	Is the equipment developmentally appropriate?	Students who are included in a high school program could participate in developmentally appropriate activities rather than simply, say, throwing beanbags at a target.
	Is the equipment safe (e.g., nonallergenic) and in good functional shape for all students?	Nonlatex equipment might be provided. The space (e.g., cafeteria) could be cleaned to avoid potential contact with allergens. Equipment is checked to ensure that it works properly.

TABLE 11.2 Thematic Inclusion Modifications

Equipment	Instruction	Environment
THROWING AND CATCHING		
• Footprints • Foam balls • Poly spots • Textured balls • Hoops for large targets • Beeps or other auditory signals • Carpet squares • Contrasting colors • Sequence pictures • Yarn balls • Balloons • Various weights • Velcro gloves • Various sizes • Suspended objects • Scarves • Deck rings • Balls with tails • Nonrolling balls • Balls on string • Slo-mo balls • Rubber balls (e.g., Koosh balls) • Bubbles • Scoops • Hook-and-loop vests	• Picture cues • Small groups • Task cards • Peer tutoring • Guided discovery • Mirroring • Visual or oral prompts • Task variations • Problem solving • Physical assistance • Increased time for task • Positive reinforcement • Mayer-Johnson symbols (picture communication symbols) • Parallel activities • Partner activities • Demonstration or modeling of the activity • Transition schedule	• Clearly marked boundaries • Appropriate space for assistive mobility • Suspended targets (elastic rope to allow for easy adjustment) • Minimal visual clutter • Shortened distances • Removal of obstacles in the space • Equipment placed at height accessible to student's needs
STRIKING SKILLS		
• Footprints • Beanbags • Poly spots • Textured balls • Hoops for large targets • Beeps or other auditory signals • Carpet squares • Contrasting colors • Sequence pictures • Yarn • Balloons • Various weights • Hook-and-loop gloves • Suspended objects • Large shuttles or birdies • Balloon balls • Tees or large cones • Wide nets and courts • Short and large implements • Large bats or rackets • Deflated balls	• Picture cues • Partner work • Task cards • Visual aids • Guided discovery • Mirroring • Physical assistance • Peer tutoring • Verbal commands • Problem solving • Increased time for task • Small groups • Positive reinforcement • Varying distances • Brighter lighting • Hand-over-hand (physical guidance) • Mayer-Johnson symbols • Closer bases • Parallel activities • Simplified patterns • Elimination of time limits • Modified grasps • Batter allowed to sit • Transition schedule	• Clearly marked boundaries • Minimal distraction • Preferential placement near teacher or away from distractions • Appropriate space for assistive mobility • Minimal visual clutter • Student allowed to sit • Modified station area • Success orientation • Equipment placed at height accessible to student's needs
FITNESS		
• Resistance bands • Modified jump ropes • Lighter weights	• Picture cues • Posted rules • Task cards	• Appropriate space for assistive mobility • Physical assistance

Equipment	Instruction	Environment
• Towels • Heart rate monitors • Pedometers • Therapy balls • Nonweighted bars • Small hook-and-loop hand weights • Small wedges or mats	• Visual aids • Guided discovery • Mirroring • Physical assistance • Peer tutoring • Increased time for task • Small groups • Positive reinforcement • Buddy system • Mayer-Johnson symbols • Daily take-home calendar • Brockport assessment • Modified log sheets • Transition schedule	• Minimal distractions • Success orientation • Equipment placed at height accessible to student's needs
INTEGRATED MOVEMENT		
• Wedge mats • Tunnels • Hoops • Ramps • Floor beams • Wider beams • Bells on rope • Larger bases • Heavier ropes • Balance boards • Tape lines • Long jump ropes • Shakers • Chinese jump ropes • Soft-sided flying discs • Half hoops • Various balls • Contrasting colors for bases • Modified jump ropes	• Picture cues • Modified rules • Task cards • Visual aids • Guided discovery • Mirroring • Physical assistance • Peer tutoring • Verbal commands • Small groups • Increased time for task • Tandem runs • Positive reinforcement • Cognitive cues • Shortened basepaths • Simplified dances • Specific game tasks • Reduced tempo • Mayer-Johnson symbols • Goal setting • Reduced number of steps • Transition schedule	• Appropriate space for assistive mobility • Physical assistance • Success orientation • Modified obstacle course • Minimal visual clutter • Clearly defined boundaries
GROUP INITIATIVES		
• Soft polo sticks • Task cards • Cups for stacking • Card decks • Beanbags • Deck rings • Rubber chickens or pigs • Picture cards • Long and short ropes • Parachute • Carpet squares • Buddy walkers • Poly spots • Scooter boards • Wands • Noodles • Hoops • Suspended targets	• Picture cues • Partner activities • Task cards • Visual aids • Guided discovery • Mirroring • Physical assistance • Peer tutoring • Verbal commands • Small groups • Increased time for task • Modified rules • Positive reinforcement • Adapted play area • Positions marked on field • Group participation • Mayer-Johnson symbols • Transition schedule	• Clearly defined boundaries • Minimal distraction • Preferential placement near teacher or away from distractions • Appropriate space for assistive mobility • Physical assistance • Minimal visual clutter • Success orientation • Equipment placed at height accessible to student's needs

Reprinted by permission from Harford County Public School.

CURL-UP ASSESSMENT

Name_____ Date_____

Directions

Circle the level of assistance that the person requires to perform the task. Total each level of assistance column and place the subtotals in the sum of scores row. Total the sum of scores row and place the score in the person's total score achieved row. Determine the percentage independence score based on the chart. Place number of repetitions in the product score row.

Key to Levels of Assistance

IND = Independent—the person is able to perform the task without assistance.
PPA = Partial physical assistance—the person needs some assistance to perform the task.
TPA = Total physical assistance—the person needs assistance to perform the entire task.

Curl-up	IND	PPA	TPA
1. Lie on back with knees bent	3	2	1
2. Place feet flat on the floor with legs slightly apart	3	2	1
3. Place arms straight, parallel to the trunk	3	2	1
4. Rest palms of hands on the mat with fingers stretched out	3	2	1
5. Rest head on partner's hands	3	2	1
6. Curl body in a forward position	3	2	1
7. Curl back down until head touches partner's hand	3	2	1
Sum of scores			
Total score achieved			
Total possible points	21		
Percentage independence score			
Product score			

Percentage of independence

7/21 = 33%	12/21 = 57%	17/21 = 80%
8/21 = 38%	13/21 = 61%	18/21 = 85%
9/21 = 42%	14/21 = 66%	19/21 = 90%
10/21 = 47%	15/21 = 71%	20/21 = 95%
11/21 = 52%	16/21 = 76%	21/21 = 100%

From J. Conkle, *Physical Best: Physical Education for Lifelong Fitness and Health*, 4th ed. (Champaign, IL: Human Kinetics/SHAPE America, 2020). Reprinted, by permission, from AAHPERD, 1995, *Physical best and individuals with disabilities: A handbook for inclusion in fitness programs* (Champaign, IL: Human Kinetics), 100.

FIGURE 11.3 Use paperwork such as the Curl-Up Assessment form to help you determine the level of assistance needed by students with special needs for certain activities. You can find a reproducible version of the Curl-Up Assessment form in the web resource.

Reprinted by permission from AAHPERD, *Physical Best and Individuals With Disabilities: A Handbook for Inclusion in Fitness Programs* (Champaign, IL: Human Kinetics, 1995), 100.

Teaching Strategies

The continuum of teaching strategies addressed in chapter 10 offers us a variety of options for teaching students in physical education. Included in several of these strategies is the multilevel approach, which is part of differentiated goal setting and task analysis. In the multilevel approach, all students work on the same targeted areas (e.g., flexibility), but each student works toward differentiated goals based on personal abilities and interests. For example, fourth graders without disabilities might explore various stretches for a particular area of the body, students with mild disabilities might focus on learning a new stretch in their interest area, and students with severe disabilities might work on mastering one stretch with proper technique.

Plan an activity for each level and decide which level is appropriate for each student so that the entire class is involved actively in learning. For example, figure 11.3 shows a form used to assess the level of assistance needed by a person with a disability in order to perform a curl-up. The task has been broken down into its component parts through a process known as **task analysis**. In a **traditional task analysis**, motor skills are divided into discrete and underlying parts. In an **ecological task analysis**, in addition to breaking a skill into smaller parts, consideration is given to the student's preferences related to the task and the skill, and the student's strengths as a learner (Davis & Burton, 1991). Teachers should consistently evaluate the ongoing interaction between the student, the task, and the environment and make modifications as appropriate. For instance, a student may need a task to be broken further, or not as much, depending on individual ability. You can calculate a score reflecting percentage of independence, which reflects valuable information about the level and type of support that must be provided for the student. Developing a plan for increasing independence will help participants develop their fitness abilities (Houston-Wilson, 1995).

When preparing high-quality learning activities, consider the outcomes that you are expecting students to achieve. These outcomes can guide the teaching and learning process and help you create overall goals for measuring student success. When you work with students with disabilities, expect to create and measure these outcomes for health-related and skill-related physical tasks; also consider the cognitive and affective outcomes. Chapter 13 provides more information on assessing health-related fitness. Chapter 12 provides more direction on assessing the cognitive and affective domains, which are an important and sometimes overlooked part of adapted physical education. Outcomes related to health-related content knowledge can be assessed through a variety of means. Classroom teachers and special education teachers should be able to provide physical educators with information and test results indicating a functional grade level. With this information, a physical education teacher can align the student's physical education benchmarks with the student's functional level in other academic areas. For example, an eighth grader who is functioning on a first-grade level would not be asked to "apply the principle of transfer of learning to acquire a new skill" but *would* be asked to "explain that some activities use the same movements." The student would also be expected to make gains in the cognitive and affective domains with respect to his or her functional level.

Collaboration

To fully include students with disabilities in physical education, you need to put in place a network of support systems. You can use the ideas presented here in the regular class setting or in expanded opportunities, such as before- and after-school programs. You can also use them as optional opportunities or as catch-up chances for students who are experiencing difficulties.

Collaboration can include many people, such as peer tutors, parent and community volunteers, paraprofessionals, and consultants. Choose the type of collaborator

Including Pablo

The 10th-grade weight-training class at Centerville High School included several students identified as having a disability. One of those students, named Pablo, was nonambulatory and moved in a manual wheelchair. Pablo had been in school with many of the students in the class, but it had been a long time since they had seen him out of his wheelchair. Most of the time, Pablo had participated in physical education class by serving as the referee, keeping score, being an extra person on a team, or participating in an alternative activity at the side of the gymnasium. All the students liked Pablo and interacted with him, but they were unsure of what he was capable of doing physically.

During the first week of school, an adapted physical education teacher came to the class to work with Pablo. She created a weight-training sheet similar to the one used by the class, but Pablo's activities and the weight and number of repetitions for him to complete were specifically marked. The adapted physical education teacher asked for volunteers to be Pablo's weight-training buddy. She explained that the buddy would be working at the same machine as Pablo to help him if he needed it but that the buddy would also have time to complete his own workout. The buddies would rotate so that both Pablo and the buddies would have a chance to work with other people.

The adapted physical education teacher talked with Pablo and with the buddies. She asked Pablo to demonstrate how he could independently transfer from his wheelchair to the various pieces of weight-room equipment but would need help to set the pins for the weight amount. Everyone in the class was excited that Pablo was able to transfer out of his chair; it had been a long time since they had seen him out of it while participating in physical activity. They also realized how important weight training was for Pablo. This class would help him develop strength so that he could continue to get out of his wheelchair independently.

The buddies soon became unnecessary for Pablo because everyone in the class helped with anything Pablo needed, and he needed very little. The students were happy to have Pablo as part of their class and to include in activities. The adapted physical education teacher stopped by the weight-training class periodically to see how Pablo was doing. Everyone in the class told her how well Pablo was doing and how he was improving.

This story was taken from an Adapted Physical Education Teacher who provided consultative adapted physical education in Maryland.

based on the student's needs, available resources, and the individualized education plan (IEP) or 504 plan (discussed later in this chapter). Everyone involved should be aware of all lesson objectives—for example, addressing a social skill (more on this later in this chapter) in addition to a cognitive one.

To determine the type of help that a student may need, consult with the student's direct service providers, such as classroom teachers, adapted physical education specialist, occupational therapist, physical therapist, speech-language therapist, and other related service providers. It is best for all relevant information for each student to be collected before implementing a student's program. The medical and behavioral needs of some students can be overwhelming. Information received through collaboration will directly influence the quality of instruction and physical activity for the student in question. After consulting with other professionals, organize the collected information into the student profile sheets. For many students, this profile sheet plays a vital role in the process of ensuring safety and success (see figure 11.2).

To create an inclusive environment in your physical education class, teaching assistants and volunteers must be properly trained. For example, they will need you or an adapted physical education specialist to teach them how to help a student, how to avoid doing any harm (physical or emotional), and when to call for assistance. It takes time for trainees to learn enough to be useful in a physical activity setting, so be patient with them. Include these professionals in collaborative team meetings, which can involve discussing the student's basic needs and abilities (while ensuring privacy as appropriate) and simulating learning situations. Simulations can be a good way to provide training. Students with severe disabilities need assistants who are professionally trained by those qualified to do so.

Major Areas in Which to Ensure Inclusion

People with disabilities generally display the same physiological and psychological responses to exercise found in persons without disabilities, although factors such as heat dissipation and heart rate responses may be different. To ensure an inclusive learning environment, the following considerations must be addressed: students with special needs, gender, culture, and ability levels outside the norm.

Students With Special Needs

Students who require modifications in order to participate in physical education safely and successfully should come to class with either a 504 plan or an individualized education plan (IEP). An IEP lists a student's present level of performance, identifies attainable annual goals and objectives, provides clear instructions for how much time the child will spend in regular physical education class and with what support services, and identifies the level and purpose of support services. Although being part of an IEP team is time consuming, this process is vital to the student's learning and therefore must be given proper attention.

Based on the IEP or 504 plan, curriculum and teaching methods are developed to meet the student's interests. You must have direct and repeated contact with involved special services staff, parents, and medical personnel. It is recommended that you work with an adapted physical education teacher to ensure that the student receives the needed instruction. When designing health-related fitness plans for students with disabilities, keep the following guidelines in mind (adapted from DePauw, 1996):

- Individuals with disabilities generally display the same physiological responses to exercise found in persons without disabilities. However, some people with disabilities do not respond in the same way as those without disabilities; for example, heat dissipation and heart rate response may be different for a person with a spinal cord injury. Ask the family to consult with their physician.
- Although specific disabilities may affect the intensity, duration, frequency, and type of exercise, people with disabilities can benefit from training, including improving their performance.
- Wheelchairs can be adjusted or modified (by those qualified to do so) to improve physical activity performance.
- Athletes who use wheelchairs play basketball, tennis, and many other sports.

Use this information to ensure that students with disabilities are included in class activities to the greatest extent possible. Remember that students with disabilities will benefit from their involvement in physical activity and health-related fitness activities. High levels of health-related fitness can help foster independence in students with disabilities, especially those with physical disabilities (Short, 2017).

When deciding how best to teach an individual with a disability, focus on the individual rather than on the disability. In other words, refrain from making automatic judgments about a person's condition. Look at what each child *can* do instead of assuming that the child cannot do a given activity.

Developing a Respectful Environment

The best way to develop a respectful environment is to teach it. You can do so by setting dual (or even multiple) lesson outcomes. The primary outcome is the content or skill being taught, and the embedded outcome is the social skill being addressed. In order to use this approach effectively, you must understand the stages of social skill development, through which an individual may need to progress with each new group, class, or social situation:

1. Initial—feeling embarrassed or uncomfortable
2. Phony—practicing (e.g., using the right words when the teacher is near)
3. Habitual—saying the right thing in the proper setting
4. Sympathy with caring—showing concern for others
5. Anticipating with empathy—putting oneself "in their place"
6. Leadership—helping others develop social skills

In addition, each class, team, or other group will experience collective progression, and you can build teaching strategies around these group progressions:

1. Icebreakers—making sure that students know their classmates
2. Working together—learning to cooperate with all members
3. Team building—valuing every team member
4. Trust building—counting on all members to do their best
5. The result—creating a learning community

By identifying which stage your students are in and planning progressions based on that stage, you can help students create an inclusive, respectful environment for your physical education classes. This type of environment will create better learning opportunities for all students.

Coeducation Classes

One of the most widely debated areas of equity in physical education is that of coeducational classes. In today's schools, most teachers would never think of segregating students by ethnicity, yet some still find it difficult to teach male students and female students together in the same physical education class. Since Title IX has been applied to physical education classes, recent studies have suggested that students in coeducational classes feel their experiences are more successful when students of both genders interact in coeducational classes (Woodson-Smith, Dorwart, & Linder, 2015). By preventing boys and girls from interacting with one another, segregated classes also prevent them from learning how to work and play together. Segregation by gender also limits opportunities for boys and girls to reconsider any stereotypical assumptions they may hold about the physical domain. In addition, girls still tend to have less than optimal experiences in physical education classes and therefore are in particular need of environments that inspire a focus on lifelong participation in physical activity (Azzarito, Solomon, & Harrison, 2006; Constantinou, Manson, & Silverman, 2009).

Placing boys and girls in the same physical education class is only the first step toward providing students with the opportunity to examine preconceived ideas about gender. Figure 11.4 shows five steps to equity, and you should be able to identify the step that your class currently occupies. Step 5 is characterized by complete equity, including opportunities for all students to demonstrate skills, answer questions, receive feedback, and feel respect from the teacher and other students. It also includes an environment in which the teacher uses inclusive language (referring to the class as "students" instead of "you guys") and avoids using stereotypical phrases (e.g., "You throw like a girl").

As you progress through the steps, reflect on your teaching behaviors. When boys and girls appear not to be working well together, examine the learning environment and determine what might be causing the problem. You may hear, for instance, that boys won't let girls touch the ball; to address this issue, some physical educators mandate that a girl must touch the ball before the team can score. Often, the problem does not involve all of the boys in the class—it may derive from a few aggressive players, who may also prevent other boys from touching the ball. This type of situation has little to do with coeducational physical education. The remedy is either to make a rule that everyone must touch the ball,

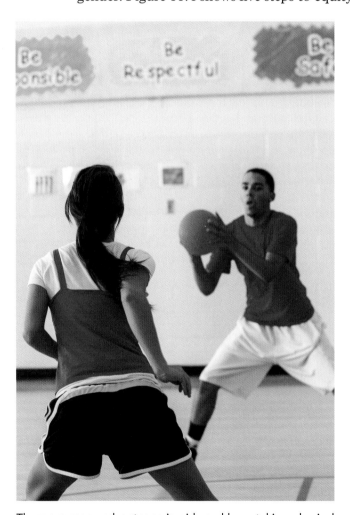

There are many advantages in girls and boys taking physical education together.

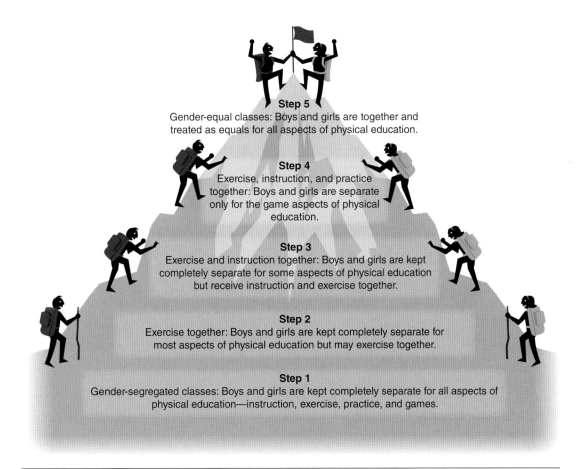

FIGURE 11.4   Coeducation classes and physical education.

Adapted by permission from B. Mohnsen, *Teaching Middle School Physical Education*, 3rd ed. (Champaign, IL: Human Kinetics, 2008).

or, better yet, to reduce the size of the teams so that everyone on the team must be involved in order for the team to succeed. In contrast, requiring that a girl must touch the ball before scoring sends the message that girls need special treatment, which only reinforces the stereotype that girls are not as competent as boys (Mohnsen, 2003).

These first three paragraphs of the Coeducation Classes section are reprinted, by permission, from B. Mohnsen, 2003, *Teaching middle school physical education*, 2nd ed. (Champaign, IL: Human Kinetics), 57.

Another persistent issue—and one that is rarely discussed in physical education (Garcia, 2011)—involves students who are discriminated against because they do not move in what are viewed as gender-typical ways. Even today, in the 21st century, sport and physical education processes are dominated by traditional conceptions of gender and the perpetuation of traditional masculinity through long-standing practices, ideals, and media portrayals. Students who move in ways that are perceived as "abnormal" may be subjected to ridicule, which can lead to a host of psychosocial and medical problems (e.g., victimization, substance abuse, suicide).

For instance, Parker and Curtner-Smith (2012) and Tischler and McCaughtry (2011) note the prevalence of homophobic and heterosexist behaviors that often go unaddressed in teaching practices. Simply put, youth, irrespective of gender or sexuality, should have the freedom to move and explore movement in all physical activities, regardless of how their movement or choice of activity is constructed by society. For LGBTQ youth, in particular, this freedom is empowering; it may also stand in contrast to the larger school culture, which for many of these students is not

The Value of Coeducational Classes

Connie Harris, 2008 NASPE District Teacher of the Year, Westlake High School, Waldorf, Maryland

If the purpose of physical education is to develop physically literate individuals, then having coeducational classes is a real-world setting. When taking an approach based on health-related fitness in class, students learn that a person does not have to be at a high level of skill to enjoy and participate in an activity with others. Placing students in situations that provide the opportunity to learn how to cooperate and involve all of their teammates, regardless of gender, leads them toward positive attitudes about themselves, others, and physical activity. Giving our students opportunities to learn social skills through activities is what sets our discipline apart from others.

Gender Equity Checklist for Physical Education

- Develop the curriculum for gender-inclusive classes.
- Provide gender-integrated classes.
- Vary teaching styles to best meet students' learning needs (for suggestions, see chapter 10).
- Use gender-inclusive language.
- Instructional materials should show male and female students actively engaged in a variety of activities.
- Monitor yourself to be conscientious of selecting all kinds of students equally for questions, discussion, demonstrations, and feedback.
- Find and use local community resources for sport and activity participation, especially those that can break gender stereotypes.
- Talk with students about gender bias and how to eliminate it.
- Set high expectations for all students; these expectations can be individualized for each student but not on the basis of gender.
- Advocate and work to promote a whole-school environment of gender equity.
- Provide useful and specific feedback to all students; avoid vague statements such as "good job."
- Change your language to gender-neutral speech (e.g., "students" instead of "you guys").

Compiled from Nilges (1996); Shimon (2005).

supportive of their experience. That lack of support can lead students to engage in self-imposed marginalization regardless of their abilities (Block, 2014).

Discussions continue about the value, or lack thereof, of separating physical education classes by gender. As with most things, there are positives and negatives. Ultimately, current research indicates that all students perform better in combined classes. Overall, if respect and acceptance of everyone are stressed in a planned curriculum, then coeducational classes are the most positive choice (McKenzie, Prochaska, Sallis, & LaMaster, 2004).

All students should experience equal opportunity in each lesson, but research has suggested that educators tend to favor boys inadvertently. In physical education, for example, boys are more likely to give and receive specific positive feedback or specific corrective feedback (e.g., "I noticed how evenly you paced your mile run" or "push off with your toes more"). Girls, in contrast, are more likely to be passive observers and to receive general feedback (e.g., "good job" or "try again"). In addition, boys are more likely to be pushed to complete a task, whereas girls may be allowed to quit (Cohen, 1993; Hutchinson, 1995; Sadker & Sadker, 1995).

Social-Emotional Learning (SEL)

There is a growing national approach to improving education for every student. This approach focuses on what is known as *social-emotional learning* (SEL), which is defined as "the process through which children and adults acquire and effectively apply the knowledge, attitudes, and skills necessary to understand and manage emotions, set and achieve positive goals, feel and show empathy for others, establish and maintain positive relationships, and make responsible decisions" (Education Week, 2016). SEL can be an important part of physical education because each portion of its definition can be applied to make all students' physical education experiences more positive.

Much of SEL relates to emotional safety and positive social interactions. Your physical education students must know that your classes are safe places for them to engage in activity without judgment or negative consequence from teachers or peers. This sense of safety can develop when you create a culture of acceptance and mutual respect. Students may not naturally have these skills; in some cases, they must be taught. You can do so by setting clear expectations for class engagement, role-modeling for students, providing guidance to correct nonsupportive words and actions, promoting behaviors such as collaboration and encouragement of others, facilitating inclusion of all types during activity, and meeting individual student needs.

Setting SEL objectives in addition to other lesson objectives can go a long way toward enhancing your students' physical education experience and therefore their learning. Gains in SEL can lead to gains in academic growth, better relationships at school, and reduced discipline problems (Dusenbury & Weissberg, 2017).

One way to monitor instruction for gender bias is to record teaching episodes. Watching or listening to the recording and scoring the type of feedback given to boys and girls can highlight instructional patterns. If you do not have access to recording equipment, ask a colleague or other trained observer to assess your instructional behaviors.

Another way to fight gender bias is to ensure that visual aids include representation of both genders participating on equal, nonstereotypical terms. You can also invite guest speakers who have crossed gender lines to play sports. Expose students to a variety of activities that develop health-related fitness, regardless of gender.

In coeducational physical education, some students may feel self-conscious about their bodies and abilities because of comments made by other students (Furrer, 2010). To minimize this risk, create a learning environment that does not tolerate speech or actions intended to judge or joke about a student's physique. Instead, model and create a learning environment in which all students feel accepted and valued.

Cultural Inclusion

Sensitivity to cultural diversity is an important skill to have in order to help students uncover what types of health-related physical activities are enjoyable for them. Culture exerts a profound influence on what students are interested in learning and what they perceive that they can accomplish. Culp (2013) notes that individuals often assess educational environments using three key questions: Can this place be mine or be adjusted to me? Can I produce results here? And can I relate to and get along with others who are here? In negotiating these questions, students initially engage in the environment based on what representations are demonstrated, taught, or portrayed in class by the teacher, peers, or in the learning environment and how this reminds them of their own experiences.

In order to uncover what these representations mean and find out what your students value in their views of sports, games, or physical activity, you must let students have a voice. One way to do so is by creating a survey. For example, it can be helpful for you to learn what cultures your students identify with and how they might view someone who holds a different view or belief. You can incorporate the information gathered from the survey into your program plans. The importance of voice has been emphasized by Lowry (1995): "If students believe that their opinions and perspectives are valued and used, then you have taken the first step in setting up a culturally sensitive environment." Another strategy is to work in tandem with teachers of other subjects to help make the health-related physical fitness curriculum more culturally inclusive. Working in this manner to incorporate physical activities, games, holidays, traditions, music, and other sounds from various cultures can provide you with a connection to each student while also promoting acceptance and understanding of all students in the class. It also shows your students that physical activity participation and health-related fitness can be achieved through a multitude of diverse means and fully individualized for every student. As the teacher, you play a vital role in fostering diverse and supportive physical activity environments.

Another way to promote a progressive, equitable, and thriving environment for all participants is through cultural negotiation (Culp, 2013; Mayes, Maile-Cutri, Goslin, & Montero, 2016). As cultural negotiators, teachers can help students explore their own and each other's cultures in a variety of ways to enrich their educational experience. Such teachers understand that their students have physical, emotional, cultural, and spiritual characteristics. They also believe that their students have multiple ways of learning and strive to create meaningful connections with them. Most important, when faced with a lack of knowledge, these educators take steps to learn while planning and reflecting often.

Banks (1988) suggests that you consider three areas when planning lessons and overall programs:

- *Integrate content.* Use activities from various cultures to achieve program goals. For example, an active game from another country can be just as good for developing cardiorespiratory endurance as a familiar game. In addition, the use of fun games can help students of different cultures adjust to their new surroundings.
- *Plan how to reduce prejudice.* Plan awareness activities that facilitate understanding among cultures, such as discussing different ways of dressing for exercise, based on cultural differences.
- *Employ culturally responsive pedagogy.* Respect differences and learn the history and meaning behind traditions and values.

You should also be ready to communicate with people outside of the teacher–student relationship. Parents and guardians of students from various cultural backgrounds should be encouraged to share their beliefs and any individual requests with you. This process sensitizes people to the philosophies and sociological issues that may affect physical education learning and attitudes toward health-related fitness. In addition, you should help your students understand that diversity in cultural values should be respected. For example, gender equity may be an offensive concept in certain cultures; in such a case, you can respect the different expectations for girls and boys in the culture in question (e.g., by allowing different attire, choice of activity, or other adaptations that do not detract from the learning process) but foster a physical education environment that allows all students to thrive and develop physical literacy. Discuss other options with the student and parents if religious or cultural beliefs need to be addressed for physical education participation. Involve a school counselor or

Teaching English as a Second Language (ESL)

North America's ethnic diversity is on the rise, as is the number people who speak languages other than English (Columna & Lieberman, 2011). Students who study English as a second language (ESL) tend to be recent newcomers to the country who do not know any English and remain silent as they negotiate the routines of a new school, environment, and culture. The "silent period" that these students experience, often for a period of months, is characterized by attempting to decode a host of verbal and nonverbal communications. Fortunately, the nature of the physical education environment lends itself to helping ESL students succeed.

Much attention has been given recently to students from immigrant, refugee, and migrant families, the vast majority of whom do not speak English. Full discussion of these groups lies beyond the scope of this chapter, but we can provide a brief overview. An *immigrant* is a person who chooses permanent residence in a foreign country and obtains the right to take up employment and seek citizenship. The largest immigrant group in the United States comes from Mexico, followed by India, China, Canada, and the Philippines. A *refugee* is an individual who has been forced to flee his or her country because of threat of war or persecution. This group can include undocumented immigrants, asylees, and individuals who have been forcibly displaced. In recent years in the United States, refugees have come largely from the Democratic Republic of the Congo, Syria, Burma, Iraq, and Somalia. A *migrant* is a person who moves from one country to another in search of access to better resources. Research on migrant youth in particular indicates that they come primarily from low-income families who live in high-poverty areas (Jaramillo & Nuñez, 2009).

Irrespective of where the student comes from, it is wise for you to invest extra time in preparing course materials, creating a safe learning environment, and increasing social interactions to overcome students' achievement gaps. For example, Sato (2010) suggests integrating students' native languages into physical education by using verbally interactive activities to promote collaboration and understanding between teachers, local students, and ESL learners. In his study, Sato found that physical education teachers saw more social interactions when they intentionally used students' native languages (e.g., greetings, numbers). With this approach as a foundation, you can also use the following strategies, which have been adapted from Columna and Lieberman (2011) and Mohnsen (2003):

- Be proactive in selecting activities that ESL learners are familiar with. You can also give assignments that call for all students to research sport and activities around the world.
- Assign an English-speaking buddy to help the non-native student. If possible, choose someone who speaks the same language as the non-English-speaking student.
- Physically move a student through a skill to help him or her comprehend what is expected.
- Use gestures and other visual aids, such as toy people and small balls.
- Use facial expressions and voice inflections to emphasize points.
- Remember to speak slowly and enunciate clearly.
- Emphasize for the student a key word or phrase associated with the target skill; ask the student's buddy to do so as well.
- Encourage the student to repeat **cue words** or phrases while executing the skill in order to learn the vocabulary that goes with the actions.
- Learn some of the important words and phrases from the child's native language.
- Use several words from ESL students during game play (e.g., words for *yes, no, pass, dribble, shoot, thank you*).

Another way to help ESL learners in the physical education environment is to seek to understand their unique situation and look for ways to make positive connections. These students may have feelings of discomfort, helplessness, frustration, fear, insecurity, uncertainty about how to behave, and anxiety about communication. They may also experience culture shock, survivor's guilt, self-doubt, anger, fatigue, hunger, and fear of victimization. As a teacher who is sensitive to the needs of your students, you will want to help them feel safe and valued in your class. To support these students, ensure that

- rules and protocols are consistent;
- the physical environment looks inclusive (e.g., in terms of images and signs) to help all students feel that they belong;
- lessons and the overall curriculum are culturally responsive;
- you are modeling the behaviors you want students to demonstrate; and
- you accentuate positive communication attempts.

administrator in the discussions. For instance, if religious beliefs mandate that girls not wear shorts, discuss appropriate alternatives with the family and agree on a way to address clothing for participation in physical activity (e.g., culottes, which look like a skirt but function like shorts). Keep in mind that not everyone in a class has to dress alike in order to benefit from physical activity. If a parent or student offers alternatives, then the student is more likely to participate; also be ready with some options of your own, and use professional social media for support. It is likely that others have already addressed most of these issues. Providing choices assists in providing an equitable environment.

Ability Inclusion

Your lessons should also be inviting and meaningful to students who are extremely talented and to those who are challenged but not classified as having a disability.

Children Who Are Physically Elite

Although Sara, who can run a mile (1.6 km) in less than six minutes, or Jimmy, who can do 150 curl-ups, may not need much of your attention, you should not neglect these students. You may in fact find that physically elite students make good peer tutors. Placing them in this role will help keep them interested in your program and may help them build social skills. Do not, however, ask them to tutor so much that their own needs go unmet or that other students sense favoritism. You can also challenge the physically gifted students in your classes to explore advanced participation in physical activity. Doing so can help those who might otherwise be bored (and, as a result, disrupt class) become assets to the class.

For example, you might ask a physically elite high school student to read a book about becoming a personal trainer and then let the student serve as an assistant by helping other students during class. You might also arrange for the student to interview a personal trainer at a local health club and write a report. It is also helpful to show interest in elite students' extracurricular sport activities and ask them to share their experiences with the class. Finally, you can encourage independence and fitness gains in elite middle school and high school students by giving them opportunities to use training principles of health-related fitness to continually challenge themselves.

Children With Developmental Delays

Some children exhibit characteristics in the psychomotor domain that are typical of being physically awkward or uncoordinated. These characteristics can go undetected, however, unless a physical education teacher, parent, or coach is attentive enough to notice differences. Wall (1982) defines a physically awkward child as one "without known neuromuscular problems who [fails] to perform . . . motor skills with proficiency." Do not assume that a child with a developmental delay will outgrow the issue on his or her own; in fact, many do not (Schincariol, 1994). Such children tend to become discouraged and consequently drop out of physical activity, never to return, which only compounds their problems.

Students should be screened for delays in motor skill development by administering an assessment of motor proficiency (Schincariol, 1994). For example, the Test of Gross Motor Development, third edition (TGMD-3; Ulrich, 2017), measures proficiency in both locomotor and objective control skills. You can administer this test, or it can be administered by an adapted physical education teacher.

Children with developmental delays often need remedial help in the form of extra practice time, instruction, and encouragement (Schincariol, 1994). These students,

Reaching Students Who Are Afraid to Try

John Hichwa, Educational Consultant,
1993 NASPE Middle School Physical Education Teacher of the Year, Redding, Connecticut

Ben came up to me after the first class and, quietly but in a serious tone, said, "Mr. Hichwa, that was a good talk, but, you know, I don't do gym." Ben informed me that he was cut from his fourth-grade travel soccer team, that his physical education experience in elementary school had been far from positive, and that he did not intend to expose himself to further failure or ridicule in the sixth grade. I thanked Ben for being so forthright and suggested that he come to our next class as an observer, which he agreed to do. At the end of that class, I asked him whether he thought he could feel comfortable taking part in class activities. Because I took the time to listen to him, showed respect for his concerns, and gave him time to feel comfortable in his new environment, Ben agreed to give it a try! Throughout the year, Ben tried his best, participated fully, and eventually learned to enjoy the many challenges.

At the beginning of sixth grade, Clare was very tall for her age, fairly heavy, and extremely clumsy. She would go through the motions, but even encouragement from her peers was construed as a personal affront and caused her great anguish. However, when activities were modified in developmentally appropriate ways, the class became less threatening to Clare. In turn, she began to experience a little success, and her self-concept began to rise. She excelled at the problem-solving initiatives and slowly gained respect from the other students. Her running times improved as she participated more enthusiastically, she didn't feel inadequate when competing with herself, and she enjoyed monitoring her progress. By eighth grade, Clare felt confident enough to demonstrate the layup shot in basketball!

From Hichwa (1998).

like those with special needs, may require one-on-one help. Arrange for such students to work with a trained volunteer, teacher's aide, or peer tutor.

Create learning situations in which children with developmental disabilities can succeed, have fun, and learn the value and benefits of physical activity. Offering choices and variety is especially critical to enticing students with developmental delays to persist in physical activity. For example, in conducting a health-related fitness circuit with a jump-rope station, offer the choice of doing step aerobics (stepping up and down) to those who are unable to jump rope. This approach allows students to participate in an activity when their lack of motor skills might otherwise prevent them from getting a good workout.

Children Who Are Obese or Low-Fit

Obesity and poor health-related fitness derive from many causes, including heredity, poor diet, socioeconomic influences, and sedentary living related to technological advancements. Thus the notion that obesity and poor fitness always arise from laziness is a misconception. More likely, younger students who are obese or low-fit have higher workload levels (i.e., to perform the same amount of work, their bodies work harder) than do students who are more fit. Of course, you want to help motivate students to strive for greater levels of physical activity, which can improve their health-related fitness. However, they may be inhibited by embarrassment or fear of failure.

For these children, a good first step is to measure their percent body fat in order to determine the severity of the problem (see the latest *FitnessGram Administration Manual*). Next, obtain assurance from the student's doctor that the student's problems do not derive from a disease, health disorder, or hereditary problem. It may help to work with the school nurse, who can help maintain a student's privacy—a high priority, along with respecting the family's wishes. Consider holding a parent–teacher–student conference to express concern and a desire to help. If medical conditions are involved, work with the student's family and doctor to establish parameters for the student's participation in class. Middle school and high school students may also benefit from sharing their negative experiences and personal concerns about physical activity and body composition. Their attitudes toward physical activity may be improved by a private conference with you or a journal-writing opportunity that lets them air their feelings.

After all medical concerns have been addressed, work with the student and family to set appropriate goals and design an individualized plan for health-related fitness. Emphasize fun and variety. Stressing the benefits of mild exercise can be an important step toward increasing physical activity. Students should have an opportunity to set an individual pace in each activity. In addition, encouraging the entire family to become more active can help increase the student's total physical activity time. Reinforce achievements by asking students to chart progress.

You must be sensitive to the issues that affect overweight or obese students. Physical activity sessions must be positive experiences for everyone. Here are some guidelines to follow:

- Treat students as individuals; do not compare them with one another.
- Encourage a range of physical activities, including non-weight-bearing exercises, such as swimming, water exercise, and cycling.
- Encourage low-impact activities (e.g., walking) and provide low-impact alternatives (e.g., marching) to high-impact exercises (e.g., jogging).
- Schedule rest periods to allow recovery from activity.
- Teach students about the principle of tolerance for exercise. This principle holds that when a person begins an exercise program, the person's tolerance for anaerobic metabolites (process by which chemical reactions provide quick energy for the body to engage in physical activity of high intensity) is low, but progressing in intensity over a period of a few weeks reduces and eliminates the discomfort.
- Encourage students not to stop during warm-up periods. The warm-up period for overweight and obese students can be more uncomfortable, but maintaining activity throughout can increase exercise tolerance and allow students to experience positive changes through aerobic activity.
- Ensure that students use correct exercise technique to minimize the risk of injury.
- Permit students to choose exercise clothing that reduces embarrassment.
- Ensure that students wear supportive footwear during weight-bearing activities; whenever possible, use soft surfaces rather than hard surfaces (e.g., concrete).
- Provide differentiated tasks to cater to a wide range of abilities, including low-level, easier tasks.
- Be aware of potential problems, such as breathing difficulties, movement restriction, edema (fluid retention resulting in swelling), chafing, excessive sweating, and discomfort during exercise.
- Encourage routine activity around the home and school.
- Where possible, provide opportunities for children who are overweight or obese to be active in a private context rather than a public one if this increases their comfort level. After school, a student might choose to walk on a tread-

mill rather than a busy outdoor trail. In physical education, this could mean allowing the student the choice of positioning in the gymnasium (back row of a yoga class) or demonstrating an evaluated routine just for the teacher instead of the entire class.

- Enable children who are obese to follow an individually designed exercise program based on their particular needs and capabilities.
- Encourage guidance and support from school staff, family members, friends, and peers.
- Always provide positive feedback and encouragement.

Reprinted by permission from J.P. Harris and J.P. Elbourn, *Teaching Health-Related Exercise at Key Stages 1 and 2* (Champaign, IL: Human Kinetics, 1997), 25-27.

Children With Other Health Concerns

A student's ability or willingness to participate fully in physical education can also be affected by other health concerns. Two conditions that many of your students may have are asthma and diabetes. It is important for you to identify these students and make accommodations based on their health conditions for the sake of their safety and comfort while participating in your class. In addition to following your school's emergency action protocols, knowing how these conditions affect students will better prepare you to meet their needs.

People who have asthma are susceptible to narrowing of the airways, which makes breathing difficult. This narrowing can be brought on by a number of factors, including irritants, allergens, weather changes, viral infections, emotions, and exercise. The factors differ among people and may vary over time.

Exercise-induced asthma may occur during or after exercise. The usual symptoms are wheezing, coughing, tightness of the chest, and breathlessness. Regular physical activity, however, offers specific benefits for students with asthma—such as decreased frequency and severity of attacks and reduced need for medication—over and above the benefits that it offers for children in general. Therefore, you should encourage students with asthma to be active, and they should be integrated as fully as possible into physical education lessons and sporting activities. Moreover, students with asthma should be able to participate in activities alongside their peers with minimal adaptation.

A student is most likely to experience exercise-induced asthma when performing continuous aerobic exercise at moderate intensity for more than six minutes in cold, dry air (for example, cross country running). Although students with asthma should be encouraged to participate in physical education as fully as possible, it is also important to be aware of possible limitations. In addition, students should have ready access to their inhalers; schools should not keep asthma medication in a central storage area.

Although you should treat each student individually and adhere to school protocols, you should also observe the following general recommendations when students exercise:

- Encourage the use of an inhaler 5 to 10 minutes before exercise.
- Encourage students to have a spare inhaler readily available for use.
- A student arriving for activity with airway constriction should be excused from participation for that session.
- Allow a gradual warm-up of at least 10 minutes.

- Permit and encourage intermittent bursts of activity interspersed with reduced intensity exercise.

- Permit lower intensity activity.

- Encourage swimming—people with asthma more easily tolerate the environmental temperature and humidity of an indoor pool.

- In cold, dry weather, encourage the wearing of a scarf or exercise face mask over the mouth and nose in the open air.

- Encourage breathing through the nose during light exercise—this method warms and humidifies the air.

- Do not permit students with asthma to exercise when they have a cold or viral infection.

- Where possible, advise students with severe asthma to avoid exercise during the coldest parts of the day (usually early morning and evening) and in times of high pollution.

- If symptoms occur, ask the student to stop exercising and encourage him or her to use an inhaler and to rest until recovery is complete.

- In the case of an asthma attack, send for medical help, contact the student's parents, give medicine promptly and correctly, remain calm, encourage slow breathing, and ensure that the child is comfortable.

Reprinted by permission from J.P. Harris and J.P. Elbourn, *Teaching Health-Related Exercise at Key Stages 1 and 2* (Champaign, IL: Human Kinetics, 1997), 25-27.

Nothing prevents most students with mild to moderate asthma from participating in a range of physical activities with minimal difficulty—if they take appropriate precautions before and during exercise.

People with type 1 or type 2 diabetes need to pay close attention to their bodies' needs before, during, and after exercise or physical activity. **Diabetes** is a condition in which the body does not produce or effectively use insulin. As a result, the body cannot metabolize carbohydrate normally and blood glucose levels can become elevated. If the condition is not properly addressed, a person with diabetes can experience **hypoglycemia** (low blood sugar), **hyperglycemia** (high blood sugar), or even death. Symptoms of hypoglycemia include fatigue, pale skin, shakiness, anxiety, sweating, hunger, irritability, tingling sensation around the mouth, confusion, abnormal behavior, visual disturbances, seizures, and loss of consciousness (Mayo Clinic, 2018b). Symptoms of hyperglycemia include frequent urination, increased thirst, blurred vision, fatigue, headache, fruity-smelling breath, nausea, vomiting, shortness of breath, dry mouth, weakness, confusion, abdominal pain, and coma (Mayo Clinic, 2018a). Look for and be able to recognize these symptoms in your students. If you have questions about whether a particular student's needs or treatment may affect the student's participation in physical education, consult the school nurse and talk with the student's parents to be better informed and prepared.

Although it may seem scary to place physical demands on the body of a student with diabetes, regular physical activity is beneficial for students with diabetes beyond the benefits provided to all participants. These additional benefits can include lower blood glucose levels, less need for insulin, and improved insulin sensitivity (Giannini, Mohn, & Chirarell, 2006). Although you as the physical education teacher will not be directly responsible for a student's diabetes treatment, it is important to be aware that a student may need to test blood glucose level before physical activity; adjust an insulin regime to meet exercise demands; and eat snacks before, during, or after exercise. The student may also have a higher risk of dehydration than other students and should not exercise if ketones are present in blood testing (Robertson, Adolfsson, Scheiner, Hanas, & Riddell, 2009). In addition, any student experiencing symptoms of hyperglycemia or hypoglycemia should stop exercising, and you should call for assistance. Take care to advise the student, parents, and school nurse if a lesson will be more strenuous than usual or if the student seems more affected by an activity than you would expect.

Summary

In health-related physical fitness education, inclusion involves making it possible for all students to succeed in and enjoy physical activity. Thus, inclusion helps all students meet the ultimate goal of becoming adults who value and pursue physical activity as a way of life. It can also teach other students valuable life lessons, such as social skills, cultural respect, and the feeling that limitations are often unfairly assigned by those with limited visions of what people can do and be.

To be inclusive (as opposed to simply going through the motions), you must make a commitment to plan and implement an inclusive program. Collaboration with both school and nonschool personnel makes the task of inclusion easier and ensures that the necessary input is available to tailor the program to the needs of all students. Simply put: If you implement a well-planned curriculum with purposeful inclusion-minded lessons that account for individual differences and the individual needs of each student, you will facilitate learning that benefits everyone.

The next chapter focuses on assessment for students with and without disabilities.

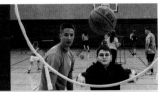

Discussion Questions

1. Define and describe the concept of inclusion as it applies to physical education.
2. Identify some of the benefits of inclusion in physical education for students with disabilities.
3. Describe some strategies for fostering inclusion in physical education for students with disabilities.
4. Identify appropriate activities that could be incorporated into a disability awareness day at your school.
5. Describe the process of task analysis and provide an example for a motor skill.
6. Describe how collaboration can help ensure successful inclusion in physical education for students with disabilities. Provide specific examples of individuals or groups with whom to facilitate collaboration.
7. Outline some strategies for creating a respectful environment for all students in your physical education classes.
8. Identify some strategies for helping students with developmental delays in the motor domain in physical education.
9. List three steps that you can take to help ensure gender equality in your physical education class.
10. Design a health-related fitness unit that promotes cultural inclusion.

PART IV

Foundations of Assessment in Health-Related Fitness and Physical Activity

Part IV provides an overview of assessment associated with health-related fitness and physical activity. Specifically, it addresses basic assessment principles, their relationship to health-related fitness teaching and learning, and their connection to developing physical literacy in your students. Chapter 12 begins by establishing a foundation for assessment of health-related fitness and physical activity based on SHAPE America's National Standards for K-12 Physical Education (2013) and their accompanying Grade-Level Outcomes (2014). It also includes recommendations for selecting assessment tools, applying them, and using assessments to shape program planning. The chapter concludes with concrete suggestions for using the appropriate tools to assess the cognitive and affective domains, as well as personal responsibility. Chapter 13 explores appropriate methods for assessing health-related fitness and physical activity and offers guidelines for assessing and sharing results in effective and helpful ways. By applying the concepts and suggestions found in part IV, you can create a program that challenges each student to develop positive lifelong health-related fitness habits.

CHAPTER 12

Assessing Student Understanding of Health-Related Fitness

Christina Sinclair

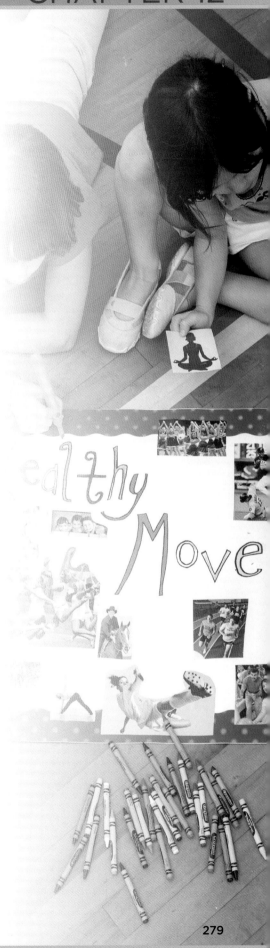

Highly effective physical education programs use assessment to support learning. In assessment for learning, assessment is designed to provide feedback, and the assessment task itself becomes a learning experience that helps the student actively construct meaning (Hay, 2006). For example, in an effective physical education class, students should expect to participate in health-related fitness assessment in order to learn how to assess their own health-related fitness, interpret their scores, understand their own health-related fitness, and develop an individualized plan to attain personal goals. This chapter explores and presents examples of appropriate strategies for using assessment and eventually assigning grades, particularly as related to the cognitive and affective domains.

Understanding Assessment

Assessment and grading have different purposes. **Assessment** involves continuous collection and interpretation of information about student performance; thus you and your students are informed through assessment. **Grades** are based on summative products and use assessments to assign value to student performance.

Student assessment is a high-stakes event. Assessment outcomes are often equated to a teachers' effectiveness; this is the case in all subjects, including physical education. In the United States, all states have adopted standards based on SHAPE America's (2014) National Standards for K-12 Physical Education and the accompanying Grade-Level Outcomes. You can use these standards and outcomes to guide your selection of content to meet your students' needs. Applied specifically to physical education, developmentally appropriate authentic assessment includes individual assessments of students as they move and participate in a variety of activities. In this way, you make comparisons not by using a single assessment score (summative evaluation) or the performance of other students in the class (norm-referenced assessment) but by examining a student's progress since the previous assessment and by examining benchmarks for growth and maturation.

Authentic assessment in physical education can include approaches such as counting daily steps using a pedometer or measuring heart rate at the beginning and end of an activity period and then reflecting on the change. In activity settings, students can use rubrics to complete partner assessments during game play in order to integrate peer assessment throughout a unit. Assessment using wearable technology (e.g., heart rate monitor, pedometer, Fitbit) can help students develop an understanding of intensity, resting heart rate, and recovery times. Together, you and your students can use such information to create an exertion chart reflecting the collective experience of the class. Based on the OMNI RPE scale of 0 to 10, a rating of 0 could represent little effort with no change in respiration and a small change in heart rate (perhaps 10 to 20 beats per minute). At the other end of the scale, a rating of 10 could represent a feeling of "Don't ask me to do one more thing until I catch my breath!" (For more information about the OMNI RPE scale, see chapter 5.) In another example, information from a pedometer can be used to track the increased number of steps that a student can take before feeling tired or how many more steps the student can take in the same amount of time.

These examples show how students can use assessment to notice their improvement in areas of health-related fitness. You can also use a tablet or desktop computer to record students' scores. Students can then use the printed results as a guide when setting personal goals; they can also include it in their journals and portfolios.

Authentic assessment in health-related fitness education should teach and motivate students to increase their physical activity in a way that benefits their overall health and wellness. Assessing student performance during activities or during play can provide valuable information. The simple act of observing a student as she or he climbs a ladder, performs locomotor movements, or executes specific health-related fitness activities (such as those found in this book's web resource) can be used to develop a health-related fitness focus that is personally informative.

Importance of Assessment

Assessment can provide the information needed to support student achievement. Assessment can be formative or summative. Formative assessment is conducted during a period of instruction (e.g., unit or semester), and it typically provides information about student mastery and helps guide content development. This type of assessment can be done at the start of the school year to determine students' developmental levels, and you can use this information to inform selection and development of content in order to address specific student needs. Formative assessment can also help you determine instructional effectiveness in terms of desired student outcomes. Summative assessment, on the other hand, is conducted at the end of an instructional period and typically combines numerous measures to provide a final unit or course grade. Summative assessment can also be used as a diagnostic tool for assessing students' health-related fitness.

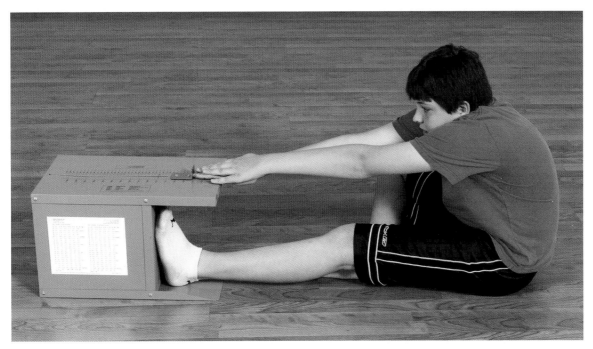

The sit-and-reach is an example of a health-related fitness assessment. When used as a formative assessment, students and teachers can gain valuable information to guide instruction and goal setting.

Assessment provides numerous useful outcomes:

- Opportunities to focus on an individual student's outcomes
- Opportunities to address the components of health-related fitness
- Specific feedback to guide each student's personal goal setting by addressing how the components of health-related fitness can be improved through specific activities and exercises
- Feedback about the teacher's effectiveness
- Feedback about overall program effectiveness
- Feedback about students' instructional needs
- Information to guide future planning
- Information for parents about the health-related fitness status of their children and what can be done to improve or maintain that fitness
- Subject matter credibility in the minds of administrators, students, and parents

According to SHAPE America (2014), "The goal of physical education is to develop physically literate individuals who have the knowledge, skills and confidence to enjoy a lifetime of healthful physical activity" (p.12). To this end, the Physical Best program focuses on a holistic approach to developing all three learning domains: psychomotor, cognitive, and affective. The **psychomotor domain** involves *skills* and motor or movement patterns. This domain is commonly assessed during drills, skill assessments, and gamelike activities. Because health-related fitness is changed through participation in physical activities, formative assessment tools can include using heart rate monitors to measure moderate and vigorous activity and using pedometers or step apps to counts steps. The **cognitive domain** involves *knowledge* of concepts related to sport, games, health-related fitness, rules, procedures, safety, and critical elements. Knowledge and understanding are most often assessed through

Examples of Learning Domain Objectives

Psychomotor Assessment

- The student is able to perform a trunk lift using the correct performance cues: lying on front, toes pointed, hands under thighs, eyes on marker, lift upper body, and hold.
- The student is able to achieve and maintain moderate-intensity physical activity as measured by the Borg Scale of Perceived Exertion, while playing a game of his or choice for 20 minutes.

Cognitive Assessment

- The student can describe at least three benefits of maintaining a physically active lifestyle.
- The student can name at least one exercise or activity that helps increase muscular endurance.
- The student can describe how to safely monitor intensity during a 30-minute walking or jogging workout.

Affective Assessment

- Students take responsibility for improving their own fitness levels by choosing to participate in health-related physical activity outside of school at least four times per week.
- Students are able to describe at least one way in which they helped a partner in class while practicing the curl-up, trunk lift, and back-saver sit-and-reach FitnessGram tests.

National Standards and Assessment

The Physical Best program is aligned with SHAPE America's *National Standards & Grade-Level Outcomes for K-12 Physical Education* (2014). Standards-based content development guides teachers' selection of developmentally appropriate activities that enable students to accomplish specific outcomes. The desired outcomes of selected activities are guided by psychomotor, cognitive, and affective objectives. Assessments shared in this chapter can be used with PE Metrics, which is the leading standards-based assessment package for cognitive and motor skills and includes evaluation tools for measuring student progress toward achieving the National Standards for K-12 Physical Education (SHAPE America, 2011) Assessments covered in this chapter focus specifically on Standard 3 ("demonstrates the knowledge and skills to achieve and maintain a health-enhancing level of physical activity and fitness"), Standard 4 ("exhibits responsible personal and social behavior that respects self and others"), and Standard 5 ("recognizes the value of physical activity for health, enjoyment, challenge, self-expression and/or social interaction") (SHAPE America, 2014, p. 12).

written assessments, oral presentations, or final projects. Students' cognitive learning outcomes can also be documented through alternative assessments, such as keeping a journal, developing a health-related fitness routine, role-playing, and engaging in peer assessment activities. The **affective domain** depends on a student's *confidence* regarding and during physical activity. Although more difficult to measure, affective behaviors can be assessed in a variety of ways, including journals and questionnaires.

Both formal and informal assessments are important to physical education programs, and they can be used for assessing learning in various domains. Informal assessment can be recurring and understood through the feedback loop: Teachers observe performance and provide feedback to encourage students. This feedback can either help students correct performance or offer information that refines performance. Informal assessment is an important teaching strategy because it provides a quick appraisal of student learning. Typically, students receive informal assessment feedback during teacher or peer observations of practice, but they can also use self-assessment skills to self-evaluate performance. Self-assessment allows students to practice strategies that they can use outside of the physical education classroom. Informal assessment takes less time and can be helpful for making decisions about pacing, selection of teaching strategies, and content modification.

Formal assessment is a more precise measure of student learning and results in recorded data that are often necessary to document final grades. Formal assessments can include teacher or student checklists, task sheets, health-related fitness rubrics, student logs, portfolios, and ActivityGram and FitnessGram printouts. These examples demonstrate the standardized, teacher-conducted nature of formal assessment.

Recommended Assessment Tools

A variety of assessment strategies are available that will enable you to gather accurate information about a student's progress. A student might find one form of assessment easier to perform and interpret than others due to individual strengths. Providing a balanced mix of assessment tools gives students a chance to excel in a variety of ways; moreover, giving students multiple opportunities to understand what they have learned can be motivating.

Each assessment strategy is designed to be developmentally appropriate, as well as reliable and valid. Assessment is designed to answer the question, "Is the student moving toward the ultimate goals of a health-related fitness education program?"

Rubrics

A **rubric** is a scoring tool that identifies the criteria used for judging student performance (Lund & Kirk, 2010). Rubrics range in complexity from checklists to tools that are holistic in nature and can be used to assess skills, attitudes, and knowledge.

ASSESSING KNOWLEDGE OF CALCULATING AND USING HEART RATE RUBRIC

Student's name _____ Date _____

Score _____ Class _____

Target component	Score 1 point	Score 2 points
Can demonstrate sites at which to count the pulse	Knows one site	Knows two sites
Understands how heart rate information indicates intensity	Some understanding	Clearly understands
Can accurately count the pulse for a fraction of a minute and then accurately calculate heartbeats per minute with a calculator	Sometimes	Most of the time
Can describe ways and reasons to increase or decrease heart rate	Some understanding	Clearly understands

From J. Conkle, *Physical Best: Physical Education for Lifelong Fitness and Health*, 4th ed. (Champaign, IL: Human Kinetics/SHAPE America, 2020).

FIGURE 12.1 Example of a rubric for assessing knowledge of calculating and using heart rate. A reproducible version of this rubric is available in the web resource.

A checklist rubric might list certain skills—for example, "Runs tall and leans slightly forward" or "Offers encouragement and support to teammates"—and include a blank where a check mark or smiley face is placed if the skill is performed correctly. A rubric might also be analytic, in which case the skills may be assigned point levels, perhaps from 1 to 5 for "never" to "always" (or for more qualitative descriptions of levels of play). Finally, rubrics may be holistic, containing paragraphs written to describe various levels of performance. Each paragraph includes several dimensions and traits (psychomotor, affective, and cognitive) and is aligned with a point value or level number.

Well-designed rubrics inform students about expectations for the quality of work necessary to reach the standard or achieve a specific grade. Teachers, students, and peers can use rubrics to score or evaluate the information gathered by most of the assessment tools described in this chapter. A rubric can also double as a task sheet to keep students focused on critical elements or knowledge concepts during class, or as an observation checklist to guide feedback given by teachers and peers. In addition, rubrics serve as a means of standardizing assessment, regardless of who uses them. This approach is one way to minimize subjectivity among different observers.

Thus, being able to create and use effective rubrics is a vital teaching and assessment skill. A sample rubric is shown in figure 12.1.

Several websites offer examples of rubrics to help you with the process of designing your own:

- PE Central: www.pecentral.org
- Physical and Health Education America: www.pheamerica.org
- supportREALteachers: www.supportrealteachers.org
- RubiStar: www.rubistar.4teachers.org
- Teach-nology: www.teach-nology.com
- Discovery Education: http://school.discoveryeducation.com
- Rubrics for Teachers: www.rubrics4teachers.com

Teacher Observation

Teacher observation is an important component in both student learning and classroom management. By circulating among students who are engaged in physical activities that integrate and apply health-related fitness concepts, you can gain information about individual student performance. Observation is also an important part of being able to adjust lessons. For example, imagine that many students are having trouble finding the proper location on the body to measure heart rate. If you identify this challenge, you can stop observing and provide clarification. Note, however, that informal teacher observation alone is not considered an adequate assessment practice. To provide useful, specific feedback to students, you need to implement formal, systematic strategies that go beyond merely observing student performance.

One observation technique that can help you assess students is that of video-recording student performance. A number of companies offer software to help you analyze movement captured on video. To find a product that meets your needs, search the web for "analysis of movement" sites or applications. Thus, periodically video-recording student performance provides opportunities for students, teachers, and parents to assess performance levels. Students should understand that personal assessment is completed to provide information about important content areas and growth in performance. The information gained can be used to develop individual health-related fitness plans through physical activity and to increase understanding and improve performance.

Self-Assessment

Teaching students how to monitor their own progress, or engage in **self-assessment**, is an important key to reaching the ultimate goal of producing adults who know how to design appropriate physical activity programs for themselves. Self-assessment also helps students focus on performance progress rather than on product, because it helps them better understand the critical elements (process components), which in turn improves performance and achievement. The following sample prompts provide students with opportunities to reflect on their learning and check for understanding:

- *Analyzing performance.* Using video and a rubric for students to self-assess or peer-assess performance provides greater accuracy in the observation of critical elements, behaviors, and events (Lacy & Hastad, 2015). For an example, see figure 12.2.

- *Recording feelings.* Ask students to record how they feel, both physically and emotionally, after physical education class and other physical activities.

- *Recording performance.* Ask students to use check marks to record the number of times they performed a health-related activity (e.g., each stretch). Young children might enjoy recording a smiley face or frowning face next to each check mark in order to indicate how they felt about each performance.

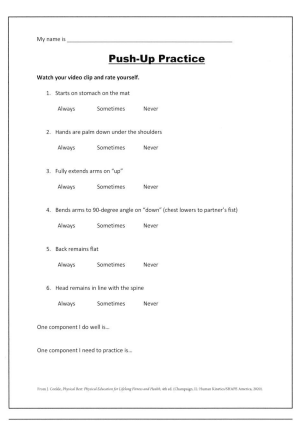

FIGURE 12.2 Push-up self-assessment for 3rd through 12th grade.

My name is _____

I helped my partner _____

Curl-Up Practice

1. Starts with back on mat

   Always   Sometimes   Never

2. Knees are bent and hands are flat on the floor

   Always   Sometimes   Never

3. Begins on command "up"

   Always   Sometimes   Never

4. Arms are straight and parallel to the body

   Always   Sometimes   Never

5. Fingertips reach to the other side of the measuring strip (approximately 3 inches) while keeping in constant contact with the mat

   Always   Sometimes   Never

6. Shoulder blades come off the mat

   Always   Sometimes   Never

7. Heels remain in contact with the floor

   Always   Sometimes   Never

8. On the "down" command, curls back down until head touches the mat

   Always   Sometimes   Never

One thing my partner does well is...

One thing my partner needs to practice is...

From J. Conkle, *Physical Best: Physical Education for Lifelong Fitness and Health*, 4th ed. (Champaign, IL: Human Kinetics/SHAPE America, 2020).

FIGURE 12.3   Curl-up peer assessment.

Peer Assessment

In **peer assessment**, students analyze each other's performances. This activity plays an important role in helping students to develop physical, cognitive, and social skills. Analyzing others' performances helps students focus on the key parts of what they need to learn, thus reinforcing their own learning. Rubrics can be used to identify specific criteria that can be used in the process of peer assessment.

Students work together in pairs or small groups to analyze each other's performances. They use the same rubrics for peer assessment that they use for self-assessment. You must teach your students specific strategies for giving helpful feedback; for instance, it can be helpful for them to role-play acceptable peer assessment behaviors. Figure 12.3 presents a peer assessment sheet that can be used to guide students as they give feedback to a partner about curl-up technique.

Logs and Journals

Log and journal entries provide a way for you to integrate writing into the physical education curriculum. Written assessments can be used to determine students' understanding of content and their ability to apply it. **Logs** provide a baseline record of behaviors and help form the basis for setting personal goals related to physical activity frequency, intensity, duration, and type. Although logs can contain brief reflections about performance, they are mainly used to record participation data. For example, students log the dates and times of each cardiorespiratory endurance activity in which they participate outside of physical education. Heart rate is recorded before, during, and after each activity, and the results are analyzed. Rating of perceived exertion can be used by students to reflect how strenuous their physical activity bouts felt. Using a 0-to-10 perceived exertion scale gives students a good idea of the intensity level and provides them with information to help them change their activity. Student reflection based on log entries can be used to explain the relationship between heart rate levels, rating of perceived exertion, and cardiorespiratory endurance development in a student journal or log.

A **journal** can include a written record that discusses how the student feels after each activity. Journals are usually designed not only as records but also as reflections. Students are encouraged to discuss their successes. Combining logging and reflective journaling gives students the opportunity to review their progress, which often motivates them to continue being physically active. Students need to be taught how to set up effective logs and journals. Figure 12.4 shows a sample log sheet for a family using pedometers to track their steps, and figure 12.5 shows a list of reflective journal questions related to the tracking.

Practical strategies for using journals can include limiting the number of questions asked and limiting the time spent on the task to two to four minutes on any one day. For example, a short reflection on the family pedometer log could be broken into two short journal times across multiple lessons:

FAMILY CHORES STEP LOG

Chore	Guardian	Guardian	Child	Child	Average chore step count
Sweeping					
Dusting					
Raking					
Washing windows					
Doing laundry					
Mowing the grass					
Individual total					

From J. Conkle, *Physical Best: Physical Education for Lifelong Fitness and Health*, 4th ed. (Champaign, IL: Human Kinetics/SHAPE America, 2020). Adapted, by permission, from R. Pangrazi, A. Beighle, and C. Sidman, 2007, *Pedometer power: 67 lessons for K-12*, 2nd ed. (Champaign, IL: Human Kinetics), 152.

Reflective Journal

Examine the Family Chores Step Log. Reflect on the log with respect to the concepts of FITT. Your reflection should consider these questions:

1. During the course of the day, which family member had the most steps? Which family member had the fewest?

2. Explain why you believe that the person with the most steps was more active.

3. Do you believe that the person who had the most steps is active enough to stay healthy? Why or why not?

4. In comparison to _____ [pick a family member], why do you think that you had fewer steps?

5. Can you think of ways to increase the number of steps you had on any of the days that you were lower? Describe the strategies you would use.

6. On which days were you most active? What did you do differently on the active days compared with the less active days?

7. Did you meet your daily goals for time?

8. Did you meet your weekly goals for frequency?

From J. Conkle, *Physical Best: Physical Education for Lifelong Fitness and Health*, 4th ed. (Champaign, IL: Human Kinetics/SHAPE America, 2020).

FIGURE 12.4   This sample log sheet shows how a family can track their steps using a pedometer. A reproducible version of the Family Chores Step Log is available in the web resource.

Adapted by permission from R. Pangrazi, A. Beighle, and C. Sidman, *Pedometer power: 67 lessons for K-12*, 2nd ed. (Champaign, IL: Human Kinetics, 2007), 152.

FIGURE 12.5   Sample reflective journal entry questions.

Three-Minute Journal (Day 1)

1. During the course of the day, which family member had the most steps?
2. Why do you think that person was more active?

Three-Minute Journal (Day 2)

1. During the course of the day, which family member had the fewest steps?
2. List some ways for that family member to increase their step count.

Reflection skills develop with guidance and practice. Encourage students to reflect on likes and dislikes, as well as positive and negative feelings about participation. Younger students can begin by logging their activities using a program such as Activity-Gram. The program is easy and fun to use, and recording information as homework may draw parents into the assignment. Encourage older students to reflect on the activities initially by using teacher-developed prompts and then by moving on to self-selected reflection content as they become more accustomed to writing reflectively. Collaborate with classroom teachers in ways that allow students to practice and get feedback on their writing skills as they reflect on their feelings about participating in physical activity. Examples of logs can be found in www.pecentral.org. Alternatively, use www.rubistar.4teachers.org and make up your own, or search "activity logs" for a wide selection of possibilities.

Rubric for Scoring Journal Entries

Scoring guidelines for journal entries:

4—Exemplary: Expresses feelings of personal participation and about sharing it with friends
3—Acceptable: Identifies feelings of personal participation
2—Needs improvement: Has difficulty expressing feelings about participation
1—Unacceptable: Does not make journal entries

Criteria for assessing journal entries	Rating			
Analyzes and expresses feelings about physical activity	4	3	2	1
Identifies evidence of success, challenge, and enjoyment present in the activity	4	3	2	1
Explains the challenge that adventure activities provide	4	3	2	1
Describes the positive effects that friends and companions bring to this experience	4	3	2	1

Adapted from NASPE (2004).

From J. Conkle, *Physical Best: Physical Education for Lifelong Fitness and Health*, 4th ed. (Champaign, IL: Human Kinetics/SHAPE America, 2020).

FIGURE 12.6   Criteria and scoring for reflective journal entries during an adventure education experience.
Adapted from NASPE (2004a).

Assessing reflective journal entries focuses on students' understanding of the assignment. Although students can be assessed on other areas of a school curriculum, such as spelling and grammar, focus here on their application and understanding of physical education content. Remember that when students share their feelings, there are no correct answers, only degrees of thoroughness and thoughtfulness. Figure 12.6 offers sample criteria and scoring guidelines for journal entries made during an adventure education experience (e.g., ropes course, wall climbing). This assessment is available in the web resource.

Student Projects

Student projects can include multiple assignments that encourage individuals, partners, or small groups to apply basic physical education knowledge in real-life settings. With your guidance, a student or group of students can learn in-depth information about their selected project topics while also developing social, technological, and research skills (Mohnsen, 2008). For example, students can investigate how muscular strength and endurance enhance performance in a particular sport. They can then formulate, assess, and report (orally or in a journal) on their findings. Projects tend to be cross-curricular in nature, bringing together content and skills developed in several subject areas. A rubric can be developed to assess each part of the project.

Follow these guidelines for developing and using projects effectively (Reeves, 2015):

- *Create a compelling problem or question.* The problem or question has to go beyond simple knowledge—it needs to require students to apply the knowledge they have gained. Examples include creation of an activity, workout, routine, or game.

- *Keep the task open ended.* Keeping the challenge or task open ended is essential; this is done best by asking students to craft something new. Instead of simply quoting back knowledge, they will be involved in inquiry and innovation.

- *Use peer feedback.* In the example of a student creating a new game, the class can be asked to play the game, which gives students more physical activity while also giving the game's creator crucial feedback about what works and what doesn't.

- *Know the educational goal.* While the student's main goal is to create and present a product, the entire project needs to align with instructional goals and relevant standards. Design projects with a clear understanding of what students will learn through the process.

Group Work Can Be Challenging

Assessment of group work requires assessing both the group's performance and each individual's performance, and designing rubrics for group projects can be difficult. At the beginning of each project, make students aware of the criteria on which their performance will be judged; to this end, it can be helpful to share the rubrics with them. Then, in addition to conducting your own assessment, consider allowing groups and individuals to assess themselves and each other. For example, if three group members each privately rate the fourth group member poorly, their appraisals may support your conclusions regarding that student. But be careful! These issues can be touchy, and a skillful teacher works to ensure that the fourth student is not embarrassed but is instead helped and encouraged to practice the targeted activity. Developing a supportive and open teaching environment is the key to helping all students do their best work. Discuss any large discrepancies with those involved, and consider using an individual accountability tool, such as a journal entry or quiz.

Cooperation with peers is essential for success. This interdependence builds social skills as well as health-related fitness skills. For example, a group might work together to design a training circuit that enhances components of health-related fitness, then oversee the circuit while another group performs the activities.

Group projects involve both a group product and individual performances. Rubrics can be developed to assess the group's efforts, and each individual can also turn in a journal entry.

Written Forms of Assessment

You may think of written assessments as objective tests (e.g., true/false, matching) or essays. Although these tests do measure some levels of student learning, authentic written assessment provides a more thorough and integrated understanding. In addition to keeping journals and logs, students can develop health-related fitness-training programs for themselves or others. They can also undertake projects that involve research and development—for example, magazine articles, video-recorded instructions for a weight training program, or pictures of appropriate or inappropriate exercises. Authentic assessments critique students' levels of understanding as well as integration and application.

Discussions

Student discussions can provide you with a wealth of information. Assessment techniques can be brief, such as conducting a check for understanding while stretching, or more thorough, such as interviewing students while they participate in stations for circuit training. Other options include pausing during a lesson and providing opportunities for whole-class discussion, both of which can be effective tools for collecting information about your students' understanding. Student discussions should be guided by objectives that state clear learning outcomes. Questions should be planned and should clearly focus on desired learning outcomes. Summarizing the discussion at the end of a lesson can provide closure as well as make effective use of time during cool-down activities (again, overlapping). You can find online resources to support effective discussions by using search phrases such as "make class discussions more exciting."

Polls

Student polls can provide some of the same information as discussions, but they use less time. Posing questions and having students vote in response provides quick information from all students. Older students can secretly mark a ballot, whereas younger students might enjoy participating in a poker chip survey (Graham, Elliott, & Palmer, 2016), in which they place one of two colors of poker chips to indicate *yes* or *no*, *true* or *false*, *disagree* or *agree*, and so on. Students can cast their votes on the way out of class. You can use the results of a poll as a group assessment to help plan and refine lessons as well as provide a point of review for ensuing lessons. One effective use of polling is to ask students, at the conclusion of a lesson, to raise their hands if they enjoyed the activity or to give a thumbs-up if they would like to play the game again in class. Polling is a quick and efficient way to assess general group enjoyment, and it avoids singling out students by requiring them to provide individual responses.

Role-Plays

Role-playing is a useful way to assess whether students can apply health-related fitness knowledge. Role-playing simulates real-life situations, giving students valuable practice. Learning activities that also provide cognitive assessment information to teachers are an efficient and effective way to use precious class time. Set up role-play situations that call for students to demonstrate competence in a real-life context. Here are some examples of role-play challenges:

- Students practice how to teach a younger student or partner to run correctly as pace changes.
- Students take the role of a teacher and demonstrate knowledge of the components of a good running stride as a means to increase their movement efficiency and cardiorespiratory endurance.
- Students work with a partner on the concept of pacing while listening to various pieces of music that incorporate different tempos.
- Students demonstrate two ways to take a pulse.
- In small groups, one student teaches three safe stretches to the rest of the group and explains what makes them safe.
- Each student pretends that a partner has sprained an ankle. The student demonstrates how to help the partner treat the injury safely following the RICES guidelines (rest, ice, compression, elevation, support).
- A student takes the role of a famous local athlete, and other students interview the person to find out what the person has done to enable such athletic achievement (adapted from National Association for Sport and Physical Education, 1995).

Role playing also offers a dynamic way to monitor students' attitudes and levels of motivation. Ask groups of students to act out how they feel about an activity or how they might change another person's opinion about physical activity. First, ask the groups to brainstorm possible actions and statements among themselves. Next, ask each group to act out its ideas for the rest of the class. Then discuss as a class which statements and actions are most likely to be helpful in a real-life situation. Ask students for suggestions of other issues that they would like to explore in this way.

Portfolios

Ongoing informal assessment, such as day-to-day observations and peer and self-assessment, should periodically be supported with formal assessments. For example, self- and peer assessments such as rubrics and class assignments can be combined to create a portfolio that provides a more complete and authentic picture of each student's progress. A portfolio provides a ready reference for assessment, grading, and parent–teacher conferences; in fact, a well-designed **portfolio** is a collection of tools that helps you assess each student. Portfolios may be presented in a three-hole binder, in a hanging file, or even as an electronic document. Because portfolios highlight student progress, they offer a powerful means for building students' self-efficacy—that is, their belief that they have the ability to learn and the competence to participate.

What should be included in a portfolio? A variety of assignments and assessments form a complete picture of each student's progress and achievements. Specifically, a portfolio might include both informal and formal assessments, such as periodic health-related fitness assessment results; rubrics that reflect affective, cognitive, and physical development; journal entries; video clips; and projects. Older students can select their own portfolio pieces (based on predetermined criteria).

Portfolios can go with students from grade to grade, and you can ask students to put two or three artifacts in their portfolio each school year, thus making it possible to monitor long-term progress. In this regard, electronic portfolios are efficient and simple to move. Portfolios can also serve as tools for monitoring a program's effectiveness in delivering a sequentially designed curriculum.

For more information, as well as strategies for using electronic portfolios, check out the PE Geek podcast and search for "portfolios" or "episode 34." This episode breaks down the various tools that physical education teachers all over the world are using to curate portfolios for their students. Resources explored in detail in this episode include Google Drive, Easy Portfolio, Easy Portfolio Site Builder, Three Ring, and FreshGrade.

Applying Assessment Tools

This section of the chapter includes numerous practical examples that demonstrate how to align assessments with standards in order to determine whether students are meeting cognitive and affective standards.

Assessing the Cognitive Domain

The cognitive domain aligns with SHAPE America's Standard 3: "demonstrates the knowledge and skills to achieve and maintain a health-enhancing level of physical activity and fitness" (SHAPE America, 2014, p.12). This standard encompasses understanding of basic training principles and nutrition. Physical Best enables students to learn along the full continuum of the cognitive domain. Lessons include learning through the simplest forms of the cognitive domain hierarchy (knowledge, comprehension, and application) as well as the most complex forms (analysis, synthesis, and evaluation). For example, activities demand that students list and define (knowledge), compute and discuss (comprehension), apply and calculate (application), analyze and differentiate (analysis), design and manage (synthesis), and evaluate and appraise (evaluation).

Figure 12.7*a* through 12.7*c* shows formative assessments, available in the web resource, that are designed to help you determine how well elementary children can identify activities for a proper warm-up and cool-down, monitor intensity levels using heart rate, and correctly identify aerobic activities. Figure 12.7*d* through 12.7*f* includes secondary-level formative and summative assessments. More specifically, the items shown in figure 12.7*d* and 12.7*e* measure students' understanding of intensity and time as they apply to the FITT principle, as well as their ability to set health-related fitness goals based on personal FitnessGram scores. Figure 12.7*f* serves as an example of a summative assessment for a yoga project.

Assessing the Affective Domain

The affective domain aligns with SHAPE America Standard 4: "exhibits responsible personal and social behavior that respects self and others" (SHAPE America, 2014, p.12). Physical Best also enables students to learn along the continuum of the affective domain. Activities include learning through the simplest form (receiving, responding) of the affective domain. For example, Physical Best activities demand that students recognize and realize (receiving) in order to cooperate and examine (responding).

Hellison's levels of personal and social responsibility also align with Standard 4 and can be used to guide development of program goals as a means to help teach students to take responsibility for their own development and contribute to the well-being of others (Hellison, 2011). Hellison defines these levels of personal and social responsibility as follows:

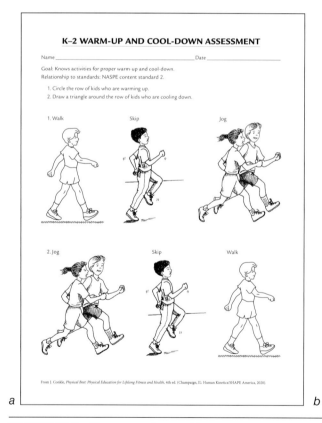

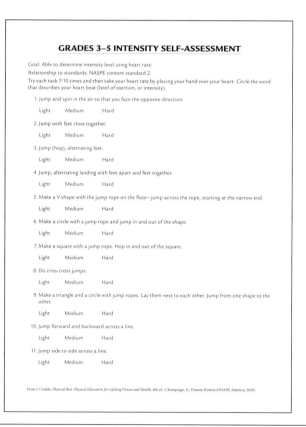

a

b

FIGURE 12.7   These sample cognitive assessments are available in the web resource.

EXIT SLIP

Name _____ Date _____

Goal: Correctly identifies aerobic activities.
Relationship to standards: NASPE content standard 4.
Circle the pictures of kids doing aerobic activities that will make their hearts stronger.

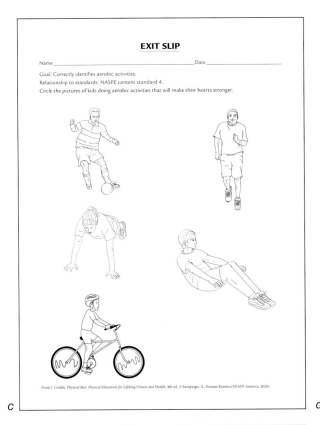

From J. Conkle, *Physical Best: Physical Education for Lifelong Fitness and Health*, 4th ed. (Champaign, IL: Human Kinetics/SHAPE America, 2020).

c

MIDDLE AND HIGH SCHOOL EXIT SLIP

Name _____ Date _____

_____ is how hard you do your physical activity. Intensity for aerobic activity can be correlated with heart rate and can affect the _____ that you are able to participate in the activity.

Hint: If you jog at the upper limits of your target heart rate range, you will not be able to jog as long as you would if you worked at the lower range of your target heart rate.

Word bank (choose from these to fill in the blanks):
  frequency
  intensity
  time
  type

From J. Conkle, *Physical Best: Physical Education for Lifelong Fitness and Health*, 4th ed. (Champaign, IL: Human Kinetics/SHAPE America, 2020).

d

GOAL-SETTING WORKSHEET

Name _____ Date _____

M = Measure and monitor
In class, my Fitnessgram scores were as follows: _____
My scores falling below the healthy fitness zone were (list) _____ .

O = Outcomes defined that are optimally challenging
Based on my Fitnessgram scores, I wish to improve fitness in the following areas:
(Example: abdominal strength and endurance)

T = Time
I will accomplish my goal in _____ weeks.

I = Individualized
I will not compare my scores to my classmates' scores.
To reach the HFZ, I need to increase my score by _____ (the exercise).
(Example: 10 curl-ups)

V = Valuable
I have chosen an important goal of _____
(Example: increasing abdominal strength)
This is important to me because . . .

A = Active
By completing this sheet, I am taking active responsibility for increasing my health and fitness. _____ (initial)

T = Type
The following types of activities will help me to reach my goal: (list several activities)
(Example: curl-ups, pelvic thrusts, oblique curls)

I = Incremental
I will add _____ (a number of exercises) to my score or add _____ minutes of _____ (activity) each week to achieve my goals.
(Example: two curl-ups each week or five minutes of jogging each week)

(continued)

From J. Conkle, *Physical Best: Physical Education for Lifelong Fitness and Health*, 4th ed. (Champaign, IL: Human Kinetics/SHAPE America, 2020). Debra Ballinger, PhD, Associate Professor, East Stroudsburg University.

e

YOGA PROJECT

Name _____ Date _____

Goal: Knows at least three cues for five yoga poses as well as health benefits of yoga.
Relationship to standards: NASPE content standards 2 and 4.

The teachers at this school want to increase their strength and flexibility levels while decreasing their stress levels. How fortunate it is that we just finished our study of yoga. A group of the teachers will be coming to the gym next week so that we can help them learn about yoga. Create five yoga pose cards that will help them learn to perform the poses correctly. You may choose to work alone, with a partner, or in a group of three.

Be sure to include the following in the yoga pose card project:
  1. Use one page for each of the five yoga poses taught in class.
  2. For each yoga pose provide a picture that demonstrates proper form using the cues learned in class. For this portion you will use a digital camera to take photos of properly performed poses.
  3. Include at least three cues for each pose.
  4. Use one page to list health benefits of yoga.

From J. Conkle, *Physical Best: Physical Education for Lifelong Fitness and Health*, 4th ed. (Champaign, IL: Human Kinetics/SHAPE America, 2020).

f

FIGURE 12.7   *(continued)*

Level IV, caring—Students at level IV, besides respecting others, participating, and being self-directed, are motivated to extend their sense of responsibility beyond themselves by cooperating, giving support, showing concern, and helping.

Level III, self-direction—Students at level III not only show respect and participation but also are able to work without direct supervision. They can identify their own needs and begin to plan and carry out their physical education programs.

Level II, participation—Students at level II not only show at least minimal respect for others but also willingly play, accept challenges, practice motor skills, and train for health-related fitness under the teacher's supervision.

Level I, respect—Students at level I may not participate in daily activities or show much mastery or improvement, but they are able to control their behavior enough that they don't interfere with the other students' right to learn or the teacher's right to teach. They do this without much prompting by the teacher and without constant supervision.

Level zero, irresponsibility—Students who operate at level zero make excuses, blame others for their behavior, and deny personal responsibility for what they do or fail to do.

Reprinted by permission from D. Hellison, *Teaching Responsibility Through Physical Activity* (Champaign, IL: Human Kinetics, 2003), 28.

Physical Best activities create opportunities for students to practice using these levels of personal and social responsibility. Figure 12.8a, 12.8b, 12.8d, and 12.8f were developed based on Hellison's levels and could be used with any number of Physical Best activities. Each of these assessments offers a way for students to reflect on their responsibility level with feedback from you.

The affective domain also aligns with SHAPE America Standard 5: "recognizes the value of physical activity for health, enjoyment, challenge, self-expression and/or social interaction" (SHAPE America, 2014, p. 12). Physical Best also enables more complex learning along the continuum of the affective domain. For example, Physical Best activities demand that students value and accept (valuing), discriminate and order (organization), and internalize and verify (characterization). The goal of this standard is for students to develop awareness of the intrinsic values and benefits of participation in personally meaningful physical activity. Students should be encouraged to enjoy movement activities and see them as a way to gain competence, take on challenges, and interact socially. Because of these intrinsic benefits of participation, they will more likely pursue lifelong activity to meet their own health-related fitness needs.

This section includes a wide variety of sample assessments designed to help you become more aware of ways to assess the affective domain. All forms are available in the web resource. Teacher observation of affective behaviors during group fitness activities can provide valuable feedback to students and inform teaching practice. Figure 12.8a provides an example of a teacher observation assessment. Accepting responsibility for personal health-related fitness is an integral part of learning to become physically active. The exit slip in Figure 12.8b could be used after students work together to practice one or more FitnessGram assessments. It is designed to allow students to reflect on how well they remained on task without close teacher monitoring and how well they helped a partner. Figure 12.8c creates an opportunity for peers to provide one another with appropriate feedback about how well they follow all safety guidelines while performing basic yoga poses. Figure 12.8d presents a sample journal entry providing evidence of student reflection on personal physical activity choices during choice time.

Figure 12.8e demonstrates how pictures and word stems can be used to help students identify feelings associated with participation in physical activities. Figure 12.8f can be used during any health-related fitness or skill development lesson to determine whether students seek challenging experiences in physical education. Figure 12.8*g* creates the opportunity for students to express thoughts and feelings related to progress on their personal health-related fitness goals.

Figure 12.8*h* includes a questionnaire that can be used to facilitate effective discussions. Figure 12.8*i* comes from the FITT Concentration activity found in the web resource. It engages students in exercise stations while assessing valuable health-related fitness information. When using this kind of assessment, place pencils at each station rather than having students move between activities carrying sharp objects. Last, figure 12.8*j* measures knowledge of yoga and the benefits of flexibility.

Assessing the Psychomotor Domain

The psychomotor domain aligns with SHAPE America Standard 3: "demonstrates the knowledge and skills to achieve and maintain a health-enhancing level of physical activity and fitness" (SHAPE America, 2014, p.12). Specifically, this standard addresses the psychomotor aspect of measuring personal health-related fitness and physical activity. When developing content, teachers may ask, "What is the appropriate age for health-related fitness assessment to begin? What type of cardiorespiratory endurance assessment should be administered? How many curl-ups represent the healthy fitness zone for a high school student?" These and many other questions are addressed in chapter 2 and in FitnessGram materials (Cooper Institute, 2016). Detailed information about assessing the psychomotor domain is provided in the next chapter.

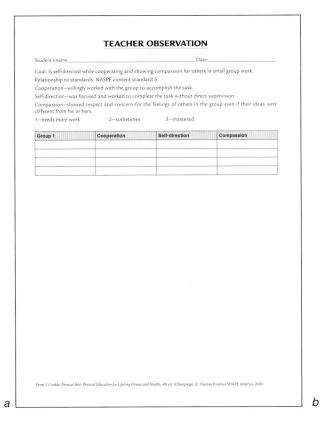

a *b*

(continued)

FIGURE 12.8 These sample affective assessments are available in the web resource.

Figure 12.8g is reprinted by permission from V. Melograno, *Professional and student portfolios for physical education* (Champaign, IL: Human Kinetics, 1998), 128. Figure 12.8h is reprinted by permission from G. Graham, *Teaching children physical education* (Champaign, IL: Human Kinetics, 1992), 159.

PEER OBSERVATION

Name _____ Date _____

Goal: Follows all safety guidelines.
Relationship to standards: NASPE content standard 5.

Today at the yoga stations, my fitness partner
   a. followed all safety rules
   b. followed safety rules sometimes
   c. forgot to follow the safety rules

To help my partner be safe, I told him or her _____
_____ .

From J. Conkle, *Physical Best: Physical Education for Lifelong Fitness and Health*, 4th ed. (Champaign, IL: Human Kinetics/SHAPE America, 2020).

c

JOURNAL ENTRY

Name _____ Date _____

Goal: Reflects on personal physical activity choices during choice time.
Relationship to standards: NASPE content standard 5.
During free choice time I _____
_____ .

My top three reasons for choosing to _____ are
1.
2.
3.
Next free choice period I want to _____
because _____ .

From J. Conkle, *Physical Best: Physical Education for Lifelong Fitness and Health*, 4th ed. (Champaign, IL: Human Kinetics/SHAPE America, 2020).

d

AFFECTIVE EXIT SLIP

Name _____ Date _____

Goal: Identifies feelings associated with participation in physical activities.
Relationship to standards: NASPE content standard 6.
Today's activities in physical education made me feel

I felt this way because
_____
_____
_____

From J. Conkle, *Physical Best: Physical Education for Lifelong Fitness and Health*, 4th ed. (Champaign, IL: Human Kinetics/SHAPE America, 2020).

e

AFFECTIVE ANALYTIC RUBRIC

Name _____ Date _____

Goal: Seeks challenging experiences in physical education.
Relationship to standards: NASPE content standard 6.

How much did you challenge yourself today in class?
   3—I challenged myself the whole time by trying new things even if they seemed hard.
   2—I challenged myself part of the time by trying some of the new things we learned.
   1—I need to work on challenging myself and would like help.

Next time I want to see whether I can _____
_____ .

From J. Conkle, *Physical Best: Physical Education for Lifelong Fitness and Health*, 4th ed. (Champaign, IL: Human Kinetics/SHAPE America, 2020).

f

FIGURE 12.8 *(continued)*

FITNESS JOURNAL

Name _____   Date _____

	I wish I could . . .	I predict that . . .	I feel good about . . .	My fears are . . .
Before my fitness preassessments Date _____				
After my fitness preassessments Date _____				
One month after my fitness program Date _____				
Two months after my fitness program Date _____				
Three months after my fitness program Date _____				

From J. Conkle, *Physical Best: Physical Education for Lifelong Fitness and Health*, 4th ed. (Champaign, IL: Human Kinetics/SHAPE America, 2020). Reprinted, by permission, from V. Melograno, 1998, *Professional and student portfolios for physical education* (Champaign, IL: Human Kinetics), 128.

g

THINKING ABOUT PHYSICAL FITNESS AND ACTIVITIES

Name _____   Date _____

1. I would rather exercise or play sports than watch TV.	Yes	No
2. People who exercise regularly seem to have a lot of fun doing it.	Yes	No
3. In school, I look forward to attending physical education class.	Yes	No
4. During physical education class at school, I usually work up a sweat.	Yes	No
5. When I grow up, I will probably be too busy to stay physically fit.	Yes	No
6. How do you feel about your ability to strike a ball with a racket?	☺	😐	☹
7. How do you feel about your ability to kick a ball hard and hit a target?	☺	😐	☹
8. How do you feel about your ability to run a long distance without stopping?	☺	😐	☹
9. How do you feel about your ability to play many different games and sports?	☺	😐	☹
10. How do you feel about your ability to participate in gymnastics?	☺	😐	☹
11. How do you feel about your ability to participate in dance?	☺	😐	☹

From J. Conkle, *Physical Best: Physical Education for Lifelong Fitness and Health*, 4th ed. (Champaign, IL: Human Kinetics/SHAPE America, 2020). Reprinted, by permission, from G. Graham, 2008, *Teaching children physical education*, 3rd ed. (Champaign, IL: Human Kinetics), 159, 208.

h

FITT CONCENTRATION

Name _____   Date _____

You will be performing a fitness activity and running to various stations to fill in your activity card. When instructed to go to a station, quickly run and write down the definition. Return to your roll call line for the next exercise. When you have completed each station, you will get into small groups and answer the questions for each category. At the end of the activity, turn in your paper for daily participation points!

Station 1: Principle of Progression
Definition:

Question: How can you apply the principle of progression to muscular strength?

Station 2: Principle of Specificity
Definition:

Question: What component of health-related fitness does core training focus on?

Station 3: Intensity
Definition:

Question: Compute your target heart rate zone using this formula:
208 − (.7 x your age) = _____ (max heart rate)
Threshold heart rate   Target ceiling heart rate
Max HR: _____   Max HR: _____
(x) .65   (x) .90

Station 4: Principle of Overload

Definition:

Question: How can you apply the principle of overload to biceps curls?

Station 5: Frequency
Definition:

Question: What is the recommended number of times to exercise during the week?

Station 6: Time
Definition:

Question: What is the recommended time to exercise for a cardiovascular benefit to occur?

(continued)

From J. Conkle, *Physical Best: Physical Education for Lifelong Fitness and Health*, 4th ed. (Champaign, IL: Human Kinetics/SHAPE America, 2020).

i

YOGA EXIT SLIP

Name _____   Date _____

Goal: Knows three cues for the warrior yoga pose and three flexibility health benefits.
Relationship to standards: NASPE content standards 2 and 4.

Today we added the warrior pose to our yoga session. Name three cues or tips that are important to performing this pose correctly and safely.

1.

2.

3.

Name three flexibility health benefits discussed in class.

1.

2.

3.

From J. Conkle, *Physical Best: Physical Education for Lifelong Fitness and Health*, 4th ed. (Champaign, IL: Human Kinetics/SHAPE America, 2020).

j

FIGURE 12.8   *(continued)*

Top 10 Lists

The creation of top 10 lists by teachers and students is one example of a fun and practical way to enhance communication between teacher and student about expectations for each other. Such discussions allow for student input about their own participation and may therefore empower students in ways that lead to increased motivation to participate.

John Hichwa asked his students to create a list of the top 10 reasons that they enjoy physical education, and he then created his own list of what he believed were the 10 most important aspects of effectively teaching physical education.

Students' Top 10 List

10. We get to grade ourselves.
 9. We are taught to make goals for ourselves and to try our hardest to achieve them.
 8. We have plenty of supplies.
 7. The activities are challenging.
 6. Physical education relieves stress from our day.
 5. We are always doing different things, so it's interesting, and you never get bored.
 4. Teachers are supportive, understanding, and are easy to get along with.
 3. We get a good workout.
 2. We are always active.
 1. Teachers make physical education fun!

Teachers' Top 10 List

10. Have enough equipment for each student.
 9. Chart each child's progress and motivate him or her to do his or her personal best.
 8. Play the game.
 7. Make lessons interesting, progressive, and challenging.
 6. Keep the development of self-responsibility as a top priority.
 5. Develop individual and cooperative skills.
 4. Provide equipment that is developmentally appropriate.
 3. Present a variety of offerings so that each child can experience success.
 2. Keep students physically active as much as possible.
 1. Treat each child fairly and with respect.

Reprinted by permission from J. Hichwa, *Right Fielders are People Too* (Champaign, IL: Human Kinetics, 1998), 54-55.

Using Assessments for Program Planning

A central reason for conducting regular assessments is to use the information to tailor your program so that it meets individual student needs. Assessment should not result in diminished activity time. Lectures have their place in a health-related fitness education program, but the goal is to keep students as physically active as possible. Your students can learn through doing. If students are having trouble learning how to pace themselves while running the mile, design an active game that teaches this concept in order to make the connection more explicit. Remember that students generally enjoy moving. If they do not enjoy a particular physical activity, then they are less likely to pursue it as a lifestyle choice. If you include a variety of movement forms in addition to health-related fitness and sport activities—for example, dance, outdoor pursuits, and adventure programming—you can spark interest in physical activity in otherwise reluctant students.

Motivating Through Assessment

Knowing *how* to be physically active for life is not enough: Students must also *want* to pursue a physically active lifestyle. Giving them the responsibility for tracking their own progress is highly motivating (Hellison, 2011). Avoid making comparisons among students; instead, focus on helping students set goals for personal improvement so that they are more likely to feel successful each time they participate in physical activity. Even a very young child can set a simple goal, such as playing physically active games after school three times a week instead of watching television.

Goals should be set based on current levels of personal health-related fitness, feelings of self-efficacy, knowledge of the FITT guidelines and training principles, access to various types of programs and activities, and the purposes that you have established for setting goals.

To guide goal setting and self-assessment, set benchmarks (i.e., the healthy fitness zones) by which students can monitor their own progress. This process makes students more accountable for their own learning and progress. It is also in keeping with the philosophy of helping students move from depending on your guidance to pursuing health-related fitness independently as a way of life.

Specifically, students may be motivated by carefully monitoring self-recorded progress toward goals that they set with their teacher. To enable this approach, give students sufficient time to allow for progress. Focus on small steps toward improvement or toward the goal. The small steps that can be seen in the student's own writing are the most motivating—they become fuel for developing a sense of competence. (For goal-setting strategies and guidelines, refer to chapter 2.)

Making Assessment Practical

Time constraints and large class sizes can make assessment difficult. To overcome such barriers, consider these tips:

- *Make assessment part of instruction.* Use stations during a lesson, and, at one or more stations, leave pencils and short exit slips that allow opportunities for assessment. Assessment can also be combined or embedded within activity through the use of self- and peer assessment, as well as projects. This approach also helps ensure that assessment enhances instruction.

- *Assess in waves.* Avoid trying to assess all students in all classes at the same time. When using exit slips, logs, journals, or portfolios, avoid having all classes use them at the same time. For example, use logs and journals with two or three classes while using more informal checks for understanding with other classes, then rotate. In this way, you read logs and journals for only two or three classes at any one time.

- *Use systematic observation.* When using teacher observation assessments, watch only small groups of students at any one time. While observing, rate only those students who did not reach proficiency, then fill in the other ratings after class. Keep in mind that it is okay not to assess all students on the same day.

- *Establish routines.* Establish efficient routines for ensuring that students get pencils, papers, and so on. Keep sharpened pencils or crayons in several tennis ball cans or other containers that can be placed around the gym where students can pick them up quickly without your taking time to pass them all out individually. Using several cans scattered around the gym also prevents students from mobbing one can of pencils, which not only wastes time but may lead to further management problems. Paper and pencils could also be placed in hoops along a wall.

- *Be purposeful and collaborate.* Establish a plan and continue trying new time-saving ideas to keep assessment practical. Collaborate with other professionals to share and gain new ways to make assessment work for you.

Summary

Assessment can take many forms. In physical education, authentic assessment offers the most value because it creates opportunities for students to demonstrate, in real-life settings, that they are moving toward the goal of becoming physically literate adults. Physical education programs should motivate students to apply motor skills, knowledge, and key approaches, including health-related fitness knowledge, in the real world. Within the context of motivation, separate health-related fitness assessment from the grading system in physical education and provide specific feedback using alternative methods that inform students about progress toward personal goals and strategies to achieve them.

This chapter has differentiated assessment from grading, provided suggestions about what and how to assess student learning, and suggested assessment tools for doing so. It has also delineated differences between traditional and authentic, formative and summative, and formal and informal assessment. Chapter 13 elaborates on some of the tools discussed in this chapter and their application to assessing health-related fitness and physical activity.

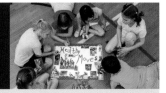

Discussion Questions

1. Why is assessment important in physical education?
2. What is assessment for learning?
3. Explain the difference between assessment and grading.
4. Define authentic assessment and provide three examples of it in physical education.
5. Explain the purpose of a rubric.
6. Describe authentic assessments that could be used to determine the extent to which students meet SHAPE America's Standard 3 ("demonstrates the knowledge and skills to achieve and maintain a health-enhancing level of physical activity and fitness").
7. Describe authentic assessments that could be used to determine the extent to which students meet SHAPE America's Standard 4 ("exhibits responsible personal and social behavior that respects self and others").
8. Describe authentic assessments that could be used to determine the extent to which students meet SHAPE America's Standard 5 ("recognizes the value of physical activity for health, enjoyment, challenge, self-expression and/or social interaction."
9. Describe best practice for making assessment in physical education practical.
10. Discuss ways in which assessment can be used to appropriately and effectively motivate students.

CHAPTER 13

Assessing Health-Related Fitness and Physical Activity

Lynn V. Johnson and Christina Sinclair

The authors gratefully acknowledge the contribution made by Jan Bishop to this chapter.

Helping students become physically literate is a primary goal of physical education programs, and meeting that goal depends in part on helping students become physically active. This chapter addresses specific strategies for assessing students' levels of physical activity and health-related fitness, both in the physical education setting and outside of school. National and state standards for physical education emphasize the ability to assess health-related fitness and to use such assessments to set personal goals for physical activity and health-related fitness. By the time your students graduate from high school, they should be able to use the results of health-related fitness assessments to design an individualized program for health-related fitness that aligns with life and career goals (SHAPE America, 2014, p. 58).

Effective health-related fitness assessments should be used to communicate each person's level of health-related fitness—not to compare students' health-related fitness or activity levels with those of others. Appropriate health-related fitness assessment includes a variety of tests designed to measure cardiorespiratory endurance, body composition, muscle strength, muscular endurance, and flexibility. New research indicates that it is also appropriate to assess power as part of health-related fitness (SHAPE America, 2017). Preassessment strategies provide students with the baseline information that they need in order to establish personal goals for improving or maintaining specific areas of physical activity and health-related fitness that are associated with good health. Once these goals have been set, periodic assessment of students' health-related fitness (conducted by the teacher or via self-assessment) provides each student with specific information about progress made toward meeting personal goals. Because the focus is on personal goals rather than on peer competition, students experience feelings of success based on their own achievements.

FitnessGram

FitnessGram is the most widely used tool in the world for assessment, education, and reporting related to youth physical fitness. Developed by the Cooper Institute, **FitnessGram** uses **criterion-referenced health standards,** which are associated with good health; in other words, it uses scientific information to determine the amount of fitness needed in order to meet minimum health levels. FitnessGram delineates **healthy fitness zones (HFZs)** to indicate the range of fitness scores associated with good health; the healthy fitness zones are based on age- and gender-appropriate fitness levels that a child needs for good health. **Normative standards** (e.g., percentiles) provide comparisons relative to other youth in a group but do not provide information about how the values relate to individual health (Corbin & Pangrazi, 2008).

FitnessGram assesses five components of health-related fitness: aerobic capacity, muscular strength, muscular endurance, flexibility, and body composition. It also provides at least two assessments for each component, which allows teachers and students to individualize the process in order to best meet students' needs. Personalized reports, such as the one shown in figure 13.1, provide objective feedback and positive reinforcement, both of which are vital to changing behavior. These reports also serve as communications links between teachers, parents, and students.

FitnessGram is designed for self-assessment and institutional assessment of personal health-related fitness, as well as parental reporting and personal tracking. Its main focus is self-assessment, and teachers must help students learn how to evaluate their scores. Specifically, students must learn how to compare their scores with the healthy

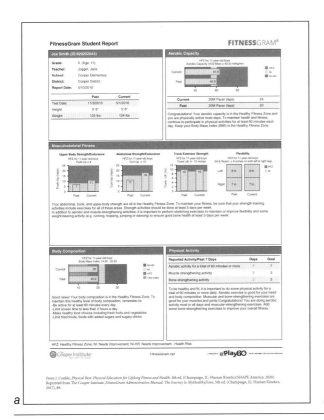 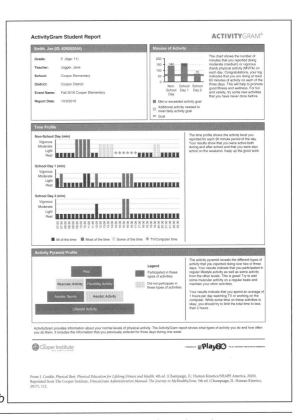

FIGURE 13.1   FitnessGram and ActivityGram provide students with individualized reports based on their assessment scores for health-related fitness.

Reprinted by permission from The Cooper Institute, *FitnessGram Administration Manual,* 5th ed. (Champaign, IL: Human Kinetics, 2017), 89.

fitness zones, which indicate fitness levels required for good health, and then use their results to develop personal programs for improvement and maintenance. Scores that fall below the HFZs are categorized as "needs improvement" to indicate that they need to be brought into the healthy fitness zone. For body composition and aerobic capacity, the "needs improvement" zone is further divided into two parts: "needs improvement" and "needs improvement—health risk" to enable more specificity in health-related fitness levels.

As part of the FitnessGram report, students receive scores, interpretations of the scores, and individualized recommendations to help them improve in any areas where their scores fall below the HFZ (figure 13.1). Immediate feedback based on personal scores for health-related fitness can help students understand how their scores relate to the achievement of a healthy lifestyle. To further encourage students to continue their positive patterns, use reinforcing statements about their healthy behaviors.

Health-related fitness assessment that is developmentally appropriate and conducted in an effective physical education program helps teach students how to be fit and healthy throughout their life span. Moreover, it provides a snapshot of each student's current health-related fitness, which allows both you and the student to plan for improvement. In this way, health-related fitness assessment can be a positive experience for students—as long as they understand the purpose, how the scores will be used, and the fact that, in the end, they can develop and sustain a healthy lifestyle.

Appropriate Uses for FitnessGram

Appropriate Use

- Conducting personal assessment to help students evaluate their level of health-related fitness
- Conducting institutional assessment to allow teachers to view group data (for curriculum development)
- Conducting personal-best assessment to allow individual students to determine performance levels privately
- Teaching students about criterion-referenced health standards and the types of activities needed to reach them
- Helping students track health-related fitness over time (for example, in portfolios)
- Documenting that FitnessGram is administered in a school and that students' self-assessments are tracked over time

Inappropriate Use

- Evaluation of individual students in physical education (grading)
- Evaluation of teacher effectiveness
- Evaluation of overall physical education quality

From The Cooper Institute 2007.

Guidelines for Assessing Health-Related Fitness

Appropriate health-related fitness and physical activity assessment should be both formative and summative and should include both process and product measurements that document students' progress toward demonstrating healthy behaviors. **Process measurements** assess the use of correct form or technique, whereas **product measurements** score the outcome or result of the assessment performance (Lund & Veal, 2013). Assessment is an integral component of a physical education curriculum, and assessments that measure knowledge and levels of health-related fitness and physical activity form important pieces of the assessment process.

Fitness education, however, involves more than testing (SHAPE America, 2017), and student assessment should be embedded into instruction as a learning experience rather than conducted as a separate event that is unrelated to instructional objectives. Indeed, students should spend the majority of their time being active and being educated about health-related fitness on the day an assessment is scheduled in physical education (SHAPE America, 2017). The following suggestions can be used to connect health-related fitness assessment to the overall physical education curriculum.

- Formal assessment of health-related fitness should not occur until the fourth grade; prior to that, however, both informal and formal assessments can be used to demonstrate understanding of the importance of physical activity and health-related fitness components.
- Teach and ask students to practice proper procedures for conducting health-related fitness assessments; help students understand the value of these assessments and the importance of each health-related fitness component that is assessed.
- Provide opportunities for students to practice conducting health-related fitness assessments with their peers. Students can evaluate each other on following

proper procedures and give appropriate feedback to each other. This peer evaluation process gives students additional opportunities to demonstrate their understanding of the assessment protocol.

- Teach the process of self-assessment and provide opportunities for students to self-assess so that they can receive feedback at any time about their progress toward meeting their goals. As students become more skilled in self-assessment, provide more opportunities for individualizing instruction and improved sequencing of learning.

- Talk with students about the importance of getting accurate measurements; reiterate the fact that scores are personal and that students should not compare scores with other students.

- Teach students the principles of goal setting and ask them to practice using scores from a teacher-measured preassessment or peer assessment.

- Teach the process of reflecting on and modifying goals based on the results of periodic health-related fitness assessment; provide opportunities for students to practice the process.

- Teach students how assessment and goal setting for levels of health-related fitness and physical activity can be integrated into lifestyle changes.

- Give students opportunities to demonstrate behaviors that support their peers as they work to meet their personal goals.

As students develop their understanding and skills, they become more independent. In this vein, the ultimate goal of physical education is to produce physically literate individuals who can conduct their own health-related fitness assessments in the context of self-designed and self-selected physical activity programs.

You can introduce the concept of physical literacy as early as kindergarten. The first step in helping students understand the importance of physical activity and health-related fitness is to encourage them to be active, both in and beyond physical education. You can progressively introduce the components of health-related fitness during grades K through 3. Then, starting in third grade, teach students the process of assessing their level of health-related fitness and setting personal goals (Standard 3.E5, or S3.E5); be aware that doing so requires a high degree of direction and supervision. By the time your students leave middle school, they will likely be capable of designing programs to remediate and improve health-related fitness based on their personal goals (S3.M15 and M16.8) and of cycling through the first three steps (teacher-directed self-assessment practice; formal teacher-administered assessment; and informal self-checks). High school students should be able to progress to formal self-assessment and to use the resulting information to design and implement a health-related fitness plan that supports their personal goals and enhances their lifestyle (S3.H11.L1 and L2). By teaching students to self-assess their levels of health-related fitness and physical activity—and to use the resulting information to inform goal setting—you will help perpetuate a continuous cycle that includes assessment, goal setting, and participation in physical activity, all with the ultimate goal of improving health-enhancing behaviors.

Planning for Health-Related Fitness Assessment

Planning for assessment and attainment of health-related fitness needs to begin well before any assessment takes place. In early elementary (K-2) physical education, students should be provided with opportunities to participate in a variety of activities that address the components of health-related fitness. Think about how you can integrate the concepts of health-related fitness into multiple aspects of your program; do not align health-related fitness exclusively with fitness assessment. The Physical Best activities provide ready-to-use activities for health-related fitness that can be incorporated into a variety of units.

When the time comes to formally assess health-related fitness in the fourth grade, the assessment must provide feedback that helps shape a health-related fitness education program. Assessment results for health-related fitness can be used to help you and your students plan for future learning and health-related fitness gains. For example, if assessment shows that students are making little or no progress in muscular strength and endurance, then you can include more activities to enhance these areas. More mature students can be involved in problem-solving tasks related to their scores for personal health-related fitness. Encourage students to set specific process-oriented goals related to the targeted areas, such as "I will do upper-body weight training two or three times per week on nonconsecutive days. In addition, each week, I will increase the number of push-ups I do by at least one repetition until I reach my healthy fitness zone. I will then continue this training program to maintain upper-body strength in the healthy fitness zone." This kind of goal setting helps students tailor their personal programs for health-related fitness to their specific needs. To keep things on a good path, check in with students regularly to monitor progress and provide suggestions for modifications.

Involving Students

Most people learn best by doing. Therefore, in order to develop students who can self-direct their own physically active lifestyles, you must involve them in each part of health-related fitness assessment. Students become more willing to accept responsibility when they begin to understand the purpose of assessment and relate their scores to what they do and what they do not do. You can help your students develop their skills of personal responsibility by using the following steps:

- Teach students proper procedures and provide opportunities for them to practice self-assessment and peer assessment.
- Encourage students to regularly assess themselves on individual components of health-related fitness while remembering that it is not necessary to complete all FitnessGram assessment components at the same time.
- Give students multiple opportunities to learn self-assessment procedures.
- Ask students to keep logs of their results to help them make improvement plans for personal health-related fitness.
- Provide students with guidance and feedback that allows them to practice goal setting for each component of health-related fitness at the appropriate grade level.

Effective Practice

For optimal performance, students need to have adequate and appropriate opportunities to practice each item repeatedly. Students who have difficulty performing a particular item (e.g., curl-up, push-up) should be given progressive practice tasks (e.g., reverse sit-up, bent-knee push-up) to help them develop the strength to perform the item appropriately. Here are some simple suggestions for developing effective practice opportunities:

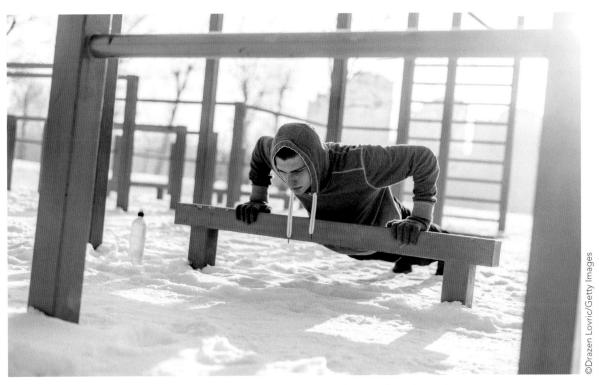

Mature students should be encouraged to set goals related to their health-related fitness.

- Discuss and demonstrate the correct techniques (critical elements) involved in each assessment item. Deliver this information in multiple forms—for example, posters, critical steps listed in word or picture form, and checklists of assessment steps for self- and peer checking.
- Ask students to practice with a friend. Provide rubrics for them to use during this practice so that the partners can provide feedback regarding technique as well as motivational support. Repeated practice will help ensure success.
- Make assessment stations available during class time or use as them instant activities to allow students to self-assess on a regular basis. Facilitate self-assessment by providing opportunities for students to review video of themselves performing tasks.
- Encourage students to give their best effort when they practice an assessment.
- Assign fitness homework that involves parents or guardians.
- Focus on personal improvement and carefully guard student privacy. Health-related fitness assessment is not a competitive sport, and a student's performance should never be compared with that of another student; nor is it acceptable to judge student effort. Provide encouragement or incentive for those who try their best regardless of their scores.
- Teach through assessment by explaining the concepts behind each assessment and talking with students about their individual results.

Students can benefit from practice through both peer and self-assessment. Practice sessions provide students with opportunities to understand health-related fitness concepts and develop personal goals to improve their health-related fitness. Appropriate practice settings provide student-friendly opportunities that focus on personal improvement.

Assessment Protocols

FitnessGram protocols are thoroughly detailed in the test manual, and it is essential that you train students to administer the protocols in order to develop a student-centered environment that provides opportunities for students to take personal responsibility for their health-related fitness development. The following strategies can increase students' adherence to proper protocols, help students become more skillful at self- and peer assessment, and help make health-related fitness assessment a positive experience for both teacher and students.

- Devote multiple days to explaining the protocols and their purposes to students and providing students with opportunities to practice. Students need to practice, practice, practice. Review the protocols and purposes again on assessment days.

- On assessment day, use the same informational posters, rubrics, and task cards (listing the critical elements or common errors) as during practice sessions.

- At each station, place drawings or diagrams depicting correct form and common errors.

- Announce assessment days in advance. Unannounced health-related fitness assessment can lead to negative attitudes toward both health-related fitness and physical activity. If preparation and practice are sufficient, students' anxiety will decrease. Encouragement can motivate students to do their best.

- Encourage students to dress appropriately for the assessment. Provide water before, during, and after strenuous assessments, such as the PACER or one-mile run. If the environment is too hot or too cold, postpone the assessment.

- Encourage parents to volunteer to help assess and record scores so that assessment day proceeds smoothly. In addition to facilitating assessment procedures, parent or guardian volunteers will develop a clearer understanding of health-related fitness assessment.

Appropriate practice is essential if student health-related fitness scores are to be valid and reliable. The more students practice the assessments, the more comfortable they become with how FitnessGram is administered.

SHAPE America (2017) has developed a position paper on appropriate and inappropriate uses of fitness testing. The paper provides valuable information for teachers to understand appropriate and inappropriate practices but also to have support of a respected national organization when detailing these practices to others, such as parents and administrators. This document is available in the web resource (figure 13.2) as well.

There is also a chart (see figure 1.2) that addresses instructional practices for an eight-step fitness education process (SHAPE America, 2016), which can help teachers and others to understand how assessing health-related fitness is an integral part of the fitness education process.

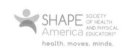

SHAPE America
SOCIETY OF HEALTH AND PHYSICAL EDUCATORS®
health. moves. minds.

Position Statement

Appropriate and Inappropriate Practices Related to Fitness Testing

SHAPE America's Position
Fitness testing is a valuable part of fitness education when integrated *appropriately* into a comprehensive physical education curriculum, and students' fitness scores should *not* be used to grade students or to evaluate physical education teachers.

Rationale
Fitness education is an important part of a comprehensive physical education program that is designed to teach students why they should and how to participate in physical activity on a regular basis, in addition to adopting other health-enhancing behaviors. Also, fitness education plays an integral role in empowering students to be physically active and to make the healthy choices that contribute to their pursuit of a lifetime of physical activity, which is an important element of SHAPE America's 50 Million Strong by 2029 commitment "to empower all students to live healthy and active lives through effective physical and health education programs."

Fitness testing, as part of fitness education, is woven into many of SHAPE America's curriculum-support resources. For example, fitness is addressed in all five of SHAPE America's National Standards for K-12 Physical Education (2013) and their corresponding Grade-Level Outcomes for K-12 Physical Education (2013), and is featured in Standard 3: the physically literate individual demonstrates the knowledge and skills to achieve and maintain a health-enhancing level of physical activity and fitness.

In addition, SHAPE America's Instructional Framework for Fitness Education in Physical Education (2012) features grade-level benchmarks for fitness education.

An Eight-Step Fitness Education Process
Figure 1 on page 2 outlines an eight-step process that demonstrates the practices necessary for providing students with meaningful fitness instruction (Corbin, Welk, Corbin & Welk, 2016). This fitness education process gives students the knowledge and skills necessary for attaining and maintaining a health-enhancing level of physical activity and fitness.

© 2017, SHAPE America – Society of Health and Physical Educators • www.shapeamerica.org
1900 Association Drive, Reston, VA 20191 • 703.476.3400 • membership@shapeamerica.org

FIGURE 13.2 Visit the web resource to see the full version of Appropriate and Inappropriate Uses of Fitness Testing (SHAPE America, 2017).

Strategies for Making Health-Related Fitness Assessments Manageable

Health-related fitness assessment can be overwhelming to teachers, especially when their time with students is limited. With that reality in mind, here are some practical ways to complete assessments both effectively and efficiently.

Elementary School

Train an older student or a parent to help you with assessments. Instead of trying to do them all at once, incorporate a health-related fitness assessment as part of your learning tasks. Students can rotate in and out of the station while you continue with the lesson. Each day, students will be assessed on a different component while you continue with your curriculum.

If it is not possible for you to have someone helping you with assessment, you can use stations as an efficient way to assess. Create four or five stations and identify one as the assessment station. The other stations can address health-related fitness or review skills or concepts from the current unit or a past one. Students rotate through the stations and perform the identified assessment when they arrive at the assessment station. Depending on the class size and the length of the class, it may be possible to complete two or more assessments in a day.

Middle School and High School

At this point, students should be able to self-assess, and they should be held responsible for following assessment protocols. The station approach could be used at this level as well, but it should not require teacher oversight. If you want to be sure that protocols are followed, you can video-record the assessments.

Spreading Out Health-Related Fitness Assessments

Laura Borsdorf, Professor, Exercise and Sport Science Department, Ursinus College, Collegeville, Pennsylvania

Instead of administering an entire assessment battery for health-related fitness at one time, you can incorporate health-related fitness assessment into other units and activities throughout the school year. Specifically, if you assess various components of health-related fitness when the assessments match concepts that the students are studying, you help connect assessment to students' lives. As a result, students are more motivated to self-assess because they see the connections between concepts, class activities, and assessment, including self-assessment. Thus, this method can be more beneficial than a formal assessment session, and it saves time as well.

Tailoring Health-Related Fitness Assessment

FitnessGram is designed to meet the needs of a diverse range of student abilities by providing multiple assessment items for each health-related fitness component. For instance, aerobic capacity can be measured by completing the 20-meter PACER test, the one-mile run, or the walk test for students above the age of 13. The results of these tests are reported in terms of $\dot{V}O_2$max so that, regardless of which test is used, the results are consistent. You can work with individual students to decide which aerobic capacity test would be most appropriate.

Given that the goal is for each student to be as successful as possible, it is important for students to feel comfortable and confident when participating in the test. Students have a wide range of cardiorespiratory endurance levels, and if all students are forced to participate in, say, the mile run, then those who are less fit often stop running long after the more aerobically fit students have completed the test. As a result, those who are less fit may feel extremely self-conscious. In the PACER assessment, in contrast, students stop at various times, and those who are more aerobically fit finish last. Thus, students with lower scores are far less likely to be spotlighted. In addition, the PACER provides opportunities for goal setting in a user-friendly way that students can relate to. Younger students may find it easier to envision improving their PACER scores by one or two laps than achieving an intangible time improvement for the mile run. Space is usually not an issue with the PACER, but teachers working in smaller instructional spaces have the option of using the 15-meter PACER. Note, however, that because of increased fatigue from making more stops and turns, the 15-meter version can lead to extra fatigue and decreased performance, so it should be used only by elementary students whose scores are not recorded.

On the other hand, students who are more aerobically fit may enjoy the mile run and perform at a higher level if that test is used. To some degree, using staggered starts for the mile run can camouflage students who run more slowly. Another idea is to have students of similar ability run in small groups, at different times, or on different days. Ideally, students would choose which aerobic capacity assessment they prefer, which not only increases their autonomy but also motivates them to do their best.

Options are also available for most of the other components of FitnessGram. For instance, body composition can be assessed by means of skinfold measurements or body mass index. At times, body composition is the most sensitive of assessments. There may be some resistance to having teachers take skinfold measurements; if so, body mass index may be an easier and less sensitive option for you to use. Similarly, upper-body strength and endurance can be assessed using the push-up, the modified pull-up, or the flexed-arm hang. The options for flexibility include the back-saver sit-and-reach and the shoulder stretch.

The two components for which alternatives are not available are abdominal strength and endurance (via the curl-up) and trunk extensor strength and flexibility (via the trunk lift). Because these two components do not provide testing options, it is particularly important for you to provide students with progressive practice opportunities that allow them to develop the appropriate strength or flexibility to perform the test correctly and with some level of success.

Elementary School Students

Elementary students should be taught about fitness and the health-related fitness components beginning as early as kindergarten. Students in grades K-2 should learn about the importance of physical activity, which activities help improve health-related fitness, and, in simple terms, the physiological responses to physical activity, such as faster heartbeat and harder breathing (SHAPE America, 2014). Although specific FitnessGram assessment items do not need to be introduced until third grade, students in grades K-2 should participate in activities with the potential to increase muscular strength and endurance, flexibility, and cardiorespiratory endurance. These activities might include, for example, using a parachute to develop arm strength and endurance, engaging in activities that require moving parts of the body through their full range of motion (e.g., making shapes with the body), and participating in moderate to vigorous physical activities. By third grade, students can begin to practice individual FitnessGram assessment items under your supervision.

The goal is to expose younger students to the various assessment items. Because health-related fitness is not strongly linked to physical activity in young children, FitnessGram is recommended as a formal assessment tool for those in the fourth grade and beyond. Younger students should practice so that they become familiar with the various parts of health-related fitness and self-assessment, but scores should not be recorded. Standards of performance are not reliable before fourth grade.

As mentioned earlier, introducing, teaching, and practicing each assessment item before the official assessment day will benefit your students and help them better understand the importance of each component of health-related fitness. You can begin by integrating one assessment item into each instructional unit. For example, focusing on flexibility (e.g., back-saver sit-and-reach assessment item) would be appropriate during an educational gymnastics unit. During a fleeing and dodging unit, the health-related fitness focus might be placed on cardiorespiratory endurance and heart-rate recovery time. This approach helps students become familiar with each assessment item and teaches them how each health-related fitness component relates to an applied setting. For instance, you might turn on the PACER for a one-minute warm-up activity or use the curl-up test as a station. Students need to be formally taught how to complete the assessments, but they also need multiple opportunities to practice them. For this age group, the key is to make practice opportunities enjoyable and to give students options if they have difficulty performing an assessment so that they can progress to the point where they are able to correctly perform the assessment task.

Middle School and High School Students

Older students should be given increased responsibility for personal assessment with adequate supervision. Over-directing students sends the message that they may not be able to assess themselves or their peers independently. However, when properly trained in the protocols for assessing health-related fitness, middle school and high school students can often display responsible and mature behavior. Each student must develop complete understanding of the purpose of health-related fitness, as well as respect for the privacy of peers. Careful consideration must be given to the maturity and knowledge of each student. When students do take on increased responsibility, you become a facilitator and supervise the assessment environment. Providing students with opportunities to control the assessment environment reinforces the concept that they need to take personal responsibility for assessing and maintaining their personal health.

Reluctant or Overanxious Students

Some students may have had negative experiences with health-related fitness assessment in the past or may simply be more reserved or private than others. Moreover, reluctance and anxiety are common emotions in every assessment situation, but a positive environment for health-related fitness assessment can help prevent these emotions from developing further. One key to reducing these behaviors is to give students opportunities to practice each assessment item frequently over an extended period in a relaxed and safe atmosphere. Students may also feel more at ease if they are given a choice of assessment items that measure the same component—such as the PACER, the one-mile run, and the walk test for assessing cardiorespiratory endurance (for middle school or high school students)—and when they are given multiple opportunities to develop their capability in these areas. Student privacy must be ensured in regard to assessment scores, and students' feelings should be treated sensitively to reassure them that the focus is on personal achievement. Students will gain much from self-assessment practice but will gain little from being forced to perform in formal assessments, which could result in negative feelings about physical activity.

Students With Disabilities

In general, the definitions, components, assessment items, and standards of health-related fitness used for students with disabilities should be the same as for students without disabilities (Lacy & Hastad, 2007). When necessary, FitnessGram can be modified for students with disabilities, and information about how to do so can be found in chapter 4 of the *FitnessGram/ActivityGram Test Administration Manual* (Meredith & Welk, 2017).

As a complement to FitnessGram, the Brockport Physical Fitness Test (BPFT) assesses the health-related fitness of people with a wide range of physical and cognitive disabilities (Winnick & Short, 2014). The Brockport test was developed through Project Target, a research study funded by the U.S. Department of Education. It is a criterion-referenced assessment of health-related fitness for children of ages 10 through 17 and includes 27 assessment items specific to the areas of aerobic functioning, body composition, and musculoskeletal functioning. Many of the assessment items can be used as alternative items for standard health-related fitness assessments. Always review each student's IEP and consult with relevant service providers, such as physical, occupational, and speech therapists, so that you know the student's medical background.

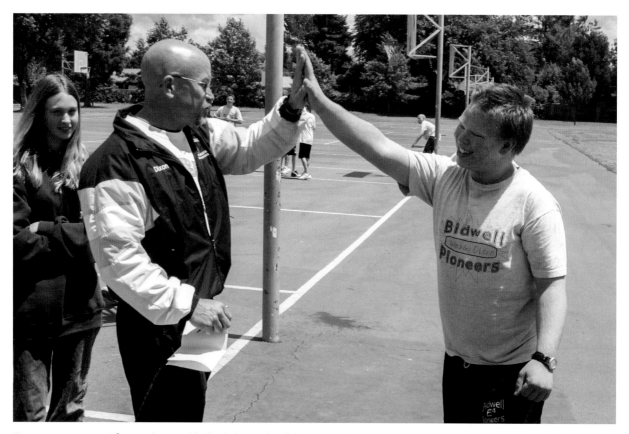

Fitness assessment for students with disabilities should measure the student's ability to function in everyday activities and should take into account the student's interests.

The *Brockport Physical Fitness Test Manual* (Winnick & Short, 2014) includes video clips, reproducible forms, and online calculators. For more information or to order the manual or other adapted physical education resources, contact Human Kinetics at 800-747-4457 or www.HumanKinetics.com.

When designing an individualized program for health-related fitness for a student with disabilities, remember that one major reason for health-related fitness assessment should be to measure a person's ability to function in everyday activities. Look at each individual, assess needs and limitations, and design alternatives to bypass those limitations. Take into account a person's interests as well. For example, if a person who uses a wheelchair would like to be able to play wheelchair basketball more proficiently and with greater stamina, then the fitness program should enhance the person's abilities in this area. Health-related fitness assessment should then discern whether the person is making progress in areas relevant to enjoying the chosen interest. It is also recommended that you personalize the assessment. You can identify each student's health-related concerns and then work with the student to select areas for assessment and decide which assessment items to use (Winnick, 2005).

Using Health-Related Fitness Results Appropriately

The main purposes of assessing health-related fitness are to teach students about health-related fitness and to use the assessment results to help set personal goals for health-related fitness and physical activity—not to grade students in physical education. To some extent, health-related fitness performance may be out of a student's control; in that case, holding the student accountable for that performance is inappropriate (Meredith & Welk, 2017). Both students and parents should understand the ways in which health-related fitness scores will, and will not, be used.

Student grades can be based on age-appropriate ability to self-assess, interpret assessment results, and set goals based on the results. Grading criteria might also include demonstrating understanding of health-related fitness concepts and principles, the importance of an active lifestyle, and knowing which activities contribute to health-related fitness. Table 13.1 provides a continuum of options that may be used either as formative assessments or as summative assessments (for use in determining a grade). These assessments include opportunities to demonstrate understanding of the importance of physical activity, which activities contribute to health-related fitness, and how to set goals and plan personal programs.

Such emphases help students become adults who are physically active for life in enjoyable, self-designed programs for health-related fitness. In contrast, grades based solely on assessment results are likely to discourage students from continuing to be physically active after they leave your program. Moreover, if you give credit for showing improvement in assessment scores for health-related fitness, remember that improvements will come in smaller increments for students who have already achieved a high level of health-related fitness; in other words, your grading system should not penalize high-fit students. Consider reporting the accomplishment of health-related fitness goals as the measure of success and the achievement of a health-enhancing level of physical activity as the basis for feedback to parents. Many teachers send home a grade for physical education and attach a separate FitnessGram report as the feedback related to health-related fitness. This method requires no extra work and is an authentic and appropriate means for reporting student assessment results.

TABLE 13.1   Sample Continuum of Health-Related Fitness Assessment

Grade	Sample lesson objectives	Alignment with National Standards and Grade-Level Outcomes	Sample goal	Possible assessment strategies
K–1	1. Demonstrate being moderate to vigorously physically active in physical education class. 2. Identify how the body responds to physical activity (e.g., faster heartbeat, harder breathing, increased strength).	S3.E2.1* S3.E3.K S3.E3.1*	To develop a basic understanding of the importance of a physically active lifestyle	• Informal: student self-rating of physical activity; checking for understanding (e.g., through use of handouts, verbal response) • Demonstration of activities that develop components of health-related fitness
2	1. Demonstrate being engaged and active in physical education class. 2. Demonstrate basic understanding of concepts of muscular strength, muscular endurance, and flexibility and ways to use the body to develop them. 3. Identify physical activities that contribute to fitness.	S3.E2.2* S3.E3.2a* S3.E3.2b*	To broaden understanding of health-related fitness and the importance of a physically active lifestyle	• Informal: self-reporting physical activity levels • Formal: demonstration of using the body as resistance to develop muscular strength; using the body to make a variety of shapes to maintain flexibility; handouts that allow students to select activities that contribute to health-related fitness
3	1. Demonstrate full participation in physical education class and participation in physical activity outside of physical education class. 2. Demonstrate basic understanding of the concept of health-related fitness and activities that enhance it. 3. Begin being able to demonstrate health-related fitness components by performing appropriate activities.	S3.E2.3* S3.E3.3* S3.E5.3*	To introduce health-related fitness components and ways to record physical activity participation outside of physical education class	• Formal: demonstration of understanding which activities enhance each type of health-related fitness; demonstration of each health-related fitness component; logging of physical activity outside of physical education class
4	1. Demonstrate active participation in physical education class and look for opportunities to increase participation in physical activity outside of class. 2. Demonstrate ability to identify health-related fitness components. 3. Introduce health-related fitness assessment (FitnessGram) administered by teacher. 4. Introduce ways to use fitness assessment results to determine what areas need improvement with teacher assistance.	S3.E1.4 S3.E2.4* S3.E3.4* S3.E5.4*	To introduce the testing procedure for health-related fitness (teacher administered) and ways to use results for remediation To provide accurate baseline data for fitness	• Formal or informal: paper-and-pencil identification of health-related fitness components; selection of appropriate activities aligned with health-related fitness components; teacher-assisted analysis of fitness assessment results; logging or journaling

Grade	Sample lesson objectives	Alignment with National Standards and Grade-Level Outcomes	Sample goal	Possible assessment strategies
5	1. Continue to participate actively in physical education and log and analyze physical activity outside of physical education in terms of benefits for health-related fitness. 2. Introduce informal self-testing checked by peer. 3. Introduce ways to use fitness testing results (self-assessed or teacher-assessed) to analyze results by comparing to Healthy Fitness Zones (FitnessGram). 4. With teacher assistance, introduce goal setting by identifying areas needing improvement and setting strategies for progress.	S3.E1.5 S3.E2.5* S3.E5.5a* S3.E5.5b*	To compare baseline data, provide more testing data, and ensure accuracy of self-testing To set physical activity and fitness goals based on results	• Formal or informal: peer analysis of self-testing; comparison of results with healthy fitness zones; development of goals (with teacher assistance) for areas needing improvement and setting of strategies for progress; logging and analysis of physical activity outside of physical education class
6	1. Continue to participate actively in physical education and in a variety of self-selected activities (including aerobic, lifetime, or recreational activities; team sports; outdoor pursuits; or dance outside of physical education). 2. Introduce informal self-testing of health-related fitness components checked by peer and teacher. 3. Begin to set and monitor physical activity goals based on current fitness level as determined by self-testing.	S3.M2.6 S3.M3.6 S3.M4.6 S3.M5.6* S3.M15.6*	To begin to use data for setting physical activity goals	• Formal: physical activity logs, goal setting, log that illustrates monitoring of goals; reflection
7	1. Continue to actively participate in physical education and in a variety of self-selected lifetime activities (e.g., sport, individual, dance, outdoor, aquatic) and health-related fitness activities outside of physical education. 2. Complete formal self-testing of health-related fitness components (checked by teacher). 3. Adjust physical activity goals based on current level of health-related fitness.	S3.M2.7 S3.M3.7 S3.M4.7 S3.M5.7* S3.M15.7*	To adjust physical activity goals based on current fitness levels	• Formal: physical activity logs; goal setting and analysis; appropriate adjustments based on current fitness level; reflection

(continued)

Table 13.1 *(continued)*

Grade	Sample lesson objectives	Alignment with National Standards and Grade-Level Outcomes	Sample goal	Possible assessment strategies
8	1. Continue to actively participate in physical education and in a variety of self-selected lifetime activities (e.g., sport, individual, dance, outdoor, aquatic) and health-related fitness activities outside of physical education. 2. Complete formal self-testing of health-related fitness components (not checked by teacher). 3. Demonstrate understanding of the overload principle and ability to adjust physical activity goals based on the FITT formula.	S3.M2.8 S3.M3.8 S3.M4.8 S3.M5.8* S3.M11.8*	To adjust physical activity goals using the overload principle and FITT formula	• Formal: physical activity log; goal setting that demonstrates adjustment of physical activity goals based on FITT formula; reflection
9-12	1. Continue to actively participate in physical education and in a variety of self-selected lifetime activities (e.g., dance, health-related fitness activity) outside of school. 2. Continue to formally self-test health-related fitness components (not checked by teacher). 3. Develop and implement individualized health-related fitness plan, including improvement goals, activity plan, and testing plan with timeline for improvement.	S3.H6.L1* S3.H12.L1 S3.H12.L2*	To develop and implement individualized fitness plan	• Formal: log and reflection on value of being physically active; development of individualized health-related fitness plan; implementation record or log of individualized health-related fitness plan

*The lesson objectives have been aligned with the appropriate Standard 3 Outcomes to illustrate consistency with the National Standards for K-12 Physical Education (SHAPE America, 2014).

Sharing Health-Related Fitness Information With Students and Parents

When sharing assessment feedback, use a balance of assessment tools across all domains so that students and parents can see how knowledge and appreciation can enhance physical development. Emphasize intrinsic over extrinsic motivators and handle affective assessment data in a sensitive manner so that students will feel comfortable and communicate honestly.

Approaching Parent–Teacher Conferences

Parent–teacher conferences provide an excellent way to share information. Interaction with parents or guardians provides the chance to convey information in a positive and caring manner. Conferences can be used to brainstorm ways to help the student and to identify types of physical activity that the whole family can enjoy. This element can be important in developing a program that holds value for students and their families.

Focus discussion on strategies to support student learning and on equipping parents with knowledge and suggestions for how to help their children learn.

When preparing for parent–teacher conferences consider the following tips (Harvard Family Research Project, 2010):

- *Send invitations.* Disseminate information about conferences to families using available sources such as newsletters, the school website, and email. Include information about the timing and goals of the conferences, as well as any alternative scheduling options.

- *Review student work.* Be prepared to go over student data, assignments, and assessments during the conferences. Think of what more you would like to learn about your students from their parents.

- *Prepare thoughts and materials.* Create an agenda or list of key issues you want to discuss about each student's progress and growth. Also consider creating a portfolio of student work to walk through with families during the conferences.

- *Send reminders.* The week before the conferences, send home a reminder of when and where they will be held. You may also want to include an outline of your agenda to prepare parents for the conferences.

- *Create a welcoming environment.* Make your gym or office comfortable for families by displaying student work, arranging seating in circles (with adult chairs, if possible), and establishing a private space for the conferences.

Remember that the parent–teacher conference provides an opportunity not only for parents to learn from you but also for you to learn from them. Their insights into their child's strengths and needs, learning styles, and nonschool learning opportunities can help you improve your instructional methods. At the same time, your effort to understand parents' perspectives makes them feel respected and builds trust. Remember also to emphasize the child's strengths and accomplishments; doing so shows parents that you value the unique strengths of their children and have high expectations for the child's ability to succeed in both school and life.

When reviewing assessment results with students and parents, take time to explain the reasons for the assessments and the significance of the results. With students, this discussion can be part of a **set induction** at the beginning of the lesson. Before conducting assessments, notify parents by means of a letter that explains the philosophy, approach, and use of the results. Reassure both students and parents that student privacy will be respected. Share the forms used to record and interpret the assessment results; the relevant forms are provided in the *FitnessGram/ActivityGram Test Administration Manual* (Meredith & Welk, 2017) and the associated software. Consider also holding a parent night that introduces the assessment protocols and sets the stage for clear, productive communication before and after assessment. To keep parents informed, you can include all of this information, as well as regular updates, on your physical education website. Parents can also obtain access to the 2015 FitnessGram software at www.MyHealthyZone.FitnessGram.net and logging in to access the parent dashboard. You can also have FitnessGram reports emailed directly to parents. For more information, go to https://help.fitnessgram.net/reports/generate-reports/.

Blank FitnessGram forms can be used to review the purpose and meaning of the assessment items and results. Distribute individual report forms privately—for instance, in a sealed envelope or during a student–teacher or parent–teacher conference. Another option is to set up a station in a physical activity circuit at which you privately discuss assessment results while the rest of the student's group participates in an activity. Along with providing assessment results and interpretations, you can also provide information and guidance to both students and parents about steps to take in order to maintain or improve health.

After health-related fitness testing, send home current FitnessGram and Activity-Gram printouts to provide information that links assessment to strategies and goals for each child. This information will help parents and guardians learn what they need to know in order to help their children accomplish personal goals. These strategies help individualize your approach. You can help students set goals based on feedback and on the student's personal objectives (see chapters 2 and 12). Brainstorming with the family to find ways to increase physical activity also opens lines of communication. Finally, sharing FitnessGram reports and goal setting can help parents and guardians become advocates for effective physical education.

Guidelines for Assessing Physical Activity

Assessing physical activity levels in physical education can be challenging. Perhaps as a result, many teachers report grading students on administrative tasks, such as dressing for activity, attendance, and participation (Young, 2011). Other studies show that effort is also included as a component of the grade in physical education. These practices lack reliability and consistency because students' assessment results for health-related fitness may vary widely even if they exhibit similar levels of effort, participation, attendance, and dressing appropriately for activity. Conversely, some students exhibit lower levels of effort, participation, attendance, or dressing appropriately for activity yet have assessment results in the healthy fitness zone. Students should be encouraged to set physical activity goals and should be rewarded and praised for achieving them or making progress toward achieving them. The FITT elements—frequency, intensity, time, and type—can be quantified and evaluated effectively through the review of student reflection, achievement of goals, and records of intensity and duration of activity.

There are a variety of ways to effectively monitor physical activity, whether it is performed in or outside of physical education. Pedometers are a common means of monitoring the total amount of physical activity (e.g., walking, running, skipping) performed daily. Many pedometers measure steps and physical activity time, and these measurements can provide students with accurate information for goal setting. In other words, students can use personalized scores to help them establish meaningful goals. Achieving these goals can be motivating. Other, more sophisticated means of tracking physical activity are also available, including heart rate monitors and accelerometers. Many of these devices come with software that can track heart rate over time and provide you and your students with real-time intensity levels during class. Others can count the number of steps taken or stairs climbed, as well as intensity levels. This information should be used to help students understand the effect of physical activity intensity levels on the heart rate or to set goals for increasing physical activity. These types of devices have also been shown to be effective in extrinsically motivating students to be active in physical education (Partridge, King, & Bian, 2011).

The **ActivityGram** portion of FitnessGram helps students understand how activity behaviors outside of school contribute to personal health and wellness. It is available within the student version of the FitnessGram software. ActivityGram helps students self-monitor their physical activity patterns so that they can see how active they truly are (Corbin et al., 2013, pp. 2-19, in Plowman & Meredith, 2013). ActivityGram provides a report that includes information about student activity levels over time, such as when they are most active and in what activities they regularly participate. These reports provide students, parents, and teachers with information that can be used to set goals for individualized activity plans. By self-managing their activity levels, students begin to learn skills that are essential to lifetime physical activity adherence (Dale & Corbin, 2000).

Physical activity assessments were added to FitnessGram to emphasize to students the importance of developing lifetime habits of regular physical activity. Although students' health-related fitness is important, they cannot maintain it unless they remain physically active. The ActivityGram assessment involves a recall of the student's physical activity, based on a validated physical activity instrument known as the Previous Day Physical Activity Recall (PDPAR; Weston, Petosa, & Pate, 1997). In the assessment, the student reports his or her activity levels for each 30-minute block of time during the day. The format uses a three-day recall consisting of two school days and one nonschool day. ActivityGram can be used with elementary, middle, and high school students, but because it requires self-reporting, the results are more accurate at the middle school and high school levels. However, it can still be used effectively at the elementary level to teach students the importance of self-tracking their activity levels (Meredith & Welk, 2017).

The online reporting system provides detailed information about the student's activity habits and prescriptive feedback about how active she or he should be. Students should begin using the ActivityGram program in the fifth grade.

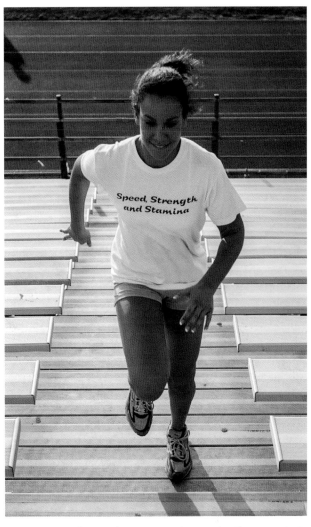

It's important for students to monitor and self-assess their physical activity outside of class as well as in class.

The goal of a physical education program is to develop a lifelong pattern of physical activity. But when it comes to health-related fitness measures, scores today do not necessarily indicate long-term results. A fifth grader born with the right genes might score well on the one-mile run without much effort, whereas a classmate might make a great effort but still record a slow time. However, if the student with the good mile-run time eventually becomes a couch potato, and the student with the poor time continues to spend time participating in a variety of activities, the latter student will likely live a healthier life.

Ultimately, physical educators want a nation of healthy, physically active citizens—not of ex-athletes who follow a couple of years of excellent health-related fitness levels with 50 years of sedentary behavior resulting in declining health, high medical bills, and poor productivity. Reward time or persistence in physical activity; in the long run, that is what results in lifelong health and fitness.

Encourage both results and time spent in physical activity. The FitnessGram criteria help teachers obtain appropriate results for a broad range of students. In addition, consider the following: Did the student with the best one-mile run time in class spend as much time in a target heart rate zone as the student who took longer to complete the same distance? Challenge the high-achieving students to do even better, to set higher goals for time and distance. Challenge each student to be his or her individual physical best and reward physical activity time.

Tools for Assessing Physical Activity

Effective strategies for assessing physical activity link the activity to health-related fitness concepts, such as overload. Students may appear to be active when you are casually observing them, but closer assessment of activity data is necessary to determine whether they are truly applying the fitness principles of overload, intensity, and specificity to make progress toward their goals for lifetime health-related fitness.

Logs and Journals

Logging physical activity information in a table, chart, or journal provides evidence of total time spent in physical activity. By itself, however, time does not necessarily demonstrate appropriate activity levels. Ratings of perceived exertion can be used by students to reflect how strenuous their physical activity bouts were. Using a 0-to-10 scale gives students a good idea of intensity level and provides them with information on which to base changes in their activity levels to reach desired outcomes. (See chapter 5 for information about the OMNI RPE scale.) Teach students that what matters are their personal feelings of effort—not how they compare with other students. Use the following strategies to gain student physical activity information:

- Teach students to use the rating of perceived exertion scale so that they can record this data in their logs or journals.
- Graph intensity levels with duration of activities. Encourage students who do not demonstrate changes over time to reexamine their goals and revise their strategies.
- Incorporate technology by asking students to use heart rate monitors and pedometers. Record indicators of intensity, such as heart rate or steps taken, over time.
- For younger students, the use of pictures (either drawings or photographs) can replace written physical activity logs.
- Involve parents or guardians by asking them to sign off periodically on their child's log or journal.

Heart Rate Monitors

Students can use **heart rate monitors** to assess the intensity of physical activity more accurately and to gain individualized feedback (Kirkpatrick & Birnbaum, 1997). Heart rate monitors can be used as tools for self-assessment of cardiorespiratory endurance. For example, a high school student may use the information from a heart rate monitor to determine that his or her heart rate is below the target heart rate during moderate walking. Learning that he or she can no longer elevate the heart rate into the target heart rate zone by walking fast, this student would be encouraged to choose a more intense level of activity. The student can determine how intensity needs to be adjusted in order to perform more vigorous cardiorespiratory endurance activity, such as jogging or in-line skating, to participate in the target heart rate zone.

Target heart rate zones are not effectively used for younger children (elementary through middle school), but heart rate monitors can still provide a way to motivate young students. For instance, they can examine resting heart rate before an activity and then compare it with their heart rate during exercise. Intermediate students can also participate in "Mini Triathlon" (available in the web resource) to compare resting and active heart rates and learn about the effects of activity on heart rate. Monitors differ in cost, accuracy, and ease of use. Pulse monitors are the least expensive and easiest to use. They work by completing an electrical circuit from one hand to another or one finger to another, thereby monitoring the heartbeat, which is displayed. Your approach with this sort of device can be as economical as buying one monitor for the whole class or providing individual monitors for students to wear on their wrists. These models are losing favor, however, to more accurate types.

More popular heart-rate monitors with photo plethysmography use a green light on the skin at the wrist to detect changes in capillary blood flow. The monitor uses light detectors to measure how much light is absorbed—the more absorbed, the higher the blood volume and the faster the heartbeat (for more detail, see the Fitbit website at https://www.fitbit.com/technology).

More accurate models use EKG technology by placing a transmitter on the chest, which sends information to a wrist receiver. This setup requires the use of a chest strap and therefore is more complicated to use. Any given chest strap should either be used by only one person or be cleaned between uses by different people.

Projection systems are available for both the photo plethysmography and the EKG types of monitors. This extension allows the heart rate to be projected to a remote screen, either individually or as a class. Various other features are also available to monitor steps, kilocalories, miles, sleep, energy balance, and sport-specific parameters. Although sophisticated devices are not necessary for teaching students about the components of health-related fitness, they can enable interactive and meaningful lessons.

Pedometers

Pedometers can provide authentic evaluation of daily physical activity (Pangrazi, Beighle, & Sidman, 2007). Specifically, they can be used as motivational tools to provide feedback about the duration (distance) or intensity (distance over time) of a physical activity. In terms of duration, Rowlands and Eston (2005) concluded that 8- to 10-year-old girls who accumulated 13,000 steps per day and boys who accumulated 12,000 steps per day engaged in sufficient amounts of physical activity to meet the 60-minute standard for a health-enhancing level of activity. However, because step counts vary greatly from day to day, monitoring weekly rather than daily can help prevent feelings of failure.

To begin, ask students to keep track of their daily step counts in a journal and average the counts from the first three days. Then ask them to use this average as a baseline for setting personal goals for their walking program. They can work up to the long-range goals established by the President's Challenge of 11,000 steps per day for girls (ages 6 through 17) and 13,000 steps per day for boys (also ages 6 through 17). In addition, children can encourage their family members to set daily step goals (generally, 10,000 steps per day for adults, or 12,000 if weight loss is a personal goal). This encouragement may increase family activity outside of school time. To help students set step goals, refer to table 13.2.

Pedometers may report steps taken, distance covered, calories burned, time spent exercising, or heart rate averaged over time. The simplest ones only count steps. Some have the capacity to be adjusted for stride length. For an average adult, 10,000 steps translates to about 3 miles (4.8 km), but the distance will differ for children. Teachers can instruct students about how to determine the number of steps per mile or kilometer. To find the number of steps in a mile, mark off a distance of 100 feet and ask students to count the number of steps that they take in that distance. Find the distance between two heel strikes, or **stride length**, by dividing 100 feet by the number of steps taken. Then divide 5,280 feet by the stride length to estimate the

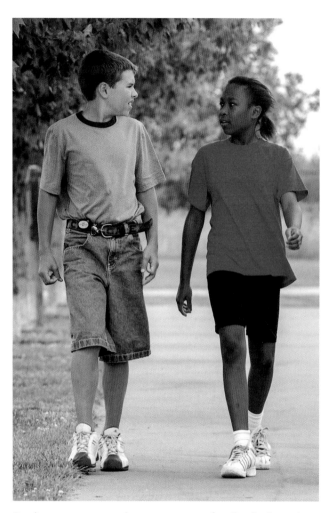

Students can use pedometers to get feedback about how much physical activity they are getting.

student's number of steps per mile. Similarly, to find the number of steps taken in a kilometer, mark off 30 meters and ask students to count the number of steps that they take to cover that distance. Find stride length, or the distance between two heel strikes, by dividing 30 meters by the number of steps taken. Then divide 1,000 meters by the stride length to estimate the student's steps per kilometer. Providing the formula and task to the math teacher is an excellent strategy for sharing content across the curriculum and informing other teachers about quality physical education at the same time.

Note that the distance measured by a pedometer is based on the number of steps taken and the stride length programmed into the device. Therefore, error can sneak in if stride length changes with the speed of a walk or run. In addition, spring-loaded pedometers tend to underestimate the number of steps taken at a slow pace—that is, about 2 miles per hour (54 m/min) (Crouter et al., 2003; Le Masurier, Lee, & Tudor-Locke, 2004). At a slow pace, people may not produce enough vertical motion to trigger a step count (Beets, Patton, & Edwards, 2005; Crouter et al., 2003). Therefore, teachers who encourage their students to move briskly help ensure a more accurate step count. Young children with less bounce in their steps may still lose steps, as will those with unusual gait patterns. If a pedometer is ineffective with a student's gait pattern (or use of a wheelchair), the student can be paired with another, and the count from the student with the

typical gait can be used for both students. Additionally, students in wheelchairs can use accelerometers instead of pedometers as a means to measure physical activity and energy expenditure (Gendle et al., 2011).

The recommended location for a pedometer is at the waistline, directly in line with the midpoint of the front of the thigh. However, if abdominal fat or a loose waistband allows a spring-loaded pedometer to tilt forward 10 degrees or more, then the step count will become less accurate and an alternative location may work better (Crouter, Schneider, & Bassett, 2005; Duncan et al., 2007). One solution for this problem is to place the pedometer on an elastic belt, which also solves the problem of fitting the pedometer clip over a waistband edge that is too thick. A student can also move the pedometer to the side or to the small of the back. Count steps and check the pedometer to see which location gives the most accurate count. In some cases, moving the pedometer to the side or back may solve the problem of pedometer tilt but leave the student unable to read the pedometer independently.

To test pedometer placement and accuracy, Cuddihy, Pangrazi, and Tomson (2005) recommend placing the pedometer on the waistband above the midpoint of the right thigh, walking 100 steps, and then checking the pedometer count. If the pedometer count is off by 3 or more steps, place it more to the right (slightly in front of or over the hip) and repeat the test. If the count is still off by 3 or more steps, place the pedometer on the waistband to the back or on an elastic belt. This test assumes that the pedometer is accurate within 3 steps when properly placed. In one study, three

TABLE 13.2 Setting Step Goals

Start point	Goal	How to reach goal	Time needed
<2,500 steps	5,000 steps per day	Increase by 250 steps per day.	10-20 days
2,501-5,000 steps	7,500 steps per day	Increase by 300 steps per day.	8-16 days
5,001-7,500 steps	10,000 steps per day	Increase by 400 steps per day.	6-12 days
7,501-10,000 steps	12,500 steps per day	Increase by 500 steps per day.	5-10 days
10,001-12,501 steps	15,000 steps per day	Increase by 500 steps per day.	5-10 days

From Sportline's Guide to Walking (Sportline, Inc., Campbell, CA)

styles of voice-announcement pedometers (for students with visual impairments) worked best when worn on the right side (Beets et al., 2007).

Pedometers currently available offer a variety of tracking features, including steps, distance, calories, continuous-minute bouts, and total activity time. Select a pedometer type based on the reliability of the features used most. Then put them to use; many creative, instructional, and motivating lessons can be generated using pedometers (Lubans, Morgan, & Tudor-Locke, 2009; Pangrazi, Beighle, & Sidman, 2007).

Physical Activity Trackers

Trackers of health-related fitness and physical activity offer another means of assessing physical activity levels, both at home and in physical education. More and more trackers have come onto the market that are designed specifically for children (ages four and up) and can be used by school-age students to track their physical activity while at home. Common features include the capacity to track activity time and steps, and some include swim tracking, reminders, and rewards. While these devices can serve as effective tools for motivating and assessing physical activity outside of physical education, more sophisticated models can monitor heart rates and activity levels during class and may include software for monitoring of health-related fitness levels, record keeping, and assessment. These devices can be used to motivate students, make them accountable, and, more important, help students learn to self-manage their physical activity, which can lead them toward a healthy and physically active lifestyle.

Step-count wristbands use more sophisticated motion detectors and often offer other features such as GPS and heart rate monitoring. Wearable technology not only provides integrated information and quick activity logging but also links to social media, thus allowing students to compete with or cheer on classmates.

One of the biggest drawbacks of pedometers and some wristbands consists of their inability to estimate intensity; for example, 1,000 walking steps count the same as 1,000 running steps despite the obvious difference in intensity. To address this lack, some devices now allow students to collect not only the number of steps taken but also the amount of time (minutes) for which they are active. Older students can be taught to divide their total number of steps by the number of minutes for which they are active in order to determine their steps per minute (SPM). Extending our example of 1,000 steps, a student might take 1,000 steps in 10 minutes (1,000/10 = 100 SPM) or 1,000 steps in 20 minutes (1,000/20 = 50 SPM). The assumption is that the more steps a person takes per minute, the more intense the activity is during that session.

Tracking both step count and heart rate offers an ideal way to combine the concepts of time (distance traveled) with intensity. Increasing either the number of steps or the heart rate provides the overload needed for appropriate progressions to enhance cardiorespiratory endurance.

In one study, Graser, Pangrazi, and Vincent (2009) tested 10- through 12-year-olds walking on a treadmill at moderate to vigorous paces and determined that a range of

120 to 140 SPM for both sexes serves as a reasonable measure of moderate to vigorous physical activity. However, members of certain populations, such as those with high levels of body fat, may benefit more from trying to improve their SPM than from using the 120 to 140 guideline. Devices with the steps-per-minute feature offer an excellent way to teach all students about intensity, baseline recording, and goal setting.

Summary

When teachers authentically assess health-related fitness and physical activity, students can begin to see that health and physical activity are related. You can use each component to monitor students' health-related fitness and help them reduce risk factors. Involve students in recording time, duration, intensity, and type of physical activity to encourage self-assessment. Teach students how to use the results of assessments for health-related fitness and physical activity to set goals for improving their health-related fitness and increasing their physical activity. When you use assessment to help students learn about their own health-related fitness—and how to maintain or make improvements in their level of physical activity—you help them become their physical best and guide them toward physical literacy.

Discussion Questions

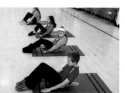

1. List four characteristics of the FitnessGram assessment that make it an appropriate choice for assessing students in grades 4 through 12.
2. How can teachers help students develop personal responsibility and become self-directed in living a physically active lifestyle?
3. Describe ways in which a teacher can create effective practice opportunities to help students improve performance assessment items for health-related fitness.
4. List and explain four strategies that physical education teachers can use to increase student adherence to protocols for health-related fitness assessment.
5. For each of the following scenarios, identify which assessment item or items for cardiorespiratory endurance would be the most appropriate and why:
    1. Student who is very aerobically fit
    2. Student who has a low level of aerobic fitness
    3. Limited space in which to implement the PACER test
6. List two alternative means of assessment for each of the following:
    1. Body composition
    2. Upper-body strength and endurance
7. Describe ways in which K-2 physical educators could introduce health-related fitness concepts to their students.
8. Describe ways in which grade 4 physical educators could introduce FitnessGram to their students.
9. Discuss appropriate and inappropriate ways to use health-related fitness assessment in grading.
10. Select a grade level and discuss ways in which you would assess your students' level of physical activity both in and beyond physical education class.

Glossary

active stretch—Stretch in which the person who is stretching provides the force by contracting the opposing (antagonist) muscle.

ActivityGram—Feature of FitnessGram that provides physical activity assessments, including detailed information about the student's activity habits and prescriptive feedback about how active he or she should be.

aerobic activity—Activity that requires the use of oxygen to produce energy for movement.

aerobic capacity—The maximum amount of oxygen that the body is able to use to produce work.

affective domain—One's attitudes, values, and sense of personal responsibility regarding physical activity.

anaerobic activity—Activity that consists of movements fueled by energy stored in the body.

anorexia nervosa—Potentially fatal disease characterized by self-induced starvation and extreme weight loss.

assessment—Continuous collection and interpretation of information about student behaviors to facilitate students' improvement in specific areas.

ballistic stretching—Stretching that involves moving quickly, bouncing, or using momentum to produce the stretch.

binge eating—Eating disorder not otherwise specified and characterized by recurrent binge eating without regular use of compensatory measures to counter the eating.

biological age—Age as an indicator of a student's developmental status.

bodybuilding—Sport in which competitors are judged on muscle size, symmetry, and definition.

body composition—Amount of lean body mass as compared with amount of body fat, typically expressed in terms of percent body weight (i.e., fat as a percent of weight).

body mass index (BMI)—Ratio of height to weight that correlates with body fat in the general population.

bran—Fiber-containing portion of a whole grain.

bulimia—Eating disorder characterized by a destructive cycle of bingeing and purging of food.

carbohydrate—Category of nutrient that provides four kilocalories per gram and is the preferred source of energy for the body, particularly the brain.

cardiorespiratory endurance—The ability to perform large-muscle, whole-body exercise at a moderate to high intensity for extended periods of time.

chronological age—Age in years.

circuit training—Training that involves several different exercises or activities and allows variation in intensity or type of activity from station to station.

cognitive domain—One's knowledge, comprehension, and ability to apply, analyze, synthesize, and evaluate.

complex carbohydrate—Foods such as whole-grain pasta, cereal, and bread that supply sustained energy.

concentric contraction—Muscle-shortening contraction.

continuous activity—Movement that lasts at least several minutes without rest.

cool-down—Period of light activity that follows more intense activity and allows the body to slow down and gradually return to near-resting levels, thus enabling proper blood flow back to the heart, reducing muscle stiffness, removing lactic acid, and preventing light-headedness, dizziness, and fainting.

cooperative learning—Teaching style that involves students in working together to complete a specified task or assignment.

criterion-referenced health standard—Standard that uses scientific information to determine the amount of fitness needed in order to meet or exceed minimal health levels.

cue word—Key term or phrase that a student repeats while executing a skill in order to learn the vocabulary that goes with the actions.

developmentally appropriate physical activity—Activity that is appropriate for a student's developmental level, age, ability, interests, knowledge, and previous experience.

diabetes—A condition in which the body does not produce or effectively use insulin.

duration—Amount of time for which an activity is or should be performed.

dynamic stretching—Movement of body parts that gradually increases range of motion, speed of movement, or both.

eating patterns—The combination of foods and beverages that a person consumes and the person's usual intake over time.

eccentric contraction—Muscle-lengthening contraction, also known as *negative exercise*.

ecological task analysis—A type of task analysis where, in addition to breaking a skill into smaller parts, consideration is given to the student's preferences related to the task, the skill, and the learner.

endosperm—The portion of a whole grain that contains mostly starch (carbohydrate) and protein.

essential nutrient—Nutrient that must be obtained from food because the body cannot make it.

exercise—Physical activity that is planned and structured and involves repetitive body movement to improve or maintain one or more of the components of health-related fitness.

exercise-induced asthma—Narrowing of the airways that is brought on by exercise and characterized by symptoms include wheezing, coughing, chest tightness, and breathlessness.

exercise prescription—The process of designing an individualized physical activity program to improve health, health-related fitness, and sport performance.

extrinsic motivation—Desire to perform a particular task based on environmental or other personal influences that promise a desired object or socially enhancing consequence, thus increasing the likelihood that a behavior will be repeated.

fartlek training—Modification of continuous training in which periods of increased intensity are interspersed into continuous activity over varying and natural terrain; also referred to as *speed play*.

fat—Category of nutrient that provides nine kilocalories per gram.

FitnessGram—Health-related fitness assessment and computerized reporting system endorsed for use with the Physical Best program.

FITT guidelines—Guidelines for safely applying the five principles of training (overload, progression, specificity, regularity, and individuality) by manipulating the frequency, intensity, time, and type of activity.

flexibility—Ability to move a joint through its complete range of motion.

frequency—How often a person performs an activity.

functional training—Training that is designed to increase muscular strength while emphasizing flexibility, balance, and coordination of movements in multiple planes.

Gardner's theory of multiple intelligences—Learning theory asserting that different individuals are strong in different intelligences, including bodily-kinesthetic, spatial, interpersonal, musical, logical-mathematical, intrapersonal, naturalistic, and linguistic.

germ—The part of a whole grain that contains most of the vitamins and minerals, plus a tiny amount of healthy fat.

grade—Value assigned to the product based on performance.

growth plate—Section of cartilage found at the end of a long bone in children.

health-related fitness—Ability to perform physical activities that is partly inherent and partly developed through regular exercise and that involves aerobic fitness, muscular strength, muscular endurance, flexibility, and body composition as they relate specifically to health enhancement.

healthy fitness zone (HFZ)—Range of fitness scores associated with good health in Fitness-Gram based on criterion-referenced standards that represent age- and gender-appropriate fitness levels for children.

heart rate monitor—Device that provides heart-rate data.

heart rate reserve (HRR)—Difference between a person's maximal heart rate and resting heart rate.

high-intensity interval training (HIIT)—A workout consisting of very hard bouts of exercise followed by a rest or active-recovery interval.

hyperextension—Movement of a joint well beyond its normal range of motion (extension), which can increase the risk of developing joint laxity and may cause injury.

hyperflexion—Movement of a joint well beyond its normal range of motion (flexion), which can increase the risk of developing joint laxity and may cause injury.

hyperglycemia—High blood sugar.

hypermobility—Excessive range of motion at a joint, which predisposes a person to injury.

hypertrophy—Increase in muscle size.

hypoglycemia—Low blood sugar.

inclusion—Process of creating a learning environment open to and effective for students whose needs and abilities fall outside the general range of similar-age children or whose cultural or religious beliefs differ from those of the majority group.

individuality principle—Principle of training that accounts for the fact that individuals begin at different levels of fitness, that each person has personal goals and objectives for physical activity and fitness, and that individuals have different genetic potentials for change.

intensity—How hard a person exercises during a given period of physical activity, the level of which should be determined based on the person's age, fitness level, and fitness goals.

interval training—Training that involves alternating short bursts of activity with rest periods.

intrinsic motivation—Internal desire to perform a particular task.

journal—Account written from the perspective of an individual and often reflecting on daily events or logged activities.

kettlebell—Ball-shaped weight that comes in any of various sizes and, when lifted and controlled, forces the muscles in the entire body (especially the core) to contract together, thus building strength and stability at the same time.

lanugo—Downy layer of hair that grows as a side effect of anorexia nervosa.

laxity—Abnormal motion of a given joint when the ligaments connecting bone to bone no longer provide stability.

log—Systematic record or accounting of behavior (usually without reflection) used mainly to record performance and participation data, thus providing a baseline record of behaviors that can be used to help set personal goals related to exercise frequency, intensity, duration, or type.

macronutrient—Any one of the three types of nutrients—carbohydrate, protein, and fat—that provide the most energy.

maximal heart rate (MHR)—Fastest rate at which a person's heart can beat, which is used to determine appropriate exercising heart rate for monitoring training intensity and is calculated through the following formula: $207 - (0.7 \times age)$.

medicine ball—Heavy ball used in muscular fitness activities that weighs between 1 and 20 pounds (0.5 and 9 kg) and is made of leather or rubber.

micronutrient—Vitamin or mineral that is required in the human diet in a very small amount.

moderate physical activity—Activity of an intensity equal to brisk walking that can be performed for a relatively long period without fatigue.

muscular endurance—Ability of a muscle or muscle group to repeatedly exert submaximal force.

muscular fitness—In the Physical Best program, a combination of muscular strength and muscular endurance.

muscular power—Ability to exert force rapidly, which can be calculated as force multiplied by distance divided by time.

muscular strength—Ability of a muscle or muscle group to exert maximal force against a resistance one time through the full range of motion.

muscular–tendon unit—Area where muscle and tendon connect to bone and which can be lengthened by stretching.

normative standard—Standard that allows comparison to others in a group but does not provide information about how the values relate to individual health.

obesity—Condition of excess body fat, typically defined as 120 percent of ideal body weight or more.

one-repetition maximum (1RM)—Amount of weight that can be lifted one time through the full range of motion; measure not recommended for children but possible to determine indirectly by performing either a 10RM or 12RM and then using a reference table to estimate the 1RM.

overload principle—Principle holding that a body system (cardiorespiratory, muscular, or skeletal) must perform at a level beyond normal in order to adapt and improve physiological function and fitness.

overtraining—Condition caused by training too much or too intensely, thus not allowing sufficient recovery time, and producing symptoms such as lack of energy, decreased performance, fatigue, depression, aching muscles, loss of appetite, and proneness to injury.

passive stretch—Stretch assisted by a force other than that of the opposing (antagonist) muscle, whether provided by the stretching person, a partner, gravity, or an implement.

peak bone mass—The maximum amount of bone a person will ever have.

pedometer—Device used to count steps taken.

peer assessment—Assessment in which students analyze the performance of other students.

performance task—A task that describes what students should know and be able to do at the end of the unit.

physical activity—Any bodily movement produced by skeletal muscle that results in expenditure of energy.

phytonutrient—Organic plant component thought to promote health and protect humans against certain cancers, heart disease, and age-related macular degeneration.

Pilates—A series of organized exercises that can improve flexibility; created by Joseph Pilates in the early 20th century.

plyometrics—Muscular fitness training technique used to develop explosive power by pre-stretching the muscle (contracting it eccentrically) before engaging in concentric contraction and often involving hops, jumps, and throws.

portfolio—Collection of a student's work, usually combining student-chosen and required material, that demonstrates achievement of program goals.

power—The peak force of a skeletal muscle multiplied by the velocity of the muscle contraction.

powerlifting—Competitive sport involving the deadlift, the squat, and the bench press.

process measurements—Measurements that assess the use of correct form or technique.

product measurements—Measurements that score the outcome or result of the assessment performance.

progression principle—Principle holding that proper progression of overload involves a gradual increase in the level of activity, which is manipulated by increasing frequency, intensity, time, or some combination of these components.

proprioceptive neuromuscular facilitation (PNF)—Static stretch that combines active and passive stretching techniques and generally involves precontraction of the muscle to be stretched and contraction of the antagonist muscle during the stretch.

protein—Type of nutrient that provides four kilocalories per gram and is used primarily for cell growth and replacement.

psychomotor domain—Skills and motor or movement patterns commonly assessed during drills, skill tests, and gamelike activities.

purging—Use of laxatives, vomiting, or diuretics to prevent absorption of calories and weight gain.

range of motion—The degree of movement that occurs at a joint.

regularity principle—Principle holding that physical activity must be performed on a regular basis in order to be effective and that long periods of inactivity can lead to loss of benefits achieved during training.

repetitions—Number of times an exercise is performed during one set.

resistance band—Elastic band or cord used to add resistance to any movement; bands can vary in length and thickness, which can change the level of resistance.

resistance training (strength training)—Systematic, planned program that uses various methods (e.g., body weight, tension bands) or kinds of equipment (e.g., machines, free weights) and progressively stresses the musculoskeletal system in order to improve muscular strength, endurance, or power.

resting energy expenditure (REE)—Energy used by the body at rest.

restrictive anorexia nervosa—A form of anorexia nervosa characterized by limited food intake without binge eating and purging.

rubric—Scoring tool, ranging in complexity from a checklist to a holistic tool, that identifies the criteria used for judging student performance and can be used to assess skills, attitudes, and knowledge.

saturated fat—Fat that tends to be hard at room temperature, comes predominantly from animal sources, and is the main contributor to high cholesterol.

self-assessment—Assessment method wherein students use rubrics, journals, or logs to monitor their own progress.

set induction—Teacher actions taken at the beginning of a learning activity to help students focus attention and understand the lesson's purpose; also known as *anticipatory set*.

simple carbohydrate—Food that is high in sugar (e.g., candy, soda pop).

skill-related fitness—Fitness consisting of components (including agility, balance, coordination, power, reaction time, and speed) that often go hand in hand with certain physical activities and are necessary for a person to accomplish or enhance performance of a skill or task; sometimes referred to as *sport-related fitness*.

skinfold—Double layer of skin and subcutaneous fat measured to assess body composition.

skinfold caliper—Device used to measure a skinfold in body composition assessment.

specificity principle—Principle holding that one must perform specific activities targeting a particular body system in order to bring about fitness changes in that area.

spotting—Technique wherein someone helps ensure the safety of a person performing an exercise or activity.

stability ball—Large, inflatable ball used as exercise equipment that is comfortable, highly supportive, generally heavy duty, and capable of holding large amounts of weight.

stages of change (transtheoretical model)—Model of behavioral change that focuses on one's motivation to change in terms of stages of readiness and awareness; identifies typical behaviors at each stage; and provides recommendations for moving through the stages, including precontemplation, contemplation, preparation, action, and maintenance.

static stretch—Slow, sustained stretch of a muscular–tendon unit that is held for 10 to 30 seconds just short of the point of mild discomfort.

stride length—Distance between two heel strikes.

target heart rate zone (THRZ)—The optimal range of exercise intensities for improving cardiorespiratory endurance when using continuous aerobic endurance training.

task analysis—Process that involves breaking a task into its component parts to help determine the level and type of support that must be provided for a person to learn the task.

tidal volume—Volume of air either inhaled or exhaled in a normal resting breath.

time—How long an activity is performed (duration).

traditional task analysis—A type of task analysis in which motor skills are divided into discrete and underlying parts.

training adaptation—Basic physiological change that occurs over the course of a training period.

training age—Age associated with how long the student has been working out with a teacher.

trans fat—Type of unhealthy fat resulting from hydrogenation of vegetable oil.

type—Mode or kind of activity that a person chooses to perform in each area of health-related fitness.

underweight—Condition in which a person weighs less than 90 percent of ideal body weight or has a body mass index lower than the 5th percentile.

unsaturated fat—Fat that is liquid at room temperature, comes from plant sources, can help lower cholesterol level, and is beneficial when consumed in moderation.

ventilation—Movement of air into and out of the lungs, the volume of which is generally expressed in liters per minute and calculated by multiplying respiratory rate by tidal volume.

vigorous physical activity—Movement that expends more energy or is performed at a higher intensity than brisk walking.

volume—In muscular fitness, the number of sets and repetitions in a workout.

warm-up—Low-intensity activity performed before a full-effort or main activity in order to prepare the body for the intense activity by improving muscle function, maximizing blood flow to the muscles, and improving flexibility.

weightlifting—Competitive sport involving maximal lifts.

yogic stretching—Unique stretching maneuvers that are mainly static and focus primarily on the trunk musculature.

References

Chapter 1

American College of Sports Medicine. (2013). *ACSM's guide to exercise prescription and testing*. Philadelphia, PA: Lippincott Williams & Wilkins.

Caspersen, C.J., Powell, K.E., & Christenson, G.M. (1985). Physical activity, exercise, and physical fitness: Definitions and distinctions for health-related research. *Public Health Report, 100*(2), 126-131.

Centers for Disease Control and Prevention. (2010a). *Strategies to improve the quality of physical education*. Atlanta, GA: U.S. Department of Health and Human Services. https://www.cdc.gov/healthyyouth/physicalactivity/pdf/quality_pe.pdf

Centers for Disease Control and Prevention. (2010b). *The association between school-based physical activity, including physical education, and academic achievement*. Atlanta, GA: U.S. Department of Health and Human Services.

The Cooper Institute. (2017). *FitnessGram administration manual* (5th ed.). Champaign, IL: Human Kinetics.

Corbin, C.B., Welk, G.J., Richardson, C., Vowell, C., Lambdin, D., & Wikgren, S. (2014). Youth physical fitness: Ten key concepts. *Journal of Physical Education, Recreation and Dance, 85*(2), 24-31.

Faigenbaum, A.D., Kraemer, W.J., Blimkie, C.J., Jeffreys, I., Michell, L.J., Nitka, M., & Rowland, T. (2009). Youth resistance training: Updated position statement paper from the National Strength and Conditioning Association. *Journal of Strength and Conditioning Research, 23*(Suppl. 5), S60-S79.

Institute of Medicine. (2012). *Fitness measures and health outcomes in youth*. Washington, DC: National Academies Press.

Institute of Medicine. (2013). *Educating the student body: Taking physical activity and physical education to school*. Washington, DC: National Academy of Sciences.

Le Masurier, G., & Corbin, C. (2006). Top 10 reasons for quality physical education. *Journal of Physical Education, Recreation and Dance, 77*(6), 44-53.

Lewallen, T.C., Hunt, H., Potts-Datema, W., Zaza, S., & Giles, W. (2015). The whole school, whole community, whole child model: A new approach for improving educational attainment and healthy development for students. *Journal of School Health, 85*(11), 729-739. https://doi.org/10.1111/josh.12310

National Association for Sport and Physical Education (NASPE). (2004). *Moving into the future: National standards for physical education* (2nd ed.). Reston, VA: Author.

SHAPE America. (2014). *National standards & grade-level outcomes for K-12 physical education*. Champaign, IL: Human Kinetics.

SHAPE America. (2015). *Position statement: Comprehensive school physical activity programs: Helping all students log 60 minutes of physical activity each day*. www.shapeamerica.org/advocacy/positionstatements/pa/index.cfm

SHAPE America. (2016). *Shape of the nation: Status of physical education in the USA*. www.shapeamerica.org/shapeofthenation

U.S. Department of Health and Human Services (USDHHS). (2008). *2008 Physical activity guidelines for Americans*. Washington, DC: Author. https://health.gov/paguidelines/guidelines

U.S. Department of Health and Human Services (USDHHS). (2014). *Healthy People 2020 leading health indicators: Progress update*. http://www.healthypeople.gov/2020/LHI/LHI-ProgressReport-ExecSum.pdf

U.S. Department of Health and Human Services (USDHHS). (2018). *2018 Physical Activity Guidelines Advisory Committee scientific report*. Washington, DC: Author.

U.S. Department of Health and Human Services, Centers for Disease Control and Prevention, National Center for Chronic Disease Prevention and Health Promotion. (1999). *Physical activity and health: A report of the surgeon general*. Atlanta, GA: Author.

Chapter 2

American Heart Association. (2015). *Physical education in public schools* [fact sheet]. Washington, DC: American Heart Association. www.heart.org/idc/groups/heart-public/@wcm/@adv/documents/downloadable/ucm_474319.pdf

Bandura, A. (1986). *Social foundations of thought and action*. Englewood Cliffs, NJ: Prentice Hall.

Batchelder, A., & Matusitz, J. (2014). "Let's Move" campaign: Applying the extended parallel process model. *Social Work in Public Health, 29*(5), 462-472. doi:10.1080/19371918.2013.865110

Birch, D.A., & Videto, D.M. (Eds.). (2015). *Promoting health and academic success: The whole school, whole community, whole child approach*. Champaign, IL: Human Kinetics.

Cardinal, B.J. (2000). Are sedentary behaviors terminable? *Journal of Human Movement Studies, 38,* 137-150.

Carlson, T.B. (1995). We hate gym: Student alienation from physical education. *Journal of Teaching in Physical Education, 14,* 467-477.

Carron, A.V., Hausenblas, H.A., & Estabrooks, P.A. (2003). *The psychology of physical activity*. New York, NY: McGraw-Hill.

Carson, R.L., & Webster, C.A. (2020). *Comprehensive school physical activity programs: Putting evidence-based research into practice*. Champaign, IL: Human Kinetics.

Centers for Disease Control and Prevention. (2013). *Comprehensive school physical activity programs: A guide for schools*. Atlanta, GA: U.S. Department of Health and Human Services.

Centers for Disease Control and Prevention. (2015). *Trends in the prevalence of physical activity and sedentary behaviors. National YRBS: 1991-2015*. https://www.cdc.gov/healthychildren and adolescents/ data/yrbs/pdf/2015/2015_yrbs-data-users-guide.pdf

Centers for Disease Control and Prevention. (2016a). *Adult obesity causes & consequences*. https:// www.cdc.gov/obesity/adult/causes.html

Centers for Disease Control and Prevention. (2016b). *Nutrition, physical activity, and obesity data, trends, and maps*. www.cdc.gov/nccdphp/DNPAO/index.html

Committee on Physical Activity and Physical Education in the School Environment; Food and Nutrition Board; Institute of Medicine; Kohl, H.W., & Cook, H.D. (Eds.). (2013a). *Educating the student body: Taking physical activity and physical education to school*. Washington, DC: National Academies Press. Available from https://www.ncbi.nlm.nih.gov/books/NBK201493/

Committee on Physical Activity and Physical Education in the School Environment; Food and Nutrition Board; Institute of Medicine; Kohl, H.W., & Cook, H.D. (Eds.). (2013b). *Educating the student body: Taking physical activity and physical education to school*. Washington, DC: National Academies Press. Available from https://www.ncbi.nlm.nih.gov/books/NBK201496/

Cox, A.E., Smith, A.L., & Williams, L. (2008). Change in physical education motivation and physical activity behavior during middle school. *Journal of Adolescent Health, 43*(5), 506-513. doi:10.1016/j.jadohealth.2008.04.020

Davies, B., Nambiar, N., Hemphill, C., Devietti, E., Massengale, A., & McCredie, P. (2015). Intrinsic motivation in physical education. *Journal of Physical Education, Recreation and Dance, 86*(8), 8-13. doi:10.1080/07303084.2015.1075922

Davison, K.K., Downs, D.S., & Birch, L.L. (2006). Pathways linking perceived athletic competence and parental support at age 9 years to girls' physical activity at age 11 years. *Research Quarterly in Exercise and Sport, 77*(1), 23-31.

Dobbins, M., Husson, H., DeCorby, K., & LaRocca, R.L. (2013). School-based physical activity programs for promoting physical activity and fitness in children and adolescents aged 6 to 18. *Cochrane Database of Systematic Reviews, 2,* article no. CD007651.

Ebert, M. (2012). Yoga in the classroom. *Green Teacher, 97,* 3-8.

Fakhouri, T.H.I., Hughes, J.P., Burt, V.L., Song, M., Fulton, J.E., & Ogden, C.L. (2014). Physical activity in U.S. youth aged 12-15 years, 2012. *NCHS Data Brief, 141*. Hyattsville, MD: National Center for Health Statistics.

Fryar, C.D., Carroll, M.D., & Ogden, C.L. (2014). Prevalence of overweight and obesity among children and adolescents: United States, 1963-1965 through 2011-2012. *Health E-Stat*. Washington, DC: National Center for Health Statistics, Department of Health and Human Services.

Gentile, D.A., Welk, G., Eisenmann, J.C., Reimer, R.A., Walsh, D.A., Russell, D.W., . . . Fritz, K. (2009). Evaluation of a multiple ecological level child obesity prevention program: Switch what you do, view, and chew. *BMC Medicine, 7*(49), 1-12.

Greenberg, J.D. (2011). Let's move! Miami. *Strategies, 24*(5), 6-7.

Herman, K.C., Reinke, W.M., Frey, A.J., & Shepard, S.A. (2013). *Motivational interviewing in schools: Strategies for engaging parents, teachers, and students.* New York, NY: Springer.

Institute of Medicine. (2013). *Educating the student body: Taking physical activity and physical education to school.* Washington, DC: Author.

Kulik, K.S., Brewer, H., Windish, L., & Carlson, H. (2017). Strategies for achieving the new SHAPE America standards and grade-level outcomes: Bringing obstacle course training into physical education. *Strategies, 30*(1), 35-42. doi.org/10.1080/08924562.2016.1251865

Kulinna, P.H., Stylianou, M., Lorenz, K.A., Conrad, C.A., Moss, R.C., Yu, H., & Mohan, A. (2016). Physical activity leaders' perceptions of comprehensive school physical activity programs. *Research Quarterly for Exercise and Sport, 87*(S2), A84.

Lewallen, T.C., Hunt, H., Potts-Datema, W., Zaza, S., & Giles, W. (2015) The whole school, whole community, whole child model: A new approach for improving educational attainment and healthy development for students. *Journal of School Health, 85*(11), 729-739. https://doi.org/10.1111/josh.12310

Luepker, R.V., Perry, C.L., McKinlay, S.M., Nader, P.R., Parcel, G.S., Stone, E.J., . . . Wu, M. (1996). Outcomes of a field trial to improve children's dietary patterns and physical activity. Child and Adolescent Trial for Cardiovascular Health. CATCH Collaborative Group. *Journal of the American Medical Association, 275,* 768-776.

McKenzie, J.F., Neiger, B.L., & Thackeray, R. (2017). *Planning, implementing, and evaluating health promotion programs: A primer* (7th ed.). Hoboken, NJ: Pearson.

Mullins, N. (2012). Obstacle course challenges: History, popularity, performance demands, effective training, and course design. *Journal of Exercise Physiology Online, 15*(2), 100-128.

National Center for Health Statistics. (2016). *Health, United States, 2015: With special feature on racial and ethnic health disparities.* Hyattsville, MD: Author.

Ogden, C.L., Carroll, M.D., Fryar, C.D., & Flegal, K.M. (2015). Prevalence of obesity among adults and youth: United States, 2011-2014. *NCHS Data Brief, 219.* www.cdc.gov/nchs/products/databriefs/db219.htm

Ogden, C.L., Carroll, M.D., Kit, B.K., & Flegal, K.M. (2014). Prevalence of childhood and adult obesity in the United States, 2011-2012. *Journal of the American Medical Association, 311*(8), 806-814.

Pate, R., Saunders, R.P., Ward, D.S., Felton, G., Trost, S.G., & Dowda, M. (2003). Evaluation of a community-based intervention to promote physical activity in youth: Lessons from Active Winners. *American Journal of Health Promotion, 17*(3), 171-182.

Prochaska, J.O., Norcross, J.C., & DiClemente, C.C. (1994). *Changing for good: The revolutionary program that explains the six stages of change and teaches you how to free yourself from bad habits.* New York, NY: William Morrow.

Prochaska, J.J., Rodgers, M.W., & Sallis, J.F. (2002). Association of parent and peer support with adolescent physical activity. *Research Quarterly in Exercise and Sport, 73*(2), 206-210.

Reis, R.S., Salvo, D., Ogilvie, D., Lambert, E.V., Goenka, S., & Brownson, R.C. (2016). Scaling up physical activity interventions worldwide: Stepping up to larger and smarter approaches to get people moving. *Lancet, 388*(10051), 1337-1348.

Sallis, J.F., Alcaraz, J.E., McKenzie, T.L., & Hovell, M.F. (1999). Predictors of change in children's physical activity over 20 months: Variations by gender and level of adiposity. *American Journal of Preventive Medicine, 16*(3), 222-229.

Sallis, J.F., McKenzie, T.L., Alcaraz, J.E., Kolody, B., Faucette, N., & Hovell, M.F. (1997). The effects of a 2-year physical education program (SPARK) on physical activity and fitness in elementary school students: Sports, Play and Active Recreation for Kids. *American Journal of Public Health, 87*(8), 1328-1334.

Sanders, G.J., Juvancic-Heltzel, J., Williamson, M.L., Roemmich, J.N., Feda, D.M., & Barkley, J.E. (2016). The effect of increasing autonomy through choice on young children's physical activity behavior. *Journal of Physical Activity & Health, 13*(4), 428-432.

Segar, M. (2015). *No sweat: How the simple science of motivation can bring you a lifetime of fitness.* New York, NY: AMACOM.

SHAPE America. (2014). *National standards & grade-level outcomes for K-12 physical education.* Champaign, IL: Human Kinetics.

SHAPE America. (2016a). *Physical education guidelines.* www.shapeamerica.org/standards/guidelines/peguidelines.cfm

SHAPE America. (2016b). *Using the whole school, whole community, whole child model to ensure student health and academic success* [Position statement]. Reston, VA: Author. www.shapeamerica.org/advocacy/positionstatements/

Siedentop, D. (2009). *Introduction to physical education, fitness, and sport* (7th ed.). Boston, MA: McGraw-Hill Higher Education.

Texas Education Agency. (2017). *Approved coordinated school health programs.* https://tea.texas.gov/Texas_Schools/Safe_and_Healthy_Schools/Coordinated_School_Health/Approved_Coordinated_School_Health_Programs/

Tingstrom, C.A. (2015). Addressing the needs of overweight students in elementary physical education: Creating an environment of care and success. *Strategies, 28*(1), 8-12. doi:10.1080/08924562.2014.980875

Trevino, R.P., Hernandez, A.E., Yin, Z., Garcia, O.A., & Hernandez, I. (2005). Effect of the Bienestar Health Program on physical fitness in low-income Mexican American children. *Hispanic Journal of Behavioral Sciences, 27*(1), 120-132.

Trost, S.G., Sallis, J.F., Pate, R.R., Freedson, P.S., Taylor, W.C., & Dowda, M. (2003). Evaluating a model of parental influence on youth physical activity. *American Journal of Preventive Medicine, 25*(4), 277-282.

U.S. Department of Health and Human Services. (2008). *Physical Activity Guidelines Advisory Committee report, 2008.* Washington, DC: Author. https://health.gov/paguidelines/report/

Weiss, M.R. (2000). Motivating kids in physical activity. *President's Council on Physical Fitness and Sports Research Digest, 3*(11), 1-8.

Chapter 3

American Heart Association. (2006). Promoting physical activity in children and youth: A leadership role for schools. *Circulation, 114*, 1214-1224.

Association for Supervision and Curriculum Development. (2014). *Whole school, whole community, whole child.* Alexandria, VA: Author.

Bailey, R. (2006). Physical education and sport in schools: A review of benefits and outcomes. *Journal of School Health, 76*(8), 397-401.

Bompa, T.O. (2000). *Total training for young champions.* Champaign, IL: Human Kinetics.

Braga, L., Elliott, E., Jones, E., & Bulger, S. (2015). Middle school students' perceptions of culturally and geographically relevant content in physical education. *International Journal of Kinesiology & Sports Science, 3*(4), 62-73.

Brooks, G., Fahey, T., & Baldwin, K. (2005). *Exercise physiology: Human bioenergetics and its applications* (4th ed.). Columbus, OH: McGraw-Hill Education.

Centers for Disease Control and Prevention. (2013). *Comprehensive school physical activity programs: A guide for schools.* Atlanta, GA: U.S. Department of Health and Human Services.

Corbin, C.B. (2014). Fitness for Life physical activity pyramid for teens [Poster]. Champaign, IL: Human Kinetics.

Faigenbaum, A.D., Kraemer, W.J., Blimkie, C.J., Jeffreys, I., Micheli, L.J., Nitka, M., & Rowland, T.W. (2009). Youth resistance training: Updated position statement paper from the National Strength and Conditioning Association. *Journal of Strength & Conditioning Research, 23*, S60-S79.

Garber, C.E., Blissmer, B., Deschenes, M.R., Franklin, B.A., Lamonte, M.J., Lee, I.M., . . . Swain, D.P. (2011). American College of Sports Medicine position stand. Quantity and quality of exercise for developing and maintaining cardiorespiratory, musculoskeletal, and neuromotor fitness in apparently healthy adults: Guidance for prescribing exercise. *Medicine and Science in Sports and Exercise, 43*(7), 1334-1359.

Graham, G., Elliott, E., & Palmer, S. (2016). *Teaching children and adolescents physical education* (4th ed.). Champaign, IL: Human Kinetics.

National Association for Sport and Physical Education. (2004). *Physical activity for children: A statement of guidelines for children ages 5-12* (2nd ed.). Reston, VA: Author.

Rowland, T. (2016). Pediatric exercise science: A brief overview. *Pediatric Exercise Science, 28*, 167-170.

Roy, B.A. (2015). Overreaching/overtraining: More is not always better. *ACSM's Health & Fitness Journal, 19*, 4-5.

SHAPE America. (2015). *Comprehensive school physical activity programs: Helping all students log 60 minutes of physical activity each day.* Reston, VA: Author.

U.S. Department of Health and Human Services. (2018). *2018 physical activity guidelines for Americans* (2nd ed.). Washington, DC: Author.

Chapter 4

American Academy of Pediatrics. (2011). *Sports drinks vs. energy drinks vs. plain water: What's best for thirsty kids?* Accessed November 15, 2018, at http://www.aappublications.org/content/32/6/32.2

American Academy of Pediatrics. (2017). *American Academy of Pediatrics recommends no fruit juice for children under 1 year.* https://www.aap.org/en-us/about-the-aap/aap-press-room/pages/American-Academy-of-Pediatrics-Recommends-No-Fruit-Juice-For-Children-Under-1-Year.aspx

American Dietetic Association. (2009). Position of the American Dietetic Association, Dietitians of Canada, and the American College of Sports Medicine: Nutrition and athletic performance. *Medicine and Science in Sports and Exercise, 41*(3), 709-731.

American Heart Association. (2016). *Health threats from high blood pressure.* www.heart.org/HEART-ORG/Conditions/HighBloodPressure/WhyBloodPressureMatters/Why-Blood-Pressure-Matters_UCM_002051_Article.jsp#.V_FoETVuOT9

Centers for Disease Control and Prevention. (2017). *Salt.* https://www.cdc.gov/salt/food.htm

Ervin, R.B., Kit, B.K., Carroll, M.D., & Ogden, C.L. (2012). Consumption of added sugar among U.S. children and adolescents, 2005-2008. *NCHS Data Brief, 87.* Hyattsville, MD: National Center for Health Statistics.

Feijo, F.M., Ballard, C.R., Foletto, K.C., Batista, B.A., Neves, A.M., Ribeiro, M.F., & Bertoluci, M.C. (2013). Saccharin and aspartame, compared with sucrose, induce greater weight gain in adult Wistar rats, at similar total calorie intake levels. *Appetite, 60*(1), 203-207.

Gardner, C., Wylie-Rosett, J., Gidding, S.S., Steffen, L.M., Johnson, R.K., Reader, D., & Lichtenstein, A.H., and on behalf of the American Heart Association Nutrition Committee of the Council on Nutrition, Physical Activity and Metabolism, Council on Arteriosclerosis, Thrombosis and Vascular Biology, Council on Cardiovascular Disease in the Young, and the American Diabetes Association. (2012). Nonnutritive sweeteners: Current use and health perspectives: A scientific statement from the American Heart Association and the American Diabetes Association. *Circulation, 126*, 509-519.

Gortmaker, S., Long, M., & Wang, C. (2009). The negative impact of sugar-sweetened beverages on children's health. *Healthy Eating Research.* http://healthyeatingresearch.org/wp-content/uploads/2013/12/HER-SSB-Synthesis-091116_FINAL.pdf

Institute of Medicine. (2010). *Dietary reference intakes for calcium and vitamin D.* Washington, DC: National Academies Press.

Institute of Medicine. (2012). *Accelerating progress in obesity prevention: Solving the weight of the nation.* Washington, DC: National Academies Press. https://doi.org/10.17226/13275

Joint Committee on National Health Education Standards. (2007). *National health education standards: Achieving excellence* (2nd ed.). Washington, DC: The American Cancer Society.

Ludwig, D.S., Peterson, K.E., & Gortmaker, S.L. (2001). Relation between consumption of sugar-sweetened drinks and childhood obesity: A prospective, observational analysis. *Lancet, 357*, 505-508.

Mayo Clinic Staff. (2016). *Added sugars: Don't get sabotaged by sweeteners.* www.mayoclinic.org/healthy-living/nutrition-and-healthy-eating/in-depth/added-sugar/art-20045328

National Heart, Lung, and Blood Institute. (2013). *Balance food and activity.* www.nhlbi.nih.gov/health/public/heart/obesity/wecan/healthy-weight-basics/balance.htm

National Institutes of Health. (2015). *Osteoporosis: Peak bone mass in women.* www.niams.nih.gov/Health_Info/Bone/Osteoporosis/bone_mass.asp

Rubio-Tapia, A., Ludvigsson, J.F., Brantner, T.L., Murray, J.A., & Everhart, J.E. (2012). The prevalence of celiac disease in the United States. *American Journal of Gastroenterology, 107*, 1538-1544.

Sacks, F.M., Bray, G.A., Carey, V.J., Smith, S.R., Ryan, D.H., Anton, S.D., . . . Williamson, D.A. (2009). Comparison of weight-loss diets with different compositions of fat, protein, and carbohydrates. *New England Journal of Medicine, 360*(9), 859-873.

Schneider, M.B., & Benjamin, H.J. (2011). Sports drinks and energy drinks for children and adolescents: Are they appropriate? *Pediatrics, 127*(6). http://pediatrics.aappublications.org/content/127/6/1182.full

U.S. Department of Agriculture. (n.d.). *USDA food composition databases.* http://ndb.nal.usda.gov/

U.S. Department of Agriculture. (2018). *Get your MyPlate plan.* https://www.choosemyplate.gov/MyPlatePlan

U.S. Department of Health and Human Services. (2018). *2018 physical activity guidelines for Americans.* Washington, DC: Author.

U.S. Department of Health and Human Services and U.S. Department of Agriculture. (2015a). *2015-2020 dietary guidelines for Americans* (8th ed.). https://health.gov/dietaryguidelines/2015/guidelines/chapter-1/a-closer-look-inside-healthy-eating-patterns/

U.S. Department of Health and Human Services and U.S. Department of Agriculture. (2015b). *2015-2020 dietary guidelines for Americans* (8th ed.), Appendix 2. Estimated calorie needs per day, by age, sex, and physical activity level. https://health.gov/dietaryguidelines/2015/guidelines/appendix-2/

U.S. Food and Drug Administration. (2018a). *Ingredients and packaging.* www.fda.gov/Food/IngredientsPackagingLabeling/default.htm

U.S. Food and Drug Administration. (2018b). *Label format examples.* www.fda.gov/Food/GuidanceRegulation/GuidanceDocumentsRegulatoryInformation/LabelingNutrition/ucm385663.htm#formats

U.S. Food and Drug Administration. (2018c). *Nutrition facts label programs and materials.* www.fda.gov/nutritioneducation

Yang, Q., Zhang, Z., Gregg, E., Flanders, D., Merritt, R., & Hu, F. (2014). Added sugar intake and cardiovascular diseases mortality among US adults. *JAMA Internal Medicine, 174*(4), 516-524.

Chapter 5

Alleyne, J.M.K. (1998). Safe exercise prescription for children and adolescents. *Paediatrics and Child Health, 3*(5), 337-342. https://www.ncbi.nlm.nih.gov/pmc/articles/PMC2851369/

American Academy of Pediatrics (AAP). (2000). Physical fitness and activity in schools. (RE9907). *Pediatrics, 105*(5), 1156-1157.

American College of Sports Medicine, & Pescatello, L.S. (2014). *ACSM's guidelines for exercise testing and prescription.* Philadelphia, PA: Wolters Kluwer/Lippincott Williams & Wilkins Health.

Bailey, R.C., Olson, J., Pepper, S.L., Porszaz, J., Barstow, T.J., & Cooper, D.M. (1995). The level and tempo of children's physical activities: An observational study. *Medicine and Science in Sport and Exercise, 27*, 1033-1041.

Bar-Or, O. (1984). Children and physical performance in warm and cold environments. In R.F. Boileau (Ed.), *Advances in pediatric sport sciences, vol. 1* (pp. 117-130). Champaign, IL: Human Performances.

Beets, M.W., Patton, M.M., & Edwards, S. (2005). The accuracy of pedometer steps and time during walking in children. *Medicine and Science in Sports and Exercise, 37*(3), 513-520.

Beighle, A., Pangrazi, R.P., & Vincent, S.D. (2001). Pedometers, physical activity, and accountability. *Journal of Physical Education, Recreation and Dance, 72*(9), 16-19.

Carson, R.L., Landers, R.Q., & Blankenship, B.T. (2010). Concluding comments and recommendations. *Journal of Physical Education, Recreation and Dance, 81*(8), 38-39. doi: 10.1080/07303084.2010.10598526

Caspersen, C.J., Powell, K.E., & Christenson, G.M. (1985). Physical activity, exercise, and physical fitness: Definitions and distinctions for health-related research. *Public Health Report, 100*(2), 126-131.

Centers for Disease Control and Prevention. (n.d.). *Physical activity and health: A report of the surgeon general.* https://www.cdc.gov/nccdphp/sgr/contents.htm

Cooper Institute. (2017). *FitnessGram administration manual: The journey to MyHealthyZone* (5th ed.). Champaign, IL: Human Kinetics.

Corbin, C.B., Welk, G.J., Richardson, C., Vowell, C., Lambdin, D., & Wikgren, S. (2014). Youth physical fitness: Ten key concepts. *Journal of Physical Education, Recreation and Dance, 85*(2), 24-31. doi:10.1080/07303084.2014.866827

Crouter, S.E., Schneider, P.L., Karabulut, M., & Bassett, D.R. Jr. (2003). Validity of 10 electronic pedometers for measuring steps, distance, and energy cost. *Medicine and Science in Sports and Exercise, 35*(8), 1455-1460.

Cuddihy, T.F., Pangrazi, R.P., & Tomson, L.M. (2005). Pedometers: Answers to FAQs from teachers. *Journal of Physical Education, Recreation and Dance, 76*(2), 36-40, 55.

Donnelly, J.E., Hillman, C.H., Castelli, D., Etnier, J.L., Lee, S., Tomporowski, P., . . . Szabo-Reed, A. (2016). Physical activity, fitness, cognitive function, and academic achievement in children: A systematic review. *Medicine and Science in Sports and Exercise, 48*(6), 1197-1222.

Fryar, C.D., Carroll, M.D., & Ogden, C.L. (September, 2018). *Prevalence of overweight, obesity, and severe obesity among children and adolescents aged 2-19 years: United States, 1963-1965 through 2015-2016.* Available from: http://www.cdc.gov/nchs/products/hestats.htm

Gomez-Pinilla, F., & Hillman, C. (2013). The influence of exercise on cognitive abilities. *Comprehensive Physiology, 3*(1), 403-428.

Greene, L.S., & Pate, R. (2014). *Training young distance runners* (3rd ed.). Champaign, IL: Human Kinetics.

Guo, S.S., Roche, A.F., Chumlea, W.C., Gardner, J.D., & Siervogel, R.M. (1994). The predictive value of childhood BMI values for overweight at age 34 y. *American Journal of Clinical Nutrition, 59*, 1810-1819.

Hatano, Y. (1993). Use of the pedometer for promoting daily walking exercise. *International Council for Health, Physical Education and Recreation, 29*, 4-8.

Heyward, V.H. (2010). *Advanced fitness assessment and exercise prescription* (6th ed.). Champaign, IL: Human Kinetics.

Hood, M.S., Little, J.P., Tarnopolsky, M.A., Myslik, F., & Gibala, M.J. (2011). Low-volume interval training improves muscle oxidative capacity in sedentary adults. *Medicine and Science in Sports and Exercise, 43*(10), 1849-1856. doi:10.1249/MSS.0b013e3182199834

Institute of Medicine. (2012). *Fitness measures and health outcomes in youth.* Washington, DC: The National Academies.

Janz, K.F., Levy, S.M., Burns, T.L., Torner, J.C., Willing, M.C., & Warren, J.J. (2002). Fatness, physical activity and television viewing in children during the adiposity rebound period: The Iowa Bone Development Study. *Preventive Medicine, 35*, 563-571.

McDowell, M.A., Briefel, R.R., Alaimo, K., Bischof, A.M., Caughman, C.R., Carroll, M.D., . . . Johnson, C.L. (1994). Energy and macronutrient intakes of persons ages 2 months and over in the United States: Third national health and nutrition examination survey, phase I, 1988-1991. *Advance Data from Vital and Health Statistics, no. 255.* Hyattsville, MD: National Center for Health Statistics.

Medina, J. (2014). *Brain rules (updated and expanded): 12 principles of surviving and thriving at work, home, and school.* Seattle, WA: Pear Press.

Milanović, Z., Sporiš, G., & Weston, M. (October, 2015). Effectiveness of high-intensity interval training (HIT) and continuous endurance training for VO2max improvements: A systematic review and meta-analysis of controlled trials. *Sports Medicine, 45*(10), 1469-1481.

National Association for Sport and Physical Education (NASPE). (2004). *Physical activity for children: A statement of guidelines for children ages 5-12* (2nd ed.). Reston, VA: NASPE.

National Association for Sport and Physical Education (NASPE). (2010). *Guidelines for participation in youth sport programs: Specialization versus multiple-sport participation* [Position statement]. Reston, VA: Author.

National Physical Activity Plan Alliance. (2018). *The 2018 United States report card on physical activity for children and youth.* Washington, DC: National Physical Activity Plan Alliance.

Office of Disease Prevention and Health Promotion (ODPHP). (2016). *Healthy People 2020.* Washington, DC: U.S. Department of Health and Human Services.

Pangrazi, R.P., Beighle, A., & Sidman, C.A. (2003). *Pedometer power: Using pedometers in school and community* (2nd ed.). Champaign, IL: Human Kinetics.

Pangrazi, R.P., & Corbin, C. (2008). Factors that influence physical fitness in children and adolescents. In G.J. Welk & M.D. Meredith (Eds.), *Fitnessgram/Activitygram reference guide.* Dallas, TX: Cooper Institute.

Pillsbury, L., Oria, M., & Pate, R.R. (2012). *Fitness measures and health outcomes in youth.* Washington, DC: National Academies Press.

Plowman, S.A., & Meredith, M.D. (2013). *FitnessGram/ActivityGram reference guide* (4th ed.). Dallas, TX: Cooper Institute.

Pontifex, M.B., Saliba, B.J., Raine, L.B., Picchietti, D.L., & Hillman, C.H. (2013). Exercise improves behavioral, neurocognitive, and scholastic performance in children with ADHD. *The Journal of Pediatrics, 162*(3), 543-551.

Ratey, J.J., & Hagerman, E. (2008). *Spark: The revolutionary new science of exercise and the brain*. New York, NY: Little, Brown.

Rowland, T.W. (1996). *Developmental exercise physiology*. Champaign, IL: Human Kinetics.

Rowland, T.W. (2005). *Children's exercise physiology*. Champaign, IL: Human Kinetics.

Rowland, T.W. (2008, August 1). Thermoregulation during exercise in the heat in children. *Journal of Applied Psychology*. https://www.physiology.org/doi/full/10.1152/japplphysiol.01196.2007

Rowland, T.W. (2016). Pediatric exercise science: A brief overview. *Pediatric Exercise Science, 28*, 167-170.

Saltin, B. (1973). Oxygen transport by the circulatory system during exercise in man. In J. Keul (Ed.), *Limiting factors of physical performance* (pp. 235-252). Stuttgart, Germany: Thieme.

Schneider, P.L., Crouter, S.E., & Bassett, D.R. Jr. (2004). Pedometer measures of free-living physical activity: Comparison of 13 models. *Medicine and Science in Sports and Exercise, 36*(2): 331-335.

Schneider, P.L., Crouter, S.E., Lukajic, O., & Bassett, D.R. Jr. (2003). Accuracy and reliability of 10 pedometers for measuring steps over a 400-m walk. *Medicine and Science in Sports and Exercise, 35*(10), 1779-1784.

SHAPE America. (2016). *Shape of the nation 2016*. https://www.shapeamerica.org/uploads/pdfs/son/Shape-of-the-Nation-2016_web.pdf

Smith, A.L., Hoza, B., Linnea, K., McQuade, J.D., Tomb, M., Vaughn, A.J., . . . Hook, H. (2013). Pilot physical activity intervention reduces severity of ADHD symptoms in young children. *Journal of Attention Disorders, 17*(1), 70-82.

Swaim, D., & Swaim, D. (2013). *Heart education: Strategies, lessons, science, and technology for cardiovascular fitness*. Champaign, IL: Human Kinetics.

Tabata, I., Nishimura, K., Kouzaki, M., Hirai, Y., Ogita, F., Miyachi, M., & Yamamoto, K. (October, 1996). Effects of moderate-intensity endurance and high-intensity intermittent training on anaerobic capacity and VO2max. *Medicine and Science in Sports and Exercise, 28*(10), 1327-1330.

Tudor-Locke, C., Pangrazi, R.P., Corbin, C.B., Rutherford, W.J., Vincent, S.D., Raustorp, A., . . . Cuddihy, T.F. (2004). BMI-referenced standards for recommended pedometer determined steps/day in children. *Preventive Medicine, 38*(6), 857-864.

U.S. Department of Health and Human Services (USDHHS). (2000). *Healthy People 2010: Understanding and improving health*. Washington, DC: U.S. Department of Health and Human Services, Government Printing Office.

U.S. Department of Health and Human Services (USDHHS). (2010). *Healthy People 2020*. Washington, DC: U.S. Department of Health and Human Services, Office of Disease Prevention and Health Promotion. https://www.healthypeople.gov/

U.S. Department of Health and Human Services (USDHHS). (2018). *Physical activity guidelines for Americans* (2nd ed.). Washington, DC: U.S. Department of Health and Human Services, Government Printing Office. https://health.gov/paguidelines/second-edition/pdf/Physical_Activity_Guidelines_2nd_edition.pdf

Virgilio, S.J. (2011). *Fitness education for children* (2nd ed.). Champaign, IL: Human Kinetics.

Welk, G.J., & Blair, S.N. (2008). Health benefits of physical activity and physical fitness in children. In G.J. Welk & M.D. Meredith (Eds.), *FitnessGram/ActivityGram reference guide* (pp. 4.1-4.12). Dallas, TX: Cooper Institute.

Welk, G.J., Differding, J.A., Thompson, R.W., Blair, S.N., Dziura, J., & Hart, P. (2000). The utility of the Digiwalker step counter to assess daily physical activity patterns. *Medicine and Science in Sports and Exercise, 32*(9 suppl), S481-488.

Winnick, J.P., & Short, F.X. (2014). *Brockport physical fitness test manual: A health-related assessment for youngsters with disabilities* (2nd ed.). Champaign, IL: Human Kinetics.

Chapter 6

Allen, D.B., Nemeth, B.A., Clark, R.R., Peterson, S.E., Eickhoff, J., & Carrel, A.L. (2007). Fitness is a stronger predictor of fasting insulin levels than fatness in overweight male middle-school children. *The Journal of Pediatrics, 150*, 383-387.

Bassali, R., Waller, J.L., Gower, B., Allison, J., & Davis, C.L. (2010). Utility of waist circumference percentile for risk evaluation in obese children. *International Journal of Pediatric Obesity, 5*(1), 97-101. doi: 10.3109/17477160903111722.

Bell, L.M., Watts, K., Siafarikas, A., Thompson, A., Ratnam, N., Bulsara, M., . . . Davis, E.A. (2007). Exercise alone reduces insulin resistance in obese children independently of changes in body composition. *The Journal of Clinical Endocrinology and Metabolism, 92,* 4230-4235.

Boreham, C.A., Twisk, J., Murray, L., Savage, M., Strain, J.J., & Cran, G.W. (2001). Fitness, fatness, and coronary heart disease risk in adolescents: The Northern Ireland Young Hearts Project. *Medicine and Science in Sports and Exercise, 33,* 270-274.

Briefel, R.R., & Johnson, C.L. (2004). Secular trends in dietary intake in the United States. *Annual Review of Nutrition, 24,* 401-431.

Campbell, W., Crim, M., Young, V., & Evans, W. (1994). Increased energy requirements and changes in body composition with resistance training in older adults. *American Journal of Clinical Nutrition, 60,* 167-175.

Centers for Disease Control and Prevention. (2012). *Anthropometric reference data for children and adults: United States, 2007-2010: Data from the National Health and Nutrition Examination Survey.* Hyattsville, MD: Author. www.cdc.gov/nchs/data/series/sr_11/sr11_252.pdf

The Cooper Institute. (2017). *FitnessGram administration manual* (5th ed.). Champaign, IL: Human Kinetics.

Faigenbaum, A.D. (2007). Resistance training for obese children and adolescents. *President's Council on Physical Fitness and Sports Research Digest, 8*(3), 1-8.

Fernandez, J.R., Redden, D.T., Pietrobelli, A., & Allison, D.B. (2004). Waist circumference percentiles in nationally representative samples of African-American, European-American, and Mexican-American children and adolescents. *Journal of Pediatrics, 145,* 439-444.

Fryar, C.D., Gu, Q., & Ogden, C.L. (2012). *Anthropometric reference data for children and adults: United States, 2007-2010: Data from the National Health and Nutrition Examination Survey.* Hyattsville, MD: Author. www.cdc.gov/nchs/data/series/sr_11/sr11_252.pdf

Going, S.B., Hingle, M., & Farr, J. (2013). Body composition. In A.C. Ross, B. Caballero, R.J. Cousins, K.L. Tucker, & T. Ziegler (Eds.), *Modern nutrition in health and disease* (11th ed., pp. 635-648). Baltimore, MD: Lippincott Williams and Wilkins.

Going, S.B., Lohman, T.G., Cussler, E.C., Williams, D.P., Morrison, J.A., & Horn, P.S. (2011). Percent body fat and chronic disease risk factors in U.S. children and youth. *American Journal of Preventive Medicine, 41*(4 Suppl. 2), S77-S86.

Haskell, W.L., Lee, I.M., Pate, R.R., Powell, K.E., Blair, S.N., Franklin, B.A., . . . Bauman, A. (2007). Physical activity and public health: Updated recommendation for adults from the American College of Sports Medicine and the American Heart Association. *Medicine and Science in Sports and Exercise, 39*(8), 1423-1434.

Heyward, V.H., & Wagner, D.R. (2004). *Applied body composition* (2nd ed.). Champaign, IL: Human Kinetics.

Institute of Medicine. (2013). *Educating the student body: Taking physical activity and physical education to school.* Washington, DC: National Academies Press.

Katmarzyk, P.T., Srinivasan, S.R., Chen, W., Malina, R.M., Bouchard, C., & Berenson, G.S. (2004). Body mass index, waist circumference, and clustering of cardiovascular disease risk factors in a biracial sample of children and adolescents. *Pediatrics, 114*(2), e198-e205.

Kim, S., & Valdez, R. (2015). Metabolic risk factors in U.S. youth with low relative muscle mass. *Obesity Research & Clinical Practice, 9*(2), 125-132.

Laurson, K.R., Eisenmann, J.C., & Welk, G.J. (2011a). Body fat percentile curves for U.S. children and adolescents. *American Journal of Preventive Medicine, 41*(4 Suppl. 2), S63-S67.

Laurson, K.R., Eisenmann, J.C., & Welk, G.J. (2011b). Development of youth percent body fat standards using receiver operating characteristic curves. *American Journal of Preventive Medicine, 41*(4 Suppl. 2), S93-S99.

Laurson, K.R., Eisenmann, J.C., & Welk, G.J. (2011c). Body mass index standards based on agreement with health-related body fat. *American Journal of Preventive Medicine, 41*(4 Suppl. 2), S100-S105.

Li, C., Ford, E.S., Zhao, G., & Mokdad, A.H. (2009). Prevalence of pre-diabetes and its association with clustering of cardiometabolic risk factors and hyperinsulinemia among U.S. adolescents: Nation Health and Nutrition Examination Survey 2005-2006. *Diabetes Care, 32*(2), 495-503.

McDowell, M.A., Fryar, C.D., Ogden, C.L., & Flegal, K.M. (2008). Anthropometric reference data for children and adults: United States, 2003-2006. *National Health Statistics Report, 10*, 1-48.

Meredith, M.D., & Welk, G.J. (Eds.). (2013). *FitnessGram/ActivityGram test administration manual* (4th ed.). Champaign, IL: Human Kinetics.

National Eating Disorders Association. (2016). Anorexia nervosa and bulimia nervosa. www.nationaleatingdisorders.org.

Ogden, C.L., Carroll, M.D., Fryar, C.D., & Flegal, K.M. (2015). Prevalence of obesity among adults and youth: United States, 2011-2014. *NCHS Data Brief, 219*, 1-8.

Ogden, C., Carroll, M.D., Lawman, H.G., Fryar, C.D., Kruszon-Moran, D., Kit, B.K., & Flegal, K.M. (2016). Trends in obesity prevalence among children and adolescents in the United States, 1988-1994 through 2013-2014. *Journal of the American Medication Association, 315*(21), 2292-2299.

Plowman, S.A., & Meredith, M.D. (2013). *FitnessGram/ActivityGram reference guide* (4th ed.). Dallas, TX: Cooper Institute.

Ross, R., Freeman, J., & Janssen, P. (2000). Exercise alone is an effective strategy for reducing obesity and related comorbidities. *Exercise and Sport Science Review, 28*, 165-170.

Shaibi, G.Q., Cruz, M.L., Ball, G.D., Weigensberg, M.J., Salem, G.J., Crespo, N.C., & Goran, M.I. (2006). Effects of resistance training on insulin sensitivity in overweight Latino adolescent males. *Medicine and Science in Sports and Exercise, 38*, 1208-1215.

Sharma, A.K., Metzger, D.L., Daymont, C., Hadjiyannakis, S., & Rodd, C.J. (2015). LMS tables for waist-circumference and waist-height ratio Z-scores in children aged 5-19 y in NHANES III: Association with cardio-metabolic risks. *Pediatric Research, 78*(6), 723-729.

Silva, A.M., Fields, D.A., & Sardinha, L.B. (2013). A PRISMA-driven systematic review of predictive equations for assessing fat and fat-free mass in healthy children and adolescents using multi-component molecular models as the reference method. *Journal of Obesity*, article ID 148696. doi: 10.1155/2013/148696.

Swanson, S.A., Crow, S.J., Le Grange, D., Swendsen, J., & Merikangas, K.R. (2011). Prevalence and correlates of eating disorders in adolescents. Results from the nation comorbidity survey replication adolescent supplement. *Archives of General Psychiatry, 68*(7), 714-723.

Talma, H., Chinapaw, M.J., Bakker, B., HiraSing, R.A., Terwee, C.B., & Altenburg, T.M. (2013). Bioelectrical impedance analysis to estimate body composition in children and adolescents: A systematic review and evidence appraisal of validity, responsiveness, reliability and measurement error. *Obesity Review, 14*(11), 895-905.

Troiano, R.P., Berrigan, D., Dodd, K.W., Masse, L.C., Tilert, T., & McDowell, M. (2008). Physical activity in the United States measured by accelerometer. *Medicine and Science in Sports and Exercise, 40*(1), 181-188. doi: 10.1249/mss.0b013e31815a51b3.

U.S. Department of Agriculture. (2013). *Diet quality of children age 2-17 years as measured by the Healthy Eating Index—2010.* https://www.cnpp.usda.gov/sites/default/files/nutrition_insights_uploads/Insight52.pdf

U.S. Department of Education. (2011). *Family Educational Rights and Privacy Act: Guidance for students.* http://www2.ed.gov/policy/gen/guid/fpco/ferpa/students.html

U.S. Department of Health and Human Services. (1999). *Promoting physical activity.* Champaign, IL: Human Kinetics.

U.S. Department of Health and Human Services. (2001). *Surgeon general's call to action to prevent and decrease overweight and obesity.* Washington, DC: U.S. Government Printing Office. www.surgeongeneral.gov/calltoaction/fact_adolscents.html

Welk, G.J., Going, S.B., Morrow, J.R., & Meredith, M.D. (2011). Development of new criterion-referenced fitness standards in the FitnessGram program. Rationale and conceptual overview. *American Journal of Preventive Medicine, 41*(4 Supp. 2): S63-S67.

Wickelgren, I. (1998). Obesity: How big a problem? *Science, 280*(May), 1364-1367.

Williams, D.P., Going, S.B., Lohman, T.G., Harsha, D.W., Srinivasan, S.R., Webber, L.S., & Berenson, G.S. (1992). Body fatness and the risk of elevated blood pressure, total cholesterol and serum lipoprotein ratios in children and adolescents. *American Journal of Public Health, 82*, 358-363.

Ziegler, E., & Filer, L. (2000). *Present knowledge in nutrition* (7th ed.). Washington, DC: International Life Sciences Press.

Additional Resources for Chapter 6

Daniels, S.R., Arnett, D., Eckel, R.H., Gidding, S.S., Hayman, L., Kumanyika, S., . . . Williams, C.L. (2005). Overweight in children and adolescents: Pathophysiology, consequences, prevention, and treatment. *Circulation, 111*, 1999-2012.

Deurenberg, P., van der Kooy, K., Leenan, R., Westrate, J.A., & Seidell, J.C. (1991). Sex and age specific population prediction formulas for estimating body composition from bioelectrical impedance: A cross validation study. *International Journal of Obesity, 15*, 17-25.

Flegal, K.M., Carroll, M.D., Ogden, C.L., & Curtin, L.R. (2010). Prevalence and trends in obesity among US adults, 1999-2008. *Journal of the American Medical Association, 303*(3), 235-241.

Guo, S.S., Roche, A.F., Chumlea, W.C., Gardner, J.D., & Siervogel, R.M. (1994). The predictive value of childhood BMI values for overweight at age 34 y. *American Journal of Clinical Nutrition, 59*, 1810-1819.

Houtkeeper, L.B., Going, S.B., Westfall, C.H., Roche, A.F., & Van Loan, M. (1992). Bioelectrical impedance estimation of fat-free body mass in children and youth: A cross-validation study. *Journal of Applied Physiology, 72*, 366-373.

Houtkeeper, L.B., Lohman, T.G., Going, S.B., & Hall, M.C. (1989). Validity of bioelectrical impedance for body composition assessment in children. *Journal of Applied Physiology, 66*, 814-821.

Kim, H.K., Tanaka, K., Nakadomo, F., Watanabe, K., & Marsuura, Y. (1993). Fat-free mass in Japanese boys predicted from bioelectrical impedance and anthropometric variables [Abstract]. *Medicine and Science in Sports and Exercise, 25*, S59.

Kushner, R.F., Schoeller, D.A., Field, C.R., & Danford, L. (1992). Is the impedance index (ht2/R) significant in predicting total body water? *American Journal of Clinical Nutrition, 56*, 835-839.

Lohman, T.G. (1992). *Advances in body composition assessment: Current issues in exercise science series.* Monograph no. 3. Champaign, IL: Human Kinetics.

Lukaski, H.C., Johnson, P.E., Bolonchuk, W.W., & Lykken, G.I. (1985). Assessment of fat-free mass using bioelectric impedance measurements of the human body. *American Journal of Clinical Nutrition, 41*, 810-817.

Ogden, C.L., Carroll, M.D., & Flegal, K.M. (2008). High body mass index for age among US children and adolescents, 2003-2006. *Journal of the American Medication Association, 299*(20), 2401-2405.

Rowland, T.W. (1990). *Exercise and children's health.* Champaign, IL: Human Kinetics.

Segal, K.R., Gutin, B., Presta, E., Wang, J., & Van Itallie, T.B. (1985). Estimation of human body composition by electrical impedance [Abstract]. *Federation Proceedings, 46*, 1334.

Segal, K.R., Van Loan, M., Fitzgerald, P.I., Hodgdon, J.A., & Van Itallie, T.B. (1988). Lean body mass estimation by bioelectrical impedance analysis: A four-site cross-validation study. *American Journal of Clinical Nutrition, 47*, 7-14.

Slaughter, M.H., Lohman, T.G., Boileau, R.A., Horswill, C.A., Stillman, R.J., Van Loan, M.D., & Benben, D.A. (1988). Skinfold equations for estimation of body fatness in children and youth. *Human Biology, 60*, 709-723.

Van Loan, M., & Mayclin, P.L. (1987). Bioelectrical impedance analysis: Is it a reliable estimator of lean body mass and total body water? *Human Biology, 59*, 299-309.

Vincent, S.D., Pangrazi, R.P., Raustorp, A., Tomson, L.M., & Cuddihy, T.F. (2003). Activity levels and body mass index of children in the United States, Sweden, and Australia. *Medicine and Science in Sports and Exercise, 35*(8), 1367-1373.

Watanabe, K., Nakadomo, F., Tanaka, K., Kim, K., & Maeda, K. (1993). Estimation of fat-free mass from bioelectrical impedance and anthropometric variables in Japanese girls [Abstract]. *Medicine and Science in Sports and Exercise, 25*, S163.

Welk, G.J., & Blair, S.N. (2008). Health benefits of physical activity and physical fitness in children. In G.J. Welk & M.D. Meredith (Eds.), *FitnessGram/ActivityGram reference guide* (pp. 4.1-4.12). Dallas, TX: Cooper Institute.

Chapter 7

American College of Sports Medicine. (2006). *ACSM's resource manual for guidelines for exercise testing and prescription* (5th ed.). Philadelphia, PA: Lippincott Williams and Wilkins.

American College of Sports Medicine (Ed.). (2014). *ACSM's health-related physical fitness assessment manual.* Philadelphia, PA: Lippincott Williams and Wilkins.

Baechle, T.R., & Earle, R.W. (Eds.). (2008). *Essentials of strength training and conditioning*. Champaign, IL: Human Kinetics.

Behm, D.G., Button, D.C., & Butt, J.C. (2001). Factors affecting force loss with prolonged stretching. *Canadian Journal of Applied Physiology, 26*(3), 262-272.

Bompa, T.O., & Haff, G.G. (2009). *Periodization: Theory and methodology of training*. Champaign, IL: Human Kinetics.

Brynzak, S.S., & Burko, S.V. (2013). Improving athletic performance of basketball student team with the classical yoga exercises. *Pedagogics, Psychology, Medical–Biological Problems of Physical Training and Sports, 10,* 3-6.

Canadian Fitness Professionals. (2016). *Foundations of professional personal training* (2nd ed.). Champaign, IL: Human Kinetics.

Ciocioi, A.F., & Macovei, S. (2016). Study about the evolution of joint mobility in pupils at the primary school level. *European Proceedings of Social & Behavioural Sciences.* https://www.futureacademy.org.uk/files/images/upload/ICPESK%202015%208_341.pdf

Corbin, C.B., Welk, G.J., Corbin, W.R., & Welk, K.A. (2009). *Concepts of fitness and wellness: A comprehensive lifestyle approach* (8th ed.). New York, NY: McGraw-Hill.

Corbin, C.B., Welk, G.J., Lindsey, R., & Corbin, W.R. (2004). *Concepts of fitness and wellness* (5th ed.). New York, NY: McGraw-Hill.

Faigenbaum, A.D., Bellucci, M., Bernieri, A., Bakker, B., & Hoorens, K. (2005). Acute effects of different warm-up protocols on fitness performance in children. *The Journal of Strength & Conditioning Research, 19*(2), 376-381.

Garber, C.E., Blissmer, B., Deschenes, M.R., Franklin, B.A., Lamonte, M.J., Lee, I.M., . . . Swain, D.P. (2011). American College of Sports Medicine position stand. Quantity and quality of exercise for developing and maintaining cardiorespiratory, musculoskeletal, and neuromotor fitness in apparently healthy adults: Guidance for prescribing exercise. *Medicine and Science in Sports and Exercise, 43*(7), 1334-1359.

Heyward, V.H., & Gibson, A. (2014). *Advanced fitness assessment and exercise prescription* (7th ed.). Champaign, IL: Human Kinetics.

Kloubec, J.A. (2010). Pilates for improvement of muscle endurance, flexibility, balance, and posture. *The Journal of Strength & Conditioning Research, 24*(3), 661-667.

Knudson, D.V., Magnusson, P., & McHugh, M. (2000). Current issues in flexibility fitness. *President's Council on Physical Fitness and Sports Research Digest, 3*(10).

Kraines, M.G., & Sherman, B.R. (2010). *Yoga for the joy of it!* Burlington, MA: Jones & Bartlett.

Chapter 8

American Academy of Pediatrics, McCambridge, T.M., & Stricker, P.R. (2008). Strength training by children and adolescents. *Pediatrics, 121,* 835-840.

American College of Sports Medicine. (2002). Strength training in children and adolescents. *Current Comment.* www.onlinehs.net/pe/m/acsm_youth_9-2002.pdf

Baechle, T.R., Earle, R.W., & Wathen, D. (2008). Resistance training. In T.R. Baechle & R.W. Earle (Eds.), *Essentials of strength training and conditioning* (pp. 381-412). Champaign, IL: Human Kinetics.

Baker, D., Mitchel, J., Boyle, D., Currell, S., & Currell, P. (2007). *Resistance training for children and youth: A position stand from the Australian Strength and Conditioning Association (ASCA).* http://www.strengthandconditioning.org

Behm, D.G., Faigenbaum, A.D., Falk, B., & Klentrou, P. (2008). Canadian Society for Exercise Physiology position paper: Resistance training in children and adolescents. *Applied Physiology, Nutrition, and Metabolism, 33,* 547-561.

Bompa, T. (2000). *Total training for young champions.* Champaign, IL: Human Kinetics.

Casa, D.J., Almquist, J., Anderson, S.A., Baker, L., Bergeron, M.F., Biagioli, B., . . . Valentine, V. (2013). Inter-Association Task Force for Preventing Sudden Death in Secondary School Athletics Programs: Best-practices recommendations. *Journal of Athletic Training, 48*(4), 546-553.

Corbin, C.B., Janz, K.F., & Baptista, F. (2017). Good health: The power of power. *Journal of Physical Education, Recreation and Dance, 88*(9), 28-35.

Corbin, C.B., Pangrazi, R.P., & Franks, B.D. (2000). Definitions: Health, fitness, and physical activity. *President's Council on Physical Fitness and Sports Research Digest, 3*(9), 1-8.

Corbin, C.B., Welk, G.J., Corbin, W.R., & Welk, K.A. (2016). *Concepts of fitness and wellness: A comprehensive lifestyle approach*. New York, NY: McGraw-Hill Education.

Chu, D., Faigenbaum, A., & Falkel, J. (2006). *Progressive plyometric training for kids*. Monterey Bay, CA: Healthy Learning Publications.

Dahab, K.S., & McCambridge, T. (2009). Strength training in children and adolescents: Raising the bar for young athletes? *Sports Health, 1*(3), 223-226.

Faigenbaum, A. (2001). Preseason conditioning for high school athletes. *Strength and Conditioning, 23*(1): 70-72.

Faigenbaum, A.D., Kraemer, W.J., Blimkie, C.J., Jeffreys, I., Micheli, L.J., Nitka, M., & Rowland, T.W. (2009). Youth resistance training: Updated position statement paper from the National Strength and Conditioning Association. *Journal of Strength and Conditioning Research, 23*(5 Suppl.), S60-S79.

Faigenbaum, A., Lloyd, R., & Myer, G. (2013). Youth resistance training: Past practices, new perspectives, and future directions. *Pediatric Exercise Science, 25*, 591-604.

Faigenbaum, A., & Micheli, L. (2017). Youth resistance training. *ACSM Sports Medicine Bulletin, 32*(2), 28.

Faigenbaum, A.D., & Myer, G.D. (2010a). Pediatric resistance training: Benefits, concerns, and program design considerations. *Current Sports Medicine Reports, 9*, 161-168.

Faigenbaum, A.D., & Myer, G.D. (2010b). Resistance training among young athletes: Safety, efficacy and injury prevention effects. *British Journal of Sports Medicine, 44*, 56-63.

Faigenbaum, A., & Westcott, W. (2000). *Strength & power for the young athlete*. Champaign, IL: Human Kinetics.

Faigenbaum, A., & Westcott, W. (2007). Resistance training for obese children and adolescents. *President's Council on Physical Fitness and Sports, 8*, 1-8.

Fragla-Pinkham, M.A., Haley, S.M., & Goodgold, S. (2006). Evaluation of a community-based group fitness program for children with disabilities. *Pediatric Physical Therapist, 18*(2), 159-167.

Goldberg, L., & Twist, P. (2007). *Strength ball training* (2nd ed.). Champaign, IL: Human Kinetics.

Hichwa, J. (1998). *Right fielders are people too: An inclusive approach to teaching middle school physical education*. Champaign, IL: Human Kinetics.

Kraemer, W.J., & Fleck, S.J. (2005). *Strength training for young athletes*. Champaign, IL: Human Kinetics.

Lloyd, R., Cronin, J., & Faigenbaum, A. (2016). National Strength and Conditioning Association position statement on long-term athletic development. *Journal of Strength and Conditioning Research, 30*(6), 1491-1509.

Lloyd, R.S., Faigenbaum, A.D., Myer, G.D., Stone, M., Oliver, J., Jeffreys, I., . . . Pierce, K. (2012). UKSCA position statement: Youth resistance training. *Professional Strength Conditioning, 26*, 26-39.

Lloyd, R.S., Faigenbaum, A.D, Stone M.H., Oliver, J.L., Jeffreys, I., Moody, J.A., . . . Myer, G.D. (2013). Position statement on youth resistance training: The 2014 international consensus. *British Journal of Sports Medicine, 48*(7), 498-505.

Myer, G., Quatman, C., Khoury, J., Wall, E., & Hewett, T. (2009). Youth vs. adult "weightlifting" injuries presented to United States emergency rooms: Accidental vs. non-accidental injury mechanisms. *Journal of Strength and Conditioning Research, 23*, 2054-2060.

Rowland, T.W. (2005). *Children's exercise physiology*. Champaign, IL: Human Kinetics.

SHAPE America. (2012). *Instructional framework for fitness education in physical education* [Guidance document]. Reston, VA: Author.

USA Weightlifting. (n.d.). [Home page.] www.teamusa.org/USA-Weightlifting

U.S. Department of Health and Human Services. (1996). *Physical activity and health: A report of the surgeon general*. Atlanta, GA: Centers for Disease Control and Prevention, National Center for Chronic Disease Prevention and Health Promotion.

Additional Resources for Chapter 8

Chu, D., & Myer, G. (2013). *Plyometrics*. Champaign, IL: Human Kinetics.

Kraemer, W., & Fleck, S. (1993). *Strength training for youth athletes*. Champaign, IL: Human Kinetics.

National Strength and Conditioning Association. *NSCA LIFTS Course*. https://www.nsca.com/education/Courses/foundations-of-coaching-lifts/

Sharkey, B., & Gaskill, S. (2006). *Sport physiology for coaches*. Champaign, IL: Human Kinetics.

Chapter 9

Centers for Disease Control and Prevention. (2006). *Physical education curriculum analysis tool.* Atlanta, GA: CDC.

Hichwa, J. (1998). *Right fielders are people too.* Champaign, IL: Human Kinetics.

Joint Committee on National Health Education Standards. (2007). *National health education standards: Achieving excellence.* Atlanta, GA: American Cancer Society.

SHAPE America. (2014). *National standards & grade-level outcomes for K-12 physical education.* Champaign, IL: Human Kinetics.

SHAPE America. (2015). *The essential components of physical education.* Reston, VA: SHAPE America.

SHAPE America. (2016). *Shape of the nation report: Status of physical education in the USA.* Reston, VA: SHAPE America.

U.S. Department of Health and Human Services (USDHHS), Centers for Disease Control and Prevention, National Center for Chronic Disease Prevention and Health Promotion. (1996). *Physical activity and health: A report of the surgeon general.* Atlanta, GA: U.S. Department of Health and Human Services, Government Printing Office.

Chapter 10

Azmin, N.H. (2015). Effect of the jigsaw-based cooperative learning method on student performance in the General Certificate of Education Advanced-Level psychology: An exploratory Brunei case study. *International Education Studies, 9*(1), 91-106.

Casey, A. (2004). Piece-by-piece cooperation: Pedagogical change and jigsaw learning. *The British Journal of Teaching Physical Education, 35*(4), 11-12.

Gardner, H. (1983). *Frames of mind: The theory of multiple intelligences.* New York, NY: Basic Books.

Gardner, H. (1993). *Multiple intelligences: The theory in practice.* New York, NY: Basic Books.

Goldberger, M. (2008). *Teaching physical education* [First On-Line Edition]. spectrumofteachingstyles.org, James Madison University.

Hedeen, T. (2003). The reverse jigsaw: A process of cooperative learning and discussion. *Teaching Sociology, 31*, 325-332.

Hensen, K.T. (1996). Teachers as researchers. In J. Sikula (Ed.), *Handbook of research on teacher education* (2nd ed., pp. 53-66). New York, NY: Simon & Schuster Macmillan.

Huang, Y.-M., Liao, Y.-W., Huang, S.-H., & Chen, H.-C. (2014). A jigsaw-based cooperative learning approach to improve learning outcomes for mobile situated learning. *Educational Technology & Society, 17*(1), 128-140.

Johnson, A.P. (2012). *A short guide to action research* (4th ed.). Old Tappan, NJ: Pearson Education.

Metzler, M.W. (2005). *Instructional models for physical education.* Scottsdale, AZ: Holcomb Hathaway Publishers.

Mosston, M., & Ashworth, S. (2010). *Teaching physical education.* Old Tappan, NJ: Pearson Education.

Rink, J.E. (2005). *Teaching physical education for learning* (5th ed.). St. Louis, MO: McGraw-Hill.

SHAPE America. (2011). *The Physical Best activity guides* (3rd ed.). Champaign, IL: Human Kinetics.

Sheehan, D.P., Katz, L., & Koorman, B.J. (2015). Exergaming and physical education: A qualitative examination from the teachers' perspectives. *Journal of Case Studies in Education, 4*, 1-14.

Chapter 11

American Alliance for Health, Physical Education, Recreation and Dance. (1995). *Physical Best and individuals with disabilities: A handbook for inclusion in fitness programs.* Reston, VA: AAHPERD.

Azzarito, L., Solomon, M., & Harrison, L. (2006). ". . . If I had a choice, I would . . .": A feminist poststructuralist perspective on girls in physical education. *Research Quarterly for Exercise and Sport, 77*, 222-289.

Banks, J.A. (1988). *Multiethnic education: Theory and practice.* Needham Heights, MA: Allyn & Bacon.

Block, B.A. (2014). Supporting LGBTQ students in physical education: Changing the movement landscape. *Quest, 66*(1), 14.

Cohen, G. (1993). *Women in sport.* Newbury Park, CA: Sage.

Columna, L., & Lieberman, L. (2011). *Promoting language through physical education: Using sign language and Spanish to engage everyone.* Champaign, IL: Human Kinetics.

Constantinou, P., Manson, M., & Silverman, S. (2009). Female students' perceptions about gender-role stereotypes and their influence on attitude toward physical education. *Physical Educator, 66*(2), 85-96.

Culp, B. (2013). Eliminating barriers to physical activity: Using cultural negotiation and competence. *Strategies, 26*(3), 35.

Culp, B. (2017). CultureNmotion.com.

Davis, W.E., & Burton, A.W. (1991). Ecological task analysis: Translating movement behavior theory into practice. *Adapted Physical Activity Quarterly, 8,* 154-177.

DePauw, K. (1996). Students with disabilities in physical education. In S. Silverman & C. Ennis (Eds.), *Student learning in physical education: Applying research to enhance instruction* (pp. 101-124). Champaign, IL: Human Kinetics.

Downing, J.E. (2002). *Including students with severe and multiple disabilities in typical classrooms: Practical strategies for teachers* (2nd ed.). Baltimore, MD: Brooks.

Dusenbury, L., & Weissberg, R. (2017, April). *Social emotional learning in elementary school.* Pennsylvania State University. https://www.rwjf.org/en/library/research/2017/04/social-emotional-learning-in-elementary-school.html

Education Week. (2016, September 20). Making SEL meaningful, measurable, and achievable under ESSA [Webinar]. http://secure.edweek.org/media/160920.presentation.pdf

Furrer, C.A. (2010). Coeducational versus single-sex physical education class: Implication on female students' self-esteem and participation. *Virginia Journal, 31*(1), 10-12.

Garcia, C. (2011). Gender expression and homophobia: A motor development and learning perspective. *Journal of Physical Education, Recreation and Dance, 82*(8), 47-49.

Giannini, C., Mohn, A., & Chirarell, F. (2006). Physical exercise and diabetes during childhood [Abstract]. *Acta Biomed, 77*(Suppl. 1), 18-25.

Houston-Wilson, K. (1995). Alternate assessment procedures. In J.A. Seaman (Ed.), *Physical Best and individuals with disabilities: A handbook for inclusion in fitness programs* (pp. 81-109). Reston, VA: AAHPERD.

Hutchinson, G.E. (1995). Gender-fair teaching in physical education. *Journal of Physical Education, Recreation and Dance, 60*(2), 23-24.

Individuals with Disabilities Education Act, 20 U.S.C. § 1400 (2004).

Jaramillo, N., & Nuñez, A.-M. (2009). The impact of being "migrant": Demographies of inequality and outcomes of possibility. *Pedagogies: An International Journal, 1*(4), 94-106.

Lieberman, L.J., & Houston-Wilson, C. (2018). *Strategies for inclusion: A handbook for physical educators* (3rd ed.). Champaign, IL: Human Kinetics.

Lowry, S. (1995). A multicultural perspective on planning. *Teaching Elementary Physical Education, 6*(3), 14-15.

Martin, N.R.M. (2005). *A guide to collaboration for IEP teams.* Baltimore, MD: Brooks.

Mayes, C., Maile-Cutri, R., Goslin, N., & Montero, F. (2016). *Understanding the whole student: Holistic multicultural education* (2nd ed.). Lanham, MD: Rowman & Littlefield.

Mayo Clinic. (2018a). *Hyperglycemia in diabetes.* https://www.mayoclinic.org/diseases-conditions/hyperglycemia/symptoms-causes/syc-20373631

Mayo Clinic. (2018b). *Hypoglycemia.* https://www.mayoclinic.org/diseases-conditions/hypoglycemia/symptoms-causes/syc-20373685

McKenzie, T.L., Prochaska, J.J., Sallis, F., & LaMaster, K. (2004). Coeducational and single-sex physical education in middle schools: Impact on physical activity. *Research Quarterly for Exercise and Sport, 75,* 446-449.

Mohnsen, B.J. (2003). *Teaching middle school physical education: A standards-based approach for grades 5-8.* Champaign, IL: Human Kinetics.

Nilges, L. (1996). Ingredients for a gender equitable physical education program. *Teaching Elementary Physical Education, 7*(5), 28-29.

Parker, M.B., & Curtner-Smith, M.D. (2012). Sport education: A panacea for hegemonic masculinity in physical education or more of the same? *Sport, Education and Society, 17,* 479-496.

Robertson, K., Adolfsson, P., Scheiner, G., Hanas, R., & Riddell, M.C. (2009). Exercise in children and adolescents with diabetes. *Pediatric Diabetes, 10*(Suppl. 12), 154-168.

Sadker, M., & Sadker, D. (1995). *Failing at fairness: How our schools cheat girls.* New York, NY: Simon & Schuster.

Sato, T. (2010). Physical educators' attitudes toward teaching students with limited English proficiency. *Research Quarterly for Exercise and Sport, 81*(1), Suppl. A-69.

Schincariol, L. (1994). Including the physically awkward child. *Teaching Elementary Physical Education, 5*(5), 10-11.

Shimon, J. (2005). Red alert: Gender equity issues in secondary physical education. *Journal of Physical Education, Recreation and Dance, 76*(7), 6-10.

Short, F.X. (2017). Health-related physical fitness and physical activity. In J.P. Winnick & D.L. Poretta (Eds.), *Adapted physical education and sport* (6th ed., pp. 439-454). Champaign, IL: Human Kinetics.

Snell, M.E., & Eichner, S.J. (1989). Integration for students with profound disabilities. In F. Brown & D.H. Lehr (Eds.), *Persons with profound disabilities: Issues and practices* (pp. 109-138). Baltimore, MD: Brooks.

Stainback, S., & Stainback, W. (1990). Inclusive schooling. In W. Stainback & S. Stainback (Eds.), *Support networks for inclusive schooling* (pp. 3-24). Baltimore, MD: Brooks.

Tischler, A., & McCaughtry, N. (2011). PE is not for me. *Research Quarterly for Exercise and Sport, 82,* 37-48.

Tomlinson, C.A. (2001). *How to differentiate instruction in mixed-ability classrooms* (2nd ed.). Alexandria, VA: Association for Supervision and Curriculum Development.

Ulrich, D.A. (2017). *Test of Gross Motor Development* (3rd ed.). Austin, TX: Pro-Ed.

U.S. Department of Education, Office of Special Education and Rehabilitative Services. (2010). *Thirty-five years of progress in educating children with disabilities through IDEA.* Washington, DC: Author.

Wall, A.E. (1982). Physically awkward children: A motor development perspective. In J.P. Das, R.F. Mulcahy, & A.E. Wall (Eds.), *Theory and research in learning disabilities* (pp. 253-268). New York, NY: Plenum Press.

Woodson-Smith, A., Dorwart, C.E., & Linder, A. (2015). Attitudes toward physical education of female high school students. *Physical Educator, 72*(3), 460-479.

Chapter 12

Cooper Institute. (2016). About FitnessGram. www.fitnessgram.net

Graham, G., Elliott, E., & Palmer, S. (2016). *Teaching children and adolescents physical education* (4th ed.). Champaign, IL: Human Kinetics.

Hay, P.J. (2006). Assessment for learning in physical education. In D. Kirk, D. MacDonald, & M. O'Sullivan (Eds.), *The handbook of physical education* (pp. 312-325). London, England: Sage.

Hellison, D. (2011). *Teaching personal and social responsibility through physical activity* (3rd ed.). Champaign, IL: Human Kinetics.

Lacy, A., & Hastad, D. (2015). *Measurement and evaluation in physical education and exercise science* (7th ed.). San Francisco, CA: Cummings.

Lund, J.L., & Kirk, M.F. (2010). *Performance-based assessment for middle and high school physical education* (2nd ed.). Champaign, IL: Human Kinetics.

Mohnsen, B.S. (2008). *Teaching middle school physical education: A standards-based approach for grades 5-8* (3rd ed.). Champaign, IL: Human Kinetics.

National Association for Sport and Physical Education (NASPE). (1995). *Moving into the future: National standards for physical education.* Reston, VA: NASPE.

Reeves, D. (2015). *Using project-based learning in physical education.* Buck Institute for Education. https://www.bie.org/blog/using_project_based_learning_in_physical_education

SHAPE America. (2011). *PE metrics: Assessing National Standards 1-6 in secondary school.* Champaign, IL: Human Kinetics.

SHAPE America. (2014). *National standards & grade-level outcomes for K-12 physical education*. Champaign, IL: Human Kinetics.

Chapter 13

Beets, M.W., Foley, J.T., Tindall, D.W.S., & Lieberman, L.J. (2007). Accuracy of voice-announcement pedometers for youth with visual impairment. *Adapted Physical Activity Quarterly, 24*(3), 218-227.

Beets, M.W., Patton, M.M., & Edwards, S. (2005). The accuracy of pedometer steps and time during walking in children. *Medicine and Science in Sports and Exercise, 37*(3), 513-520.

Cooper Institute. (2007). *Fitnessgram/Activitygram test administration manual* (4th ed.), G.J. Welk & M.D. Meredith (Eds.). Champaign, IL: Human Kinetics.

Corbin, C., & Pangrazi, R. (2008). Fitnessgram and Activitygram: An introduction. In G.J. Welk & M.D. Meredith (Eds.), *Fitnessgram/Activitygram reference guide* (pp. 1-3). Dallas, TX: Cooper Institute.

Crouter, S.E., Schneider, P.L., & Bassett, D.R. Jr. (2005). Spring-levered versus piezo-electric pedometer accuracy in overweight and obese adults. *Medicine and Science in Sports and Exercise, 37*(10), 1673-1679.

Crouter, S.E., Schneider, P.L., Karabulut, M., & Bassett, D.R. Jr. (2003). Validity of 10 electronic pedometers for measuring steps, distance, and energy cost. *Medicine and Science in Sports and Exercise, 35*(8), 1455-1460.

Cuddihy, T.F., Pangrazi, R.P., & Tomson, L.M. (2005). Pedometers: Answers to FAQs from teachers. *Journal of Physical Education, Recreation and Dance, 76*(2), 36-40, 55.

Dale, D., & Corbin, C. (2000). Physical activity participation of high school graduates following exposure to conceptual or traditional physical education. *Research Quarterly for Exercise and Sport, 71*, 61-68.

Duncan, J.S., Schofield, G., Duncan, E.K., & Hinckson, E.A. (2007). Effects of age, walking speed, and body composition on pedometer accuracy in children. *Research Quarterly for Exercise and Sport, 78*(5), 420-428.

Gendle, S.C., Richardson, M., Leeper, J., Hardin, L.B., Green, J.M., & Bishop, P.A. (2011). Wheelchair-mounted accelerometers for measurement of physical activity. *Disability and Rehabilitation: Assistive Technology, 7*(2), 139-148.

Graser, S.V., Pangrazi, R.P., & Vincent, W.J. (2009). Step it up: Activity intensity using pedometers: If you think pedometers can't measure MVPA, think again. *Journal of Physical Education, Recreation and Dance, 80*(1), 22-24.

Harvard Family Research Project. (2010). *Parent–teacher conference tip sheets*. Cambridge, MA: Harvard Graduate School of Education.

Kirkpatrick, B., & Birnbaum, B. (1997). *Lessons from the heart: Individualizing physical education with heart rate monitors*. Champaign, IL: Human Kinetics.

Lacy, A., & Hastad, D. (2007). *Measurement and evaluation in physical education and exercise science* (5th ed.). San Francisco, CA: Benjamin Cummings.

Lagally, K.M. (2013). Using ratings of perceived exertion in physical education. *Journal of Physical Education, Recreation and Dance, 84*(5), 35-39.

Le Masurier, G.C., Lee, S.M., & Tudor-Locke, C. (2004). Motion sensor accuracy under controlled and free-living conditions. *Medicine and Science in Sports and Exercise, 36*(5), 905-910.

Lubans, D.R., Morgan, P.J., & Tudor-Locke, C. (2009). A systematic review of studies using pedometers to promote physical activity among youth. *Preventive Medicine, 48*(4), 307-315.

Lund, J., & Veal, M.L. (2013). *Assessment-driven instruction in physical education*. Champaign, IL: Human Kinetics.

Meredith, M.D., & Welk, G.J. (Eds.). (2017). *FitnessGram/ActivityGram administration manual* (5th ed.). Champaign, IL: Human Kinetics.

Pangrazi, R., Beighle, A., & Sidman, C.A. (2007). *Pedometer power: Using pedometers in school and community* (2nd ed.). Champaign, IL: Human Kinetics.

Partridge, J.A., King, K.M., & Bian, W. (2011). Perceptions of heart rate monitor use in high school physical education classes. *Physical Educator, 68*(1), 30-43.

Plowman, S.A., & Meredith, M.D. (2013). *FitnessGram/ActivityGram reference guide* (4th ed.). Dallas, TX: Cooper Institute.

Rowlands, A.V., & Eston, R.G. (2005). Comparison of accelerometer and pedometer measures of physical activity in boys and girls, ages 8–10. *Research Quarterly for Exercise and Sport, 76*(3), 251-257.

SHAPE America. (2014). *National standards & grade-level outcomes for K-12 physical education.* Champaign, IL: Human Kinetics.

SHAPE America. (2016). *Shape of the nation: Status of physical education in the USA.* www.shapeamerica.org/shapeofthenation

SHAPE America. (2017). *Appropriate and inappropriate practices related to fitness testing* [Position statement]. Reston, VA: Author.

Weston, A.T., Petosa, R., & Pate, R.R. (1997). Validation of an instrument for measurement of physical activity in youth. *Medicine and Science in Sports and Exercise, 29*(1), 138-143.

Winnick, J.P. (2005). *Adapted physical education and sport* (4th ed.). Champaign, IL: Human Kinetics.

Winnick, J.P., & Short, F.X. (2014). *Brockport physical fitness test manual: A health-related assessment for youngsters with disabilities* (2nd ed.). Champaign, IL: Human Kinetics.

Young, S. (2011). A survey of student assessment practice in physical education: Recommendations for grading. *Strategies, 24*(6), 24-26.

Index

Note: The italicized *f* and *t* following page numbers refer to figures and tables, respectively.

About the Editor

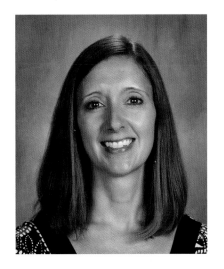

Jackie Conkle, DHEd, is a health education teacher and the wellness committee chair at Peters Township Middle School in McMurray, Pennsylvania. She also serves as the health and physical education facilitator for the K-8 staff. Jackie prides herself in providing many wellness activities during the school day for staff and students and instructing students in after-school physical activity programs. Jackie also provides CPR and first aid training to the school district's staff as an instructor for the American Red Cross. She loves working with others to improve the health of all. Jackie earned a bachelor's degree in health and physical education from the Indiana University of Pennsylvania, a master's degree in physical education teacher education from West Virginia University, and a doctoral degree in health education and administration from A.T. Still University. Jackie is a longtime member of both SHAPE America and the Pennsylvania State Association for Health, Physical Education, Recreation and Dance. For six years, she was an instructor for the National Association for Sport and Physical Education, working to improve physical education nationwide. Helping young people develop a love of movement is among her highest professional goals. When not working on professional endeavors, Jackie is happiest enjoying time with her wonderful husband and three young children in Scenery Hill, Pennsylvania. In her free time, Jackie likes to be active outdoors, especially riding her horses in barrel racing competitions.

About SHAPE America

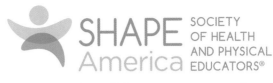

SHAPE America – Society of Health and Physical Educators is the nation's largest membership organization of health and physical education professionals. Since its founding in 1885, the organization has defined excellence in physical education, and our National Standards for K-12 Physical Education serve as the foundation for well-designed physical education programs across the country. We provide programs, resources and advocacy to support health and physical educators at every level, from preschool to university graduate programs. For more information, visit www.shapeamerica.org.

The organization has most recently created the National Standards & Grade-Level Outcomes for K-12 Physical Education (2014), National Standards for Initial Physical Education Teacher Education (2016), National Standards for Health Education Teacher Education (2017) and National Standards for Sport Coaches (2006). Also, SHAPE America participated as a member of the Joint Committee on National Health Education Standards, which published National Health Education Standards, Second Edition: Achieving Excellence (2007).

The SHAPE America website, www.shapeamerica.org, holds a treasure trove of free resources for health and physical educators, adapted physical education teachers, teacher trainers and coaches, including activity calendars, curriculum resources, tools and templates, assessments and more. Visit www.shapeamerica.org and search for Teacher's Toolbox.

Every spring, SHAPE America hosts its National Convention & Expo, the premier national professional-development event for health and physical educators.

Advocacy is an essential element in the fulfillment of our mission. By speaking out for the school health and physical education professions, SHAPE America strives to make an impact on the national policy landscape.

Our Vision: A nation where all children are prepared to lead healthy, physically active lives.

Our Mission: To advance professional practice and promote research related to health and physical education, physical activity, dance and sport.

Our Commitment: 50 Million Strong by 2029

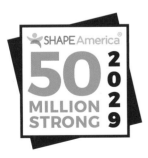

50 Million Strong by 2029 is SHAPE America's commitment to put all children on the path to health and physical literacy through effective health and physical education programs. We believe that through effective teaching, health and physical educators can help students develop the ability and confidence to be physically active and make healthy choices. As educators, our guidance can also help foster their desire to maintain an active and healthy lifestyle in the years to come. To learn more visit www.shapeamerica.org/50Million.

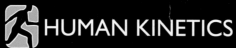

HUMAN KINETICS

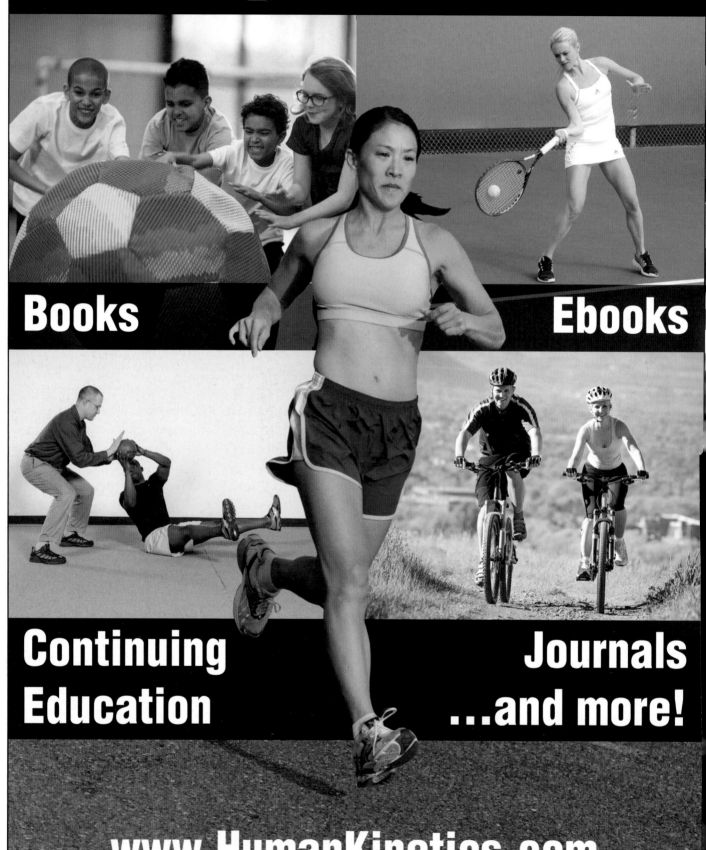

Books

Ebooks

Continuing Education

Journals ...and more!

www.HumanKinetics.com